MIX
Papier aus verantwortungsvollen Quellen
Paper from responsible sources
FSC® C105338

Joseph R Krecioch

Human Craniofacial Variation and Dental Anomalies

An anthropological investigation into the relationship between human craniometric variation and the expression of orthodontic anomalies

Anchor Academic
Publishing

Krecioch, Joseph R: Human Craniofacial Variation and Dental Anomalies: An anthropological investigation into the relationship between human craniometric variation and the expression of orthodontic anomalies, Hamburg, Anchor Academic Publishing 2014

Buch-ISBN: 978-3-95489-329-4
PDF-eBook-ISBN: 978-3-95489-829-9
Druck/Herstellung: Anchor Academic Publishing, Hamburg, 2014

Bibliografische Information der Deutschen Nationalbibliothek:
Die Deutsche Nationalbibliothek verzeichnet diese Publikation in der Deutschen Nationalbibliografie; detaillierte bibliografische Daten sind im Internet über http://dnb.d-nb.de abrufbar.

Bibliographical Information of the German National Library:
The German National Library lists this publication in the German National Bibliography. Detailed bibliographic data can be found at: http://dnb.d-nb.de

All rights reserved. This publication may not be reproduced, stored in a retrieval system or transmitted, in any form or by any means, electronic, mechanical, photocopying, recording or otherwise, without the prior permission of the publishers.

Das Werk einschließlich aller seiner Teile ist urheberrechtlich geschützt. Jede Verwertung außerhalb der Grenzen des Urheberrechtsgesetzes ist ohne Zustimmung des Verlages unzulässig und strafbar. Dies gilt insbesondere für Vervielfältigungen, Übersetzungen, Mikroverfilmungen und die Einspeicherung und Bearbeitung in elektronischen Systemen.

Die Wiedergabe von Gebrauchsnamen, Handelsnamen, Warenbezeichnungen usw. in diesem Werk berechtigt auch ohne besondere Kennzeichnung nicht zu der Annahme, dass solche Namen im Sinne der Warenzeichen- und Markenschutz-Gesetzgebung als frei zu betrachten wären und daher von jedermann benutzt werden dürften.

Die Informationen in diesem Werk wurden mit Sorgfalt erarbeitet. Dennoch können Fehler nicht vollständig ausgeschlossen werden und die Diplomica Verlag GmbH, die Autoren oder Übersetzer übernehmen keine juristische Verantwortung oder irgendeine Haftung für evtl. verbliebene fehlerhafte Angaben und deren Folgen.

Alle Rechte vorbehalten

© Anchor Academic Publishing, Imprint der Diplomica Verlag GmbH
Hermannstal 119k, 22119 Hamburg
http://www.diplomica-verlag.de, Hamburg 2014
Printed in Germany

Absract

Krecioch, Joseph R.

Human Craniofacial Variation and Dental Anomalies: An anthropological investigation into the relationship between human craniometric variation and the expression of orthodontic anomalies.

Keywords: anthropology, palaeopathology, palaeoepidemiology, craniometrics, morphology, orthodontics, dental, skull, dentition, anomalies.

Dental anomalies of number, shape, and position are frequently analysed in the orthodontic and clinical literature but are rarely discussed in an anthropological or archaeological context. While some of these anomalies are believed to follow Mendelian inheritance patterns and the importance of heredity is stressed, other developmental dental disorders are often hypothesised to be the result of a modern, urbanised lifestyle as a response to reduced masticatory stress and subsequent crowding of the dentition.

This study of 131 skulls and dentitions from 6 archaeological collections from England and Macedonia examines the relationship between craniometric variables and the expression of dental anomalies. A number of standard craniometric measurements were taken to estimate relative sizes of cranial functional complexes and determine whether or not, and to what extent, changes in the shape or size of these variables were associated with the expression of dental anomalies.

Statistical analyses determined that the null hypothesis, that there is no relationship between craniometrics and dental anomalies, can be rejected. A number of dental anomalies were found to have a relationship with reduced sizes in cranial and masticatory elements, although dental crowding was not as significant a factor in masticatory complex reduction. A cause and effect relationship cannot be determined but the data presented here suggests that both heredity and environmental causes may be influential in the expression of dental anomalies.

Acknowledgments

I would like to express my gratitude to Professor Séb Villotte and Dr Alan Ogden, as well as Dr Jo Buckberry and the Biological Anthropology Resource Centre at the University of Bradford, UK.

And I would like to thank Angela Pencheva for her help in setting up the Macedonian side, and especially Dr Fanica Veljanovksa and the Museum of Macedonia, Skopje, not only for access to the collections and assistance but also for the plentiful coffee!

CONTENTS

Absract 5
Acknowledgments 6
I. Introduction 9
    Research Questions 9
    Aims and Objectives 10
II. Literature Review 12
    Basis of Human Craniometric Variation 12
    Synopsis of Craniofacial Development 16
    Development of the Masticatory Complex 17
    Environment, Heredity, and Craniofacial Development 18
        Heritability studies 21
            Source 24
    Occlusal Variation and Dental Anomalies 25
III. Materials and Methods 35
    Materials 35
Blackfriars 36
Hickleton 37
Marvinci 37
Demir Kapija 38
        Collection 38
        Methods 38
Congenital Syndromes 42
    Statistical Analysis. 43
IV. Results 45
Frequencies and Distribution of Anomalies 45
No cases of any infracranial congenital disorder, such as cleidocranial dysplasia, were observed among any population sample. 46
    Relationships between anomalies 46
    Preliminary Craniometric Analysis 46
    Relationships between anomalies and craniometrics 48
V. Discussion 53
    Palaeoepidemiology and the analysis of dental anomalies 54
    General distribution of anomalies 55
    Hyperdontia 55
    Misshapen and peg-shaped teeth 56
    Hypodontia 57

> Transpositions 58
> Rotations and reversals 58
> Ectopic eruptions and impactions 59
> Dental Crowding 59
> Relationships between dental anomalies and craniometrics 60
> Heritability, population variation and dental anomalies 61

Mandibular and dental arch dimensions and the aetiology of dental anomalies 68

VI. Conclusion 72

REFERENCES 74

Appendices 84

List of Figures

Figure 1. Mildly rotated left mandibular premolars, Hickleton 36. 41

Figure 2. Peg-shaped left maxillary M3, Chichester 33. 42

Figure 4. Bar graph illustrating relative distribution of CBHI. 47

Figure 3. Bar graph illustrating relative distribution of TFI. 47

Figures 5, (left), 6 (right). Boxplots showing relative size differences in
mandibular features with and without tooth rotations 48

Figures 7 (left), 8 (right). Graphs showing relative frequencies of rotations
among Total Facial Index categories, English and Macedonian samples. 51

Figure 9. Scatterplot of select indices to rotation prevalence in population samples
(normal skulls). Samples with higher rates of rotations cluster among high CI,
and low CBHI and MAI. 66

Figure 10. Scatterplot indicating skulls with rotations inclined toward higher
MAX/BCDL indices and medial Facial Breadth (FB1) indices. 69

List of Tables

Table 1. Heritability estimates. 25
Table 2 Collections summary 38
Table 3 List of cranial landmark measurements. 39
Table 4 Distribution of anomalies by sex. See text. 45
Table 5 Prevalence of Anomalies by Population Sample. 45
Table 6 Summary of mean, significant difference of craniometrics with anomalies. 49
Table 7 Means of craniometric variables, any anomaly absent and present. 52
Table 8 Means of craniometric variables with crowding absent or present. 52
Table 9 Means of craniometric variables by population rotation prevalence,
    normal skulls only. 64
Table 10 Means of craniometric indices by population, normal skulls only. 65
Table 11 Means of new indices and ratios by population, normal skulls only. 65

I. Introduction

Summary

The aetiology and epidemiology of dental anomalies of shape, number, and position have significant contributions in the orthodontic clinical literature, and the heritability and variation of the human skull is a major concern of anthropology, but there appears to be little research into the relationship of these dental anomalies with cranial morphological variation. Anthropologists have had a tendency to regard specific nonmetric traits, such as Carabelli's cusp, and tooth crown metrics in studies of human variation and population distance (Scott 1988; Turner and Scott 2008), and have clarified the effects of developmental plasticity and homoplasy on such studies (von Cramon-Taubadel 2009b, 2011). The study of dental anomalies has been limited to case descriptions and only rarely mentioned in regard to demographics or relationship to morphological variation. Such analyses may not only contribute to anthropological studies of human phenotypic variation, but may help to further elucidate the multifactorial and complex aetiology of dental anomalies.

This project investigated whether there exists a relationship between variation in the size and shape of the skull and pathological dental anomalies of position, shape, and number. By examining several premodern population samples from two different geographical areas, as well as comparing variation at the local level, the research analysed the differences between normal skulls and skulls expressing dental anomalies and occlusal disorders.

Research Questions

The shape and size of the human skull is largely under genetic control but highly affected by the environment, while tooth morphology is more strictly determined by genetics. Numerous studies have associated cranial morphological variation as well as metric and nonmetric dental morphology with global migrations and genetic distance; few, however, have investigated the relationship between craniometrics and occlusal and dental variation. This project examined whether the variation in skull shape, through population distance or admixture (gene flow) or the environment (including diet), in turn affects the likelihood of nonmetric dental anomalies due to spatial changes in the masticatory complex. Further:

- Can the shape or size of the dental arch relative to the size of other cranial components contribute to dental anomalies?
- If so, are these morphological changes based on individual or population variation?
- Is population-based phenotypic variation a contributor to occlusal and dental disorders?
- Do non-syndromic dental anomalies show population variation unrelated to phenotypic variation, suggesting a more heritable component to dental anomalies?
- Is the expression of dental anomalies in congenital syndromes the result of changes to skull morphology?

Aims and Objectives

The aim is to further elucidate the aetiology of pathological dental anomalies and to bring the subject into an anthropological and archaeological context by applying a comprehensive review of the clinical literature to the analysis of archaeological populations. Anthropologically, such data may contribute to the further understanding of the interaction of genetics with the environment to produce human phenotypic variation, and the evolution and adaptation of the modern human masticatory apparatus.

Among the Objectives is the exploration of the relationship between morphologically variable functional complexes of the skull and face with the dentition, and investigating whether craniometric morphological changes lead to changes in frequencies or occurrence of dental anomalies, thus supporting or contradicting proposed theories of the aetiology of these dental anomalies.

II. Literature Review

Basis of Human Craniometric Variation

Change in the shape and size of the skull has been a hallmark of human evolution; a trajectory toward an expanded braincase and a less prognathic, smaller face has been a distinguishing feature of anatomically modern *Homo sapiens* (Lieberman et al 2002). The anteroposteriorly shortened and superoinferiorly heightened face has been hypothesized to have been a result of the increased maturation period in modern humans, the final globular shape of the adult human skull a response to increasing brain size (Bogin 2003; McBratney-Owen and Lieberman 2003). Despite the long evolutionary history of the expanding cranial vault in humans, and the clear pattern of craniofacial change from earlier hominoids, there has been continuing debate regarding the extent to which the changes are primarily genetic or environmental (Relethford 1994, 2004; Ackermann and Cheverud 2004; Roseman 2004; Roseman and Weaver 2007; Betti et al 2009, 2010). Significantly, the variation in craniometrics between modern human populations often exceeds that of the variation between species of many non-human primates (Strand Vidarsdóttir and O'Higgins 2003) and this craniometric variation has been used for decades in assessing population affinities.

The size and shape of the skull is largely polygenetic, and formed from the interaction of developmental plastic functional complexes with the environment within the constraints and parameters of genetic inheritance (Moss 1997a; Hallgrimssona et al 2007; Martínez-Abadías et al 2009, 2011), and adult skull dimensions are the result of the interplay between several functional complexes (see below; Moss and Young 1960; Moss 1997a; Bastir and Rosas 2005; Sardi and Ramírez Rozzi 2007). Thus it has been argued that geographic and climatic conditions are responsible for cranial shape rather than exclusively genetics (Relethford 2004; Betti et al 2009, 2010) although more recent studies have supported a more direct relationship between heredity and craniometrics (von Cramon-Taubadel and Smith 2012).

In a seminal work, Moss and Young stated "[t]he form of the skull is related to its *functions*... Cranial form closely reflects the functional demands of [the] soft tissues throughout life" (1960:281; emphasis in original). They went on to divide the skull into two main components, the neurocranium and the face. While still the result of evolutionary selective pressures, Moss and Young (1960:290) emphasized that the skeletal response is 'secondary' and compensatory to changes in surrounding soft tissue. Although an early reading of the description of Moss' Functional Matrix Hypothesis (FMH) leaves little room for the influence of heredity, a later synthesis emphasized the importance of epigenetic theory (Moss 1997b), which refers to the development and transmission of phenotypic features not directly the result of DNA mutations or combinations (Jaenisch and Bird 2003; Jobling et al 2004).

Moss was certainly not the first to recognize the plasticity of the human skull and its responsiveness to environmental change. Since at least the beginning of the 20th century, the effect of climate was recognized as a defining feature of cranial shape, and Boas' 1912 study of the effect of migration clearly indicated the extent to which a developing living skull adapts to a change in environmental and climatic conditions (Relethford 2004; González-José et al 2005). Boas' research showed significant divergence in the cranial measurements of American-born and foreign-born Europeans, a significant advancement of the time, but also important in general to warn anthropologists of the inherent adaptability of the skull regardless of the effect of heritability (Relethford 2004; González-José et al 2005).

Moss' FMH is important for understanding the nature of the plasticity and development of the human cranium, and most research today takes into account the functional modularity of the skull. Research into the ontogeny of craniofacial variation begins with a postulation of Moss' FMH, that once bone growth has started according to its predetermined genetic plan, the development of the elements are shaped by local extrinsic, as well as other, possibly genetic, factors (Hunt 1998). Not only is an element affected by neuromuscular activity of its functional matrix, but also by the movement or growth of associated elements, compensating for changes in shape to maintain functional integrity (Moss 1960, 1997a; Hunt 1998). Whether a functional module evolves independently or is instead integrated and coevolving with other cranial modules is the subject of recent debate, but the significance of the functional influence of cranial development remains.

Modules may be 'nested' for the purposes of analysis; Pucciarelli et al (2006) divided the neurocranium into four distinct subcomplexes (anteroneural, midneural, posteroneural, and otic), and the face into four as well (optic, respiratory, masticatory, and alveolar). Such division according to single functions is not uncommon, but in general there is a zoological tendency toward dividing the cranium into three major functional components, the splanchnocranium (face), chondrocranium (cranial base), and the dermatocranium (essentially the vault) (Kuroe et al 2004; von Cramon-Taubadel 2011a). But von Cramon-Taubadel argued that such a division does not take into account the evolutionary significance of ossification timing (von Cramon-Taubadel 2011a). Earliest ossification areas are thought to be less affected by the environment, the implication being that the early ossification and inability to deform to stress demands is the result of strong genetic control (Lieberman et al 2002; Strand Vidarsdóttir et al 2002; Strand Vidarsdóttir and O'Higgins 2003; Bastir and Rosas 2005; von Cramon-Taubadel 2011a).

Craniofacial Development

Throughout human evolution, the trend toward bipedalism and expanding brain size has left modern humans with a range of craniofacial variability based on the position and orientation of the cranial base and the large, rounded cranial vault, providing global variation by which populations can be assessed, as well as individual variation, although a prolific debate continues over to what extent individual cranial variation is determined by environmental, genetic, and epigenetic contributions (Relethford 2004; González-José et al 2005; Carson 2006; Betti et al 2009, 2010; von Cramon-Taubadel and Smith 2012; among others). Much recent data supports the theory that the bones of the cranial base and cranial vault are under stronger genetic control, and thus more informative in heritability and distance studies, than the bones of the face, which are far more influenced by environmental stress, diet, and other external factors (Lieberman 2000, 2002; Harvati and Weaver 2006; Martínez-Abadías et al 2009).

Facial growth, as emphasised by Enlow (1990) and Enlow and Hans (1996) is the result not only of this phylogenetic shaping of the cranial vault and basicranium, but is responsive and compensatory, which can result in a "normal" or ideal state, or one of malocclusion, if not abnormality. The plasticity of the human face and the continual compensatory development throughout adulthood is the basis for the field of orthodontics, which is concerned with the prevention and treatment of occlusal abnormality caused by individual variation in craniofacial development (Houston and Tulley 1989).

Synopsis of Craniofacial Development

The study of craniofacial growth saw a tremendous amount of change from the 1960s through the 1990s. Once genes were thought to singularly control entire skeletal elements, only to be seen to contribute to a relationship between tension factors and bone response, a much more multifactorial approach, largely based explanations resembling, if not derived from, the Functional Matrix Hypothesis, in which regulatory genes guide tissue through its response to surrounding tissue "input signals" (Enlow and Hans 1996). The timing of the developmental process is integral to responsiveness to environmental input. A prenatal, early ossified element is considered less likely to adapt or respond to stimuli; a number of studies have corroborated that the bones that develop the earliest have the highest heritability rates (Martínez-Abadías et al 2009; von Cramon-Taubadel 2011a). Later development of the cranial vault is largely accomplished through early brain expansion and the responses at sutures and synchondroses; the face, while influenced by this vault expansion and movement, is also affected by the development of associated functional mechanisms, for respiration, language, and diet (Enlow 1990; Enlow and Hans 1996; Sardi and Rozzi 2007).

By birth the cranial vault consists only of bony plates surrounded by and interconnected by connective tissue, which are displaced away from each other during brain growth, the tension of the strain at the sutures promoting new bone growth (deposition), thus enlarging each of the bones individually (Enlow 1990; Enlow and Hans 1996). Similarly, functional stress from the muscles involved in mastication, respiration, and language further influence growth of the temporals and occipital, causing further displacement of all of the elements of the skull (Houston and Tulley 1989). The outer and inner tables of the skull bones are acted upon independently, the inner tables shaped by the growing brain and the outer tables by the activities of attached muscles; the tables can be pulled apart in such a way as to create sinuses, as in the frontal bone (Houston and Tulley 1989). The expansion of the vault and subsequent growth of the bones of the calvarium displace the elements anterior to it, that is, the bones of the face, the maxilla and the mandible; significant temporal and frontal bone expansion push the orbits medially and vertically toward each other, subsequently reducing the space available for the olfactory complex (and, in evolutionary terms, reducing the snout) as well as for the masticatory complex, creating a shorter, more "rectangular" than "triangular" jaw than is seen in most mammals (Enlow 1996:167).

Development of the Masticatory Complex

An equally important and simultaneous effect of vault expansion in humans is the flexure of the cranial base, hypothesized to be under stronger genetic control than other features of the cranium with an intrinsic relationship to human bipedalism (Houston and Tulley 1989; Havarti and Weaver 2006; Hallgrímsson et al 2007). The growth and movement of the cranial base (away from the mammalian posterior cranium and toward the central floor, allowing the brain to 'balance' on the spine in an upright position), particularly growth and movement at the spheno-occipital synchodroses, creates the sphenoidal sinus and pushes the maxilla in an antero-superior direction *away from* the mandible (Enlow 1990; Houston and Tully 1989). Additionally, a wide cranial base angle will result in a maxilla more anteriorly placed than the mandible, and a small cranial base angle will result in a maxilla posterior relative to the mandible (Cendekiawan et al 2010).

Further alterations occur which significantly affect the human facial plan. The horizontal span of the pharynx increases with the enlargement of the middle cranial fossa, further pushing the maxillary arch, and the mandible continues compensatory growth to match the position of the maxilla (Moss and Rankow 1968; Houston and Tulley 1989; Enlow 1996). This provides the *basis for malocclusion*, or the range of occlusal variation in humans: the mandible will compensate to the movement and growth of the maxilla to maintain functional efficacy, and if successful, normal occlusion occurs (Enlow 1990; Oyen 1990). As teeth grow and erupt, alveolar remodelling drives maxillary and mandibular growth in the direction of the growing teeth, so that the dental arches are shaped by dental growth and movement; osteoblastic activity strengthens the alveolus during development and eruption of teeth; suckling in infants helps guide masticatory growth by increasing one dimensional stress (Oyen 1990).

While the cranial vault is responding largely to the expansion of the brain (encephalization), the face is not only responding to such growth and displacement, but experiencing a significant amount of stress from functional demands on associated soft tissue from mastication, respiration, olfaction, speech, expression and a number of other activities (Houston and Tulley 1989; Enlow and Hans 1996; Bishara 2001). These environmental and functional stimuli provide variation in individual as well as population-based facial development, a process which continues throughout life (Oyen 1990; Enlow and Hans 1996).

Environment, Heredity, and Craniofacial Development

Diet

The transition from a hunter-gatherer lifestyle to agriculture has been proposed to have caused a significant change in cranial morphology. Gonzalez-Jose et al's analysis of 18 South American populations of hunter-gatherers and agriculturalists found that economic strategy was a better determiner of masticatory/alveolar morphology than population distance, emphasising the role of plasticity in the human face (Gonzalez-Jose et al 2004). For several decades data has supported the idea of cranial robusticity as a result of 'hard' unprocessed diets of hunter-gatherers, and the conversely modern 'soft' diets consisting of cooked and processed foods, requiring less force and muscle strain to ingest, result in an increase in cranial gracility "and a general deterioration of dental health" (Paschetta et al 2010:298; Corruccini 1984; Ortner 2003; Varrela 1992). Studies on mice and nonhuman primates have indicated reduction in the size of masticatory elements of the skull on subjects fed a soft diet (Corruccini and Beecher 1982; Killiardis 1986; Lauc et al 2003). In humans many studies by craniometric research into the transition between archaeological hunter-gatherer and farming populations have corroborated the effects of diet change on the masticatory apparatus (Corruccini 1984; Verrala 1992; von Cramon-Taubadel 2011b). Varrela (1992) suggested that general cranial dimensions are affected by changes in diet, not only because of plastic environmental effects, but also due to selective pressures (Varrela 1992:31). Varrela also argued that changes to mandibular growth since the transition to agriculture has contributed to an increase in occlusal variation, an assertion supported by a number of studies on living and historical populations (Lavelle 1973; Harper 1994; González-José et al 2005; von Cramon-Taubadel 2011b).

With the caveat that this technological-cultural shift may have been the result of or coincident with a population admixture or even replacement, confounding craniometric change as evidence of environmental or genetic change, Paschetta et al (2010) attempted to correct for this confounding by using genetically continuous Amerindian populations during a long period that included the agricultural transition from hunter-gatherer lifestyle (Paschetta et al 2010:302). They divided the cranial measurements into the functional complexes of neurocranial, facial, alveolar, masticatory, and mandibular modules, and further divided each of these complexes into distinct morphological components, following the methods of hierarchical functional craniology (Paschetta et al 2010). Their results supported the idea that dietary softness (determined not only by cultural archaeological evidence but dental microwear analysis) can result in reduced growth of elements of the masticatory complex (in this case the attachment of the temporalis muscle, the zygomatic arch, and palate) due to reduced strain "magnitude and/or frequency" (Paschetta et al 2010:308). However, general reduction in whole skull size or relative size of face was not observed in the Ohio Valley samples, suggesting that the plastic effects of diet on craniometrics are localized to specicifc maxillofacial elements rather than general (Paschetta et al 2010:309).

Corruccini referred to modern occlusal variation as part of the epidemiological transition that includes a number of other deleterious health effects of modern lifestyle and diet (Corruccini 1984). According to Ortner (2003:598), "chewing stress stimulates mandibular more than maxillary growth". Since normal, or ideal, occlusion is dependent on the mandible "catching up" to maxillary growth and movement spurred on by encephalization and basicranial development (Moss and Rankow 1968; Enlow 1996), it is not surprising that modern dietary habits would be implicated as contributing to an increase in dental crowding and occlusal variability in modern human populations: Hillson regarded dental anomalies such as crowding as "so common as to be almost normal" (Hillson 1996:112), although he questioned the validity of a soft diet as being the prime cause of modern occlusal anomalies, considering the range of other environmental and behavioural conditions (such as mouth-breathing) that affect facial position more continuously (Hillson 1996:116).

Environmental and Climatic Effects

Changes in diet, then, are likely not the only influence upon human occlusal variation; environmental variables, particularly climate, have been proposed as a source for craniometric variation, but recent research has found such effects limited to specific areas of the face, such as the area around the nasal aperture, or as a result of extreme cold environments (Roseman 2004; Harvati and Weaver 2006; Betti et al 2009, 2010). If climate does significantly affect craniometrics, it would be expected that genetically distant populations would adapt similarly to similar environments, but a 2009 study of over 6000 skulls from modern populations throughout the world found that climatic signatures are far less significant on craniometrics than those that can be explained by geographic distance from Africa, supporting not only the hypothetical African origin of *Homo sapiens*, but reflecting the high degree of heritability of cranial morphology (Betti et al 2009, 2010). It is important to note, however, that closely related populations may inhabit, and thus adapt similarly to, similar environments (Betti et al 2010).

Heritability studies

Craniofacial metric variation is continuous and size is responsible for 10 to 36 percent of variation in the shape of the face (Hunter 1990). The continuous variability implies that it is polygenic and facial height may be the result of a variety of factors under genetic control including size of teeth, height of maxilla or mandibular symphyseal height (Hunter 1990:252), all further affected by environmental stimuli. The multifactorial, polygenic nature of craniofacial growth obfuscates the nature of craniofacial variation; even if one gene determined the size and shape of an element, the action of the growth and movement of an associated element, for instance the teeth and muscles acting upon the mandible, the final size of the mandible would appear to be a continuous, polygenetic variable trait (Hunter 1990:245).

Elements susceptible to environmentally-influenced remodelling are plastic and should not only be more variable, but less likely to recapitulate phylogeny and population history; confounding this is homoplasy, which is the morphological similarity of elements of two populations based on similar selective or adaptive pressures from similar environments (von Cramon-Taubadel 2009a). In general, the least variable skeletal traits should have higher heritabilities than such plastic traits.

Penetrance refers to the ability of a gene to be expressed in an individual; that is, the fact that not all individuals who carry a dominant allele will express the phenotype (Pritchard and Korf 2011). *Expressivity* can be variable as well, meaning that while every individual who may be carrying a specific gene expresses it phenotypically, the range of phenotypic expression varies (Pritchard and Korf 2011). Polygenetic control of a feature, that is the expression of a feature under the control of a number of genes, is more likely to be affected by the environment; not only can environmental variables contribute to the development of polygenetic traits, but some may have a *threshold* point at which the combination of genes and environmental conditions allow expression (or conversely restrict expression) of the trait (Mossey 1999a; Jobling et al 2004; Pritchard and Korf 2011).

Heritability can be described as the proportion of phenotypic variability that can be attributed to genetic control (Konigsberg 2000; Carson 2006; Pritchard and Korf 2011), and is represented statistically as an estimate, h^2, described by the formula:

(1) $$h^2 = \frac{Va}{Va+Ve} = \frac{Va}{Vp}$$

in which Va is the sum of genetic variance, Ve total environmental variance, and Vp phenotypic variability (Konigsberg 2000; Carson 2006; Pritchard and Korf 2011). This formula is an estimate of *narrow sense* heritability, leaving out the effects of dominance, which complicates phenotypic expression but is not transmitted (Konigsberg 2000). The formula for *broad sense* heritability,

(2) $$h^2 = \frac{Va+Vd}{Va+Vd+Ve} = \frac{Va+Vd}{Vp} = \frac{Vg}{Vp}$$

includes the effects of allelic dominance, Vd; craniometrics, however, is concerned with multivariate, continuous quantitative traits and relies heavily on narrow-sense heritability estimates (Hunter 1990; Konigsberg 2000; Carson 2006).

The h^2 formulae are based on twin studies, and provide a range between 0.0 and 1.0; similarly, r represents a correlation based on estimates of heritability from family studies, ranging from 0.0 to 1.0, in which 1.0 represents total heritability; the expected heritability between a parent and its offspring for any trait can be no more than 0.5, and that of monozygotic twins can be expected to reach 1.0 (Hunter 1990; Townsend et al 2009). Regardless of method, estimating heritability requires genealogical information, and a number of clinical studies have utilized radiographs of patients with known family histories to estimate heritability of craniofacial features (Watnick 1972; Hunter 1990; Harris 2008; Sherwood et al 2008; among others) or archaeological craniometrics on collections with known genealogies, such as the ossuary at Halstatt, Austria, each skull of which is labelled with the name, sex, age, marriage status and family relationships (Carson 2006; Martínez-Abadías et al 2009). Utilizing the Halstett crania, Carson carried out a heritability analysis of standard craniometric dimensions, finding that cranial length measurements tend to be more heritable than breadth measurements (see Table 1), and that overall facial metrics have lower heritability than neurocranial metrics (Carson 2006:177).

Von Cramon-Taubadel (2011a) tested seven "functional developmental modules" (FDMs) for correlations with genetic indicators of heritability, to test the hypothesis that early-forming endochondroses would be more phylogenetically informative than single-function modules (2011a:84). The results of the study, summarized in Table 1 along with a number of other estimated heritabilities, indicated that, among the 15 populations used in the study, the vault was the most directly heritable and the face much less so. This result has been obtained by other studies, some of which indicate that the temporal bone, specifically, is under the strongest genetic control, although in sharp contrast to others (see Table 1; Carson 2006; Betti et al 2009, 2010; von Cramon-Taubadel 2009b). Despite utilizing the same collection, differing results are the result of utilizing different covariates and different individuals (Martínez-Abadías et al 2009). These results generally support the significance of the effects of environment, climate, diet and other external factors that affect the plasticity of the human face and that may be mitigated by geography or cultural variation, as well as the utility of cranial vault shape as indicative of population affinity.

Element, module	Estimated heritability	Source
Vault	0.66	von Cramon-Taubadel 2011
Dermatocranium	0.62	"
Chondrocranium	0.61	"
Nasal	0.57	"
Face	0.53	"
Auditory	0.49	"
Orbit	0.25	"
Temporal	0.69	von Cramon-Taubadel 2009
Full cranium	0.64	"
Sphenoid	0.62	"
Parietal	0.60	"
Frontal	0.57	"
Maxilla	0.56	"
Occipital	0.54	"

Zygomatic	0.37	"
Nasal height (NLH)	0.73	Carson 2006
NLH	0.43	Martínez-Abadías et al 2009
Bimaxillary breadth (ZMB)	0.60	Carson 2006
ZMB	0.07	Martínez-Abadías et al 2009
Cranial length (GOL)	0.36	Carson 2006
GOL	0.31	Martínez-Abadías et al 2009
Occipital chord (OCC)	0.33	Carson 2006
OCC	0.04	Martínez-Abadías et al 2009
Parietal Chord (PAC)	0.31	Carson 2006
PAC	0.06	Martínez-Abadías et al 2009
Bizygomatic breadth (ZYB)	0.26	Carson 2006
ZYB	0.28	Martínez-Abadías et al 2009
Malar length, max (XML)	0.24	Carson 2006
XML	0.20	Martínez-Abadías et al 2009
Cranial Breadth (XCB)	0.23	Carson 2006
XCB	0.36	Martínez-Abadías et al 2009
Biauricular breadth (AUB)	0.40	Martínez-Abadías et al 2009
Foramen Magnum length (FOL)	0.38	Martínez-Abadías et al 2009
Basion-Nasion length (BNL)	0.24	Martínez-Abadías et al 2009

Table 1. Some published heritability estimates of major cranial elements, regions, or measurements (higher numbTable 1er indicates more likely neutral, that is strongly genetic control over development).

Occlusal Variation and Dental Anomalies

Like the cranial vault and base, the size and shape of teeth have been described as being significantly under genetic control (Doris et al 1981; Dempsey and Townsend 2001; Thesleff 2000; Townsend 2009; Nelson and Ash 2010; Galluccio et al 2012) and "relatively independent" of the genetic factors that guide the development of the rest of the masticatory process (Ortner 2003:598), a result of the ectodermal origin of teeth developing within mesodermal bone (Mossey 1999a). Tooth crowns are formed very early during development, and are less likely to adapt to changing environment, except for the pattern of movement and eruption (Sperber 2006; Ortner 2003), and although acted upon by external stimuli which can result in carious lesions, abrasions, and hypoplasia, teeth cannot remodel (Lycett and Collard 2005). This potential for incongruence may be the initial cause of the theorized increase in occlusal variation and dental anomalies in modern and genetically mixed populations (Mossey 1999a).

Malocclusion, crowding, and impactions

The manner in which the teeth of the maxillary arch meet the teeth of the mandibular arch is the definition of occlusion, although the term is used to indicate a range of meanings related to the closing or use of the jaws (Bishara 2001; Nelson and Ash 2010). Ideal occlusion is one in which the maxillary incisors slightly overlap their mandibular counterparts, the maxillary canines lie in between the mandibular canine and first premolar, and the posterior teeth are matched maxillary cusps for mandibular grooves (Leighton 1991; Hillson 1996; Bishara 2001; Nelson and Ash 2010). As is implied in preceding sections, a normal or ideal occlusion is considered rare in modern, industrialised societies (Hillson 1996; Corruccini 1984). Malocclusions are classified for orthodontic purposes according to severity of misalignment and need for treatment, generally relating to degree or extent of overbite, crossbite, or evidence of crowding (Bishara 2001), that is, divergence from the ideal articulation of teeth. Some researchers have linked malocclusion class with specific anomalies, which may indicate a genetic correlation between malocclusion type and a number of anomalies (Basdra et al 2001).

The environmental and dietary changes consequent of westernisation and urbanization had been thought to be responsible for the reduction in jaw sizes that have led to an increase in third molar impactions, crowding, and other anomalies (Doris et al 1981; Lombardi 1982; Corruccini 1984; Leighton 1991). Lombardi theorized that the selective pressures on the evolution of tooth size have not had time to match the quick changes in diet and compensatory reduction of jaw dimensions in modern populations (Lombardi 1982:38). Corruccini's 1984 description of malocclusion as a result of the affects of modern society argued against the idea of ethnic mixing or genetic causes for occlusal variation, finding that elements of jaw size, affected by diet and personal behaviour, rather than tooth size causes the discrepancies in the tooth-jaw relationship known in modern societies (Corruccini 1984:425).

In 1996 Hunter argued against popular assumptions that this evolutionary trend in *Homo* of decreasing mandible size has left little room for the third molar, resulting in other associated anomalies (Hunter 1996). Hunter was concerned that the assumption was often repeated without actual data to support it, in fact going so far as to claim that teeth and jaws are larger in more modern populations (Hunter 1996:263). More recent research has instead supported the original assumption.

Mossey, like Corruccini, saw ethnic mixing as part of the complex of features characteristic of westernisation, in addition to soft diet and environmental pressures, leading to the increase in dental and occlusal variation, and argued that if the jaw cannot grow to accommodate the genetically-determined size of teeth, there must be a threshold beyond which the third molar cannot develop (Mossey 1999a). While Mossey saw the size and shape of teeth and the masticatory complex as largely inherited, he emphasized the polygenetic nature of dental and maxillofacial development thus allowing modifications from environmental pressures, in the aetiology of dental anomalies and malocclusions (Mossey 1999a,b). Based on the idea that gene flow from distant ethnic groups may introduce novel metric variation, he further noted that ethnically "pure" groups are more likely to have ideal occlusion: in the "pure racial stocks, such as the Melanesians of the Philippine islands, malocclusion is almost non-existent" (Mossey 1999b:195).

Harris (2008) explained the pervasiveness of malocclusion and dental anomalies in recent times and in Western nations, agreeing with Corruccini that such occlusal and dental variation is a "disease of civilization" (Corruccini 1984:419).

According to Harris, only one in ten "youths" in the United States today has a "naturally occurring good occlusion" (Harris 2008:129). Sceptical of heritability measures, Harris maintained that malocclusions are largely environmental, despite recognizing the high heritability of skeletal arch dimensions and, without significant explanation, claimed that theories of malocclusion as the result of ethnic mixing "have been thoroughly debunked" (Harris 2008:129).

The influence of heritability over occlusion was demonstrated by Normando et al (2011) in their comparison of malocclusion between an indigenous Amazonian population that was the result of a couples' divergence from an ancestral group, resulting in a high rate of endogamy among the descendents of the new population (Normando et al 2011:1). Because the groups lived in essentially the same environment and ate the same diet, a significant increase in occlusal variation among the new group was interpreted by Normando et al as the result of polygenetic control of craniofacial and occlusal features exaggerated by inbreeding (Normando et al 2011:3). As interethnic mixing may introduce new metric variation or disorders, so endogamy can exaggerate effects of additive polygenic traits by artificially multiplying them (Luac et al 2003; Normando et al 2011). Similar effects of inbreeding were examined by Lauc et al's 2003 study of an endogamous island Croatian population, in which occlusal variables with high heritabilities, such as overjet, were significantly more common among individuals of consanguineous families than the normal population (Luac et al 2003). Luac et al go on to suggest that the genes responsible for the observed occlusal variations were of little effect, "but extremely numerous", (Luac et al 2003:307) again pointing to a polygenetic threshold model of inheritance of dental and craniofacial anomalies. Recent studies implicate more than 300 different genes in the dental development (Galluccio et al 2012).

Dental anomalies of shape, position, and number

Significant as a clinical concern, but less frequently investigated as an anthropological subject, is the expression of pathological dental anomalies of shape, position, and number. Among these anomalies is the congenital absence of teeth; ranging from agenesis, anodontia, in which an individual has no teeth; oligodontia, in which the subject is missing more than six teeth; and hypodontia if fewer than six teeth are missing (Bailleul-Forestier et al 2008a; Kouskoura et al 2011), although the term hypodontia is also used generally when at least one tooth is congenitally missing (Kirzioğlu et al 2005; Parkin et al 2009). Hypodontia is the most common dental anomaly in modern humans, and the agenesis of the third molar is by far the most common type (Vastardis 2000; Cellikoglu et al 2011). Although there is evidence for heritability of tooth agenesis, it appears to be multifactorial and is often associated with other anomalous dental structures (Hillson 1996; Vastardis 2000; Brook 2009; Parkin et al 2009; Cellikoglu et al 2011) and reduced tooth size (Brook 2009). Importantly, congenital absence of teeth (or even loss of deciduous teeth) can result in reduction of size of the developing craniofacial structures as well as malpositioning of remaining teeth (Cellikoglu et al 2011). Prevalence of hypodontia varies among the populations of the world, as well as between sexes, and has been reported to be as high as 25% of the population (Brooks 2009). Exclusive of third molar agenesis, prevalence rates seem to range between less than one percent (<1.0%) to over ten percent (>10%), depending on the population (Vastardis 2000; Celikoglu et al 2011).

The expression of extra teeth (beyond the expected complement of 32), either oddly shaped supernumeraries or supplemental, full-sized teeth, is known as hyperdontia. Less frequent in modern populations than hypodontia, hyperdontia includes the additional peg-shaped tooth in between the two central maxillary incisors, the mesiodens, as the most common form (Rajab and Hamdam 2002; Mishra 2011). Non-syndromic supernumerary teeth are associated with larger teeth, tend to be ectopic or impacted, and occur more frequently in males than females (Batra et al 2005; Brook 2009). Hyperdontia not associated with a congenital syndrome are rare; like hypodontia frequencies depend upon population, but range from 0.1% to 3.6% (Batra et al 2005). Although like most dental traits originally believed to be multifactorial and polygenetic, recent research has posited an autosomal dominant trait because of its expression in family pedigrees (Batra et al 2005), but others maintain that specific genes cannot be identified for tooth number anomalies, and suggest a complex aetiology (Galluccio et al 2012).

Supernumeraries have been associated with tooth rotations, in which a tooth erupts at angle divergent from the curve of the dental arch (Rajab and Hamdan 2002). Among the anterior teeth such rotation or 'winging' "is so common as to be almost normal" (Hillson 1996:112) and produces an overlap that is characteristic of anterior crowding (Hillson 1996). Rotations have also been described as associated with agenesis of nonadjacent teeth, suggesting a multifactorial but genetic association with other anomalies (Baccetti 1998).

Transpositions, in which two adjacent teeth have 'switched' positions, or a tooth erupts in the normal position of a nonadjacent tooth (Ely et al 2006; Papadopoulous et al 2009), also have frequency variations among populations (Chattopadhyay and Srinivas 1996; Ely et al 2006) but general frequency is around 1% (Ely et al 2006) and most commonly occurs in the maxilla (Chattopadhyay and Srinivas 1996; Babacan et al 2008). Most studies posit a multifactorial origin for transpositions, in which epigenetic factors change the path of an erupting tooth (Chattopadhyay and Srinivas 1996; Baccetti 1998; Ely et al 2006).

Dental and occlusal variation in the archaeological and anthropological context
Although the aetiology and epidemiology of dental anomalies of shape, number, and position have significant contributions in the orthodontic clinical literature, and the heritability and variation of the human skull is a major concern of anthropology, there appears to be little research into the relationship of these dental anomalies with cranial morphological variation. Anthropologists have had a tendency to regard specific nonmetric traits, such as Carabelli's cusp, and metrics in studies of human variation (Scott 1988; Turner and Scott 2008).

For the past decade a good deal of research has provided some answers to the aetiology and epidemiology of supernumerary teeth and hypodontia; the incidence of rotated or reversed teeth, however, seems less investigated and is often aggregated into general categories of malocclusion (Evensen and Øgaard 2007; Ling and Wong 2010). Dental arch dimensions and other occlusal variables have been suggested as causes or aetiologies for rotations, but rotation also appears to occur without associated anomalies, as was reported in the pygmoid *Homo sapiens* from Flores, Indonesia (Jacob et al 2006). The Flores samples otherwise do not differ significantly from modern human values for dental or craniofacial variables, including arch and tooth dimensions, other than 90° rotated 2nd premolars (Jacob et al 2006).

Non-syndromic supernumerary teeth have been reported and treated since at least as early as the 7th century AD (Rajab and Hamdam 2002; Duncan 2009), and a number of case reports from prehistoric North America have appeared in the anthropological literature (Ortner 2003), although descriptions extend to as far as far as the Australopithecines (Duncan 2009), and supernumeraries have been recorded in a number of extant and extinct anthropoids (Jungers and Gingerich 1980; Swindler 2002). Legoux (1974) described a number of dental anomalies in a small Final Gravettian population from l'Abri-Pataud, France, the most significant of which are two supernumerary teeth alongside the right upper M2 (17) in one individual and a reversed right upper PM2 (15) in another. He suggested that the rare collection of dental traits among these remains is indicative of a small endogamous population, and proposed a 'mother/child' relationship between two of them (Legoux 1974). Similarly, a description of several supernumeraries along with among a small sample from the Mayan site of Ixlú, Guatemala suggested not only the genetic aetiology of hyperdontia but the association with other anomalies, as well as the close relationship of the specimens (Duncan 2009).

Several descriptions of transpositions have been reported from North American sites, 11 cases of canine-first premolar transposition from one Pueblo site in New Mexico (Burnett and Weets 2001), and 7 cases of the same type from prehistoric Santa Cruz island, California (Sholts et al 2010). Assuming transpositions are heritable traits and not the result of occlusal disorder, the high prevalence of such a rare anomaly among one population again suggests small, endogamous populations and inbreeding or close relationships between the individuals with the anomalies (Sholts et al 2010).

Explaining crowding and malocclusions as a result of ethnic mixing and environmental or cultural changes, in which the discrepancy between genetically large teeth and smaller jaw components force the teeth to fit into anomalous positions

(Howe et al 1983; Ortner 2003), Ortner described the skull of a child from prehistoric Florida exhibiting small skeletal structure and severe displacement of several teeth "because of inadequate space in the maxilla" (Ortner 2003:602).

The "epidemiologic transition" theory of Corruccini regarding crowding in modern populations was not supported in an assessment of the relationship between medieval and modern dentitions (Harper 1994). Instead, the study found more occlusal variation and anomalies with a medieval sample from a London plague pit. These mediaeval skulls had wider dental arches and shorter arch lengths, and more crowding in the anterior mandibular dentition compared to a modern European sample (Harper 1994). Crowding and irregularity was also found to be common among a Copper Age French site, in which all of the examined skulls expressed anterior maxillary crowding, and several exhibited impacted canines (Mockers et al 2004). The average arch width in this French sample was found to be lower than in modern Caucasians, and the authors argued that the dental irregularities observed are likely the result of "normal-sized teeth erupting in undersized jaws", following from an "especially sedentary way of life" (Mockers et al 2004:155).

Infracranial Congenital Conditions

Hypodontia and hyperdontia are both commonly attributes of a number of congenital syndromes; the rare occurrence of these anomalies outside of known congenital conditions is consequently referred to specifically as "nonsyndromic dental anomalies." Although many of these syndromes consist of soft-tissue lesions, a number of the important conditions have been known to affect skeletal structures. Among these syndromes that have been described as leaving skeletal evidence linked with hypodontia are Down syndrome (Trisomy 21), holoprosencephaly, and ectodermal dysplasia; those linked with hyperdontia are Cleidocranial dysplasia

(cleidocranial dysostosis), Gardner's syndrome, and Nance-Horan syndrome
(Bailleul-Forestier et al 2008b; Aufderheide and Rodríguez-Martín 1998).

III. Materials and Methods

Materials

To examine the relationship between dental anomalies and craniometrics, a number of complete or mostly co0mplete adult skulls are required. But in order to gauge whether individual variation in the shape or size of cranial components is a result of population variation, a number of populations must be analysed. In addition, each sample must be large enough that one may expect dental anomalies to occur. Such issues are not easy to negotiate with small collections, and using the Biological Anthropology Resource Centre (BARC), University of Bradford, several samples were utilised to represent a mediaeval British population sample, and two collections from the Museum of Macedonia, Skopje, to represent an outgroup from Hellenistic and Mediaeval period Balkans. Summary table of the collections and craniometric data can be found in Appendix A.

A total of 131 individual skulls were selected following a visual examination to determine viability based on the condition of the skull, the facial and masticatory components of the large premodern collections. The specimens chosen were based on considerations of the viability of standard craniometrics and recording of dental anomalies. Sex assessments as recorded for each site were verified by the author following guidelines established by Buistra and Ubelaker (1994).

For the purposes of this study, immature skulls were disregarded because of concern that ontogenetic variability may not represent accurately adult shape, and that the deciduous or mixed dentition may give false results of anomalies number or position. At the initial stage of the investigation, skeletal reports and unpublished documents from BARC were searched for potential useable skulls and feasible archaeological site. Three of the populations (Blackfriars, Box Lane, and Hickleton) are located in Yorkshire, northern England, while Chichester is located in West Sussex, in the far south of England. Craniometric variation has been observed between geographically distant populations due to climate changes and environmental pressures as well as genetics (Howells 1973, 1989; Hanihara 1996; Relethford 2004). While Chichester is located rather distant from Yorkshire, the period of the specimens and their location within England, long after the population transitions of the Romano-British and Anglo-Saxon periods (Russell 2005), make the use of all of the four population samples reasonable to be regarded as an English sample for the sake of sample size.

The English Collections

Blackfriars

Blackfriars was a mediaeval Dominican friary in Gloucester, South Yorkshire, consisting of 192 individuals of the lay population as well as the friars. Of these 192 individual burials, 17 contained reasonably complete skulls. There is evidence that during its occupation between the 13th and 16th centuries the friary may have been used as a hospital based on the types of pathological conditions present in many of the skeletons, although many of the burials indicate a relatively healthy population without a large degree of stress related injuries or osteoarthroses (Blackburn 2010).

Box Lane

Box Lane, a mediaeval cemetery located in Pontrefract, in West Yorkshire, consisting of 88 individual skeletons of which only 9 skulls were suitable for study. The site is of some interest because very few immature remains have been recovered from Box Lane, and among the mostly mature skeletons a number of infracranial traumatic lesions as well as a prevalence of degenerative joint conditions suggest that the population was rural and accustomed to heavy labour (Blackburn 2010).

Hickleton

Hickleton, also in South Yorkshire, a small rural site consisting of 28 adult individuals from the mediaeval to post-mediaeval period, over 800 years of occupation (Stroud 1984); of these only 6 skulls of each sex, most from the medieaval period but several possibly from the 16th and 17th centuries, could be analysed.

Chichester

The Chichester sample was recovered from the cemetery of the St James and St Mary Magdalene hospital, and consists of 354 individual skeletons, largely with leprosy or similar pathological conditions (Magilton et al 2008). 25 male skulls and 11 female skulls were found to be informative for this study, although previously published reports indicate that the collection contains 132 complete skulls (Magilton et al 2008). Despite the use of the hospital as a leprosarium, many of the skeletons are non-pathological and may have originally served as the clerical staff or carers of the hospital (Magilton et al 2008); both pathological and non-pathological skulls were utilized in this project.

The Macedonian Collections

Marvinci

196 skeletons from two locations at Marvinci-Valandovo, southeastern Macedonia, had been excavated throughout the 1980s and represent populations from the prehistoric period, the Hellenistic period, and the Roman era (Veljanovska 2006). Prehistoric remains are very fragmentary and were not suitable for analysis; the

skulls used for this analysis were from Antiquity (4th century BC-4th century AD; Veljanovska 2006).

Demir Kapija

Approximately 30km northwest of Marvinci, this largely mediaeval site in the Republic of Macedonia was first excavated in the 1960s and consists of a total 505 burials in a necropolis dating from as early as the pre-Roman period (Valjanovksa 2001). Early Christian era remains were poorly preserved, and this study consists of 28 of the skulls from 305 mediaeval tombs.

Collection	Total Individuals N=	Skulls, Male N=	Skulls, Female N=	Total Skulls N=
English Samples				
Blackfriars	192	9	8	17
Box Lane	88	7	2	9
Hickleton	28	6	6	12
Chichester	354	25	11	36
Subtotal	*662*	*47*	*27*	*74*
Macedonian Samples				
Marvinci	192	15	14	29
Demir Kapija	505	14	14	28
Subtotal	*697*	*29*	*28*	*57*
Total	**1359**	**76**	**55**	**131**

Table 2 Collections summary

Methods

Standard craniometric variables along with craniofacial indices and ratios were compared between skulls with dental anomalies and normal (no dental anomalous conditions as described below) skulls from the population samples. Statistical analyses tested for significant differences between the groups.

Many orthodontic and clinical studies associate dental anomalies and pathological conditions to malocclusion types, but the nature of archaeological specimens presented the difficulty of matching mandibles correctly to the associated crania accurately enough to make a decision of occlusion type. This has led to the decision to only utilize standard craniometric indices and measurements.

Measurement	Code	Landmarks	Component
Maximum cranial length	GOL	g-op	Vault
Maximum cranial breadth	XCB	eu-eu	Vault
Cranial height	BBH	ba-b	Vault
Facial height	TFH	n-gn	Face
Facial breadth	ZYB	zy-zy	Face
Upper facial height	NPH	n-pr	Face
Upper facial breadth	FMT	fmt-fmt	Face
Maxilloalveolar length	MAXL	pr-alv	Palate, external
Maxilloalveolar breadth	MAXB	ect-ect	Palate, external
Palatal length	PL	ol-sta	Palate, internal
Palatal breadth	PB	enm-enm	Palate, internal
Bicondylar breadth	BCDL	cdl-cdl	Mandible
Bigonial breadth	BGO	go-go	Mandible
Height of ascending ramus	HAR	go-cdl	Mandible
Min breadth of ascending ramus	MBAR		Mandible
Height of mandible at symphysis	HMS	gn-ini	Manidble

Table 3 List of cranial landmark measurements.

Craniometrics.

16 standard cranial measurements were taken from the six population samples of complete or near-complete skulls with mandibles, using digital spreading and sliding calipers. The paired landmark measurements are as described by Howell 1973, Buikstra and Ubelaker 1994, and Bass 2005, and are presented in Table 3, above. A number of standard craniometrics (i.e., nasal, orbits) were disregarded due to the likelihood of taphonomic damage and the need to maintain a reasonable sample size. The landmark measurements were chosen to indicate in general the size and shape of the cranial vault, the face, and the masticatory process, and indices and ratios were calculated to gauge relative dimensions (Bass 2005; White et al 2011). Of the measurements chosen, not all could be taken from all skulls; at the very least measurements were taken from skulls that could provide measurements of masticatory features (palate, maxilla, mandible) or cranial features in skulls with analysable dentitions, but missing landmarks of the masticatory elements.

The craniofacial indices, percentage values that gauge breadth to length, used are as follows (Bass 2005):

(1) Cranial Index (CI) = (cranial breadth * 100) / cranial length

(2) Cranial Module (CM) = (length + breadth + height)/3

(3) Cranial Length-Height Index (CLHI) = (cranial height*100)/cranial length

(4) Cranial Breadth-Height Index (CBHI) = (cranial height*100)/maximum cranial breadth

(5) Total Facial Index (TFI) = (facial height * 100)/ bizygomatic breadth

(6) Upper Facial Index (UFI) = (upper facial height * 100)/bizygomatic breadth

(7) Maxilloalveolar Index (MAI)= (maxilloalveolar breadth * 100) /maxilloalveolar length

(8) Palatal Index (PI)= (palatal breadth * 100)/palatal length

In addition, unique indices and ratios will be calculated to determine relative size differences among the craniofacial complexes:

(9) Palatal/Maxillary ratio (PMR): Palatal index divided by maxilloalveolar index (PI/MAI)

(10) TFH/FMT: Index of upper facial breadth (FMT) to total facial height ([TFH*100]/FMT)

(11) UFH/FMT: Index of upper facial breadth to upper facial height ([UFH*100]/FMT)

(12) Jaw breadth index, MAXB/CDL: Index of bicondylar breadth to maxilloalveolar breadth ([MAXB*100]/BCDL)

(13) Mandibular breadth index (cdl/go): Index of bicondylar breadth to bigonial breadth ([BGB*100]/BCDL)

(14) UHTH: Index of upper facial height to total facial height ([NPH*100]/NGN)

(15) FB1: Facial breadth index 1 ([BCDL*100]/ZYB)

(16) FB2: Facial breadth index 2 ([FMT*100]/CDL)

(17) UFI/MAI ratio: Ratio of the maxilloalveolar index relative to the upper facial index, UFI/MAI

Clinical orthodontic literature often measures the dimensions of the dental arch by the use of dental crown traits or cusps as landmarks, but the nature of archaeological samples preclude the use of this method, because of ante- and postmortem loss of teeth. Instead, the dimensions of the masticatory complex will be calculated using the standard craniometrics as described above.

Dental Anomalies.

Visual examination of the dentition determined dental anomalies or significant pathological conditions. Few skulls included a complete dental arch, so placement of the available teeth into the appropriate sockets or examination of socket shape or position (expected, transposed, supernumerary, rotated, etc) as described in Burnett and Weets (2001) and Bass (2005) determined presence of anomalies. The anomalies and disorders investigated:

- Supernumerary teeth. Supernumeraries were recorded as supernumerary (not normally shaped) or supplemental (normally shaped), and the mesiodens, the commonest supernumerary. All were recorded as separate phenomena.

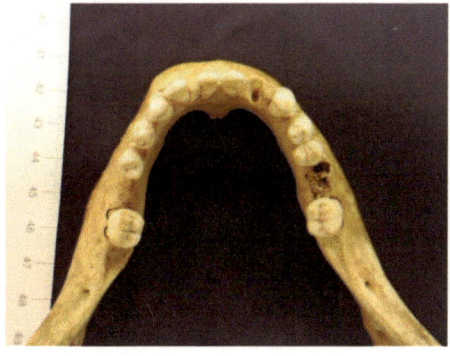

Figure1. Mildly rotated left mandibular premolars, Hickleton 36.

- Hypodontia. The congenital absence of each expected tooth was recorded, and 3rd molar agenesis regarded independently as well.
- Transposition. Any interchange of normal tooth positions was recorded, or any tooth in an unexpected socket.
- Rotations and Reversals. Lingually or labially turned teeth will be recorded along with angle, if possible. Includes winging if the winging results in angular rotation. A reversal is a completely rotated tooth, and any occurrence was recorded separately. See figure 1, right.
- Misshapen or peg-shaped teeth, unless supernumerary, were recorded. See figure 2, below.
- Impactions, ectopic and heterotopic eruptions and crowding were recorded and analysed along with anomalies.
- Other maxillofacial anomalies, pathological conditions, and infracranial syndromes with dental involvement were noted.

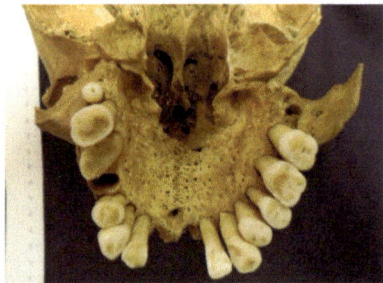

Figure 2. Peg-shaped left maxillary M3, Chichester 33.

Congenital Syndromes

Evidence for congenital syndromes and dysplasias were recorded, to be analysed separately from normal results.

Statistical Analysis.

The observations described above were recorded onto recording forms, and the data input into an IBM SPSS 18.0 database. The statistical analysis consisted of several steps:

1. Description of the frequency and distribution of the anomalies among the samples, including investigation of associations between anomalies.
2. Description of the significant differences between the craniometrics of the population samples.
3. Investigation of craniometric differences between anomalous and non-anomalous skulls, between sexes and population samples.

Skulls were examined and each possible anomaly was entered as the categorical variables 0, 'absent' or 1, 'present'. Theses variables were tested against each other using chi-square and fisher's exact tests. Distributions of continuous variables (craniometric variables, indices and ratio variables) were tested for normality and were examined against the categorical anomalies using independent samples t-tests, or Mann-Whitney tests for nonparametric data as appropriate. Other statistical tests are described in text as necessary. All statistics use $p>0.05$ as not significant, $p\leq0.05$ as significant, and $p\leq0.01$ as highly significant.

The goal of the study is to determine whether the highly heritable elements of the skull, as described in previously published research, are affected by, or conversely affect, the expression of dental anomalies. Because the formation of the dental complex has been argued to be under genetic control independent of the rest of the face (Ortner 2003, among others), and that the environment is significant in determining the shape of the face (Enlow 1990, among others), this project is investigating whether the adult shape and size of the skull (or relative sizes of cranial components) affect the expression of dental anomalies or conversely, that the presence of dental anomalies affect the shape of the face. The null hypothesis is that there is no correlation between dental anomalies and the shape or size of the skull.

IV. Results

		Female, N=55		Male, N=76		All, N=131	
		Cases	Prevalence	Cases	Prevalence	Cases	Prevalence
Any Anomaly other than Crowd	Present	30	54.5%	34	44.7%	64	48.9%
Supplemental Teeth	Present	0	.0%	2	2.6%	2	1.5%
Rotation	Present	18	32.7%	18	23.7%	36	27.5%
Reversal	Present	2	3.6%	0	.0%	2	1.5%
Peg, Misshapen	Present	0	.0%	4	5.3%	4	3.1%
Congenitally Absent Teeth	Present	2	3.6%	2	2.6%	4	3.1%
M3 Congenitally Absent	Present	5	9.1%	7	9.2%	12	9.2%
Ectopic, heterotopic, impaction	Present	7	12.7%	9	11.8%	16	12.2%
Crowding	Present	10	18.2%	21	27.6%	31	23.7%

Table 4 Distribution of anomalies by sex. See text.

Frequencies and Distribution of Anomalies

Summary statistics for all anomalies are available in Appendix B, Section 1. Prevalence rates of anomalies are listed in Table 4, above, and divided by population sample in Table 5, below. No significant correlations exist between any anomaly and sex or population. The most common dental disorder among all populations is rotation, at 27.5%, followed by crowding, at almost 24%. Although not statistically significant, prevalence does vary among the populations, with crowding among the Marvinci sample reaching almost 45%, and only around 12% among the Blackfriars sample.

	Supplemental Supernumeraries		Rotations		Reversals		Peg, Misshapen		Congenitally Absent Teeth		M3 Congenitally Absent		Ectopic, heterotopic, impaction		Crowding	
	Cases	%	Cases	%	Cases	%	Cases	%	Cases	%	Cases	%	Cases	%	Cases	%
Blackfriars, N=17	0	.0%	2	11.8%	0	.0%	1	5.9%	0	.0%	2	11.8%	1	5.9%	2	11.8%
Box Lane, N=9	1	11.1%	1	11.1%	0	.0%	1	11.1%	1	11.1%	2	22.2%	2	22.2%	2	22.2%
Chichester, N=36	1	2.8%	13	36.1%	0	.0%	2	5.6%	1	2.8%	3	8.3%	3	8.3%	7	19.4%
Demir Kapija, N=28	0	.0%	6	21.4%	0	.0%	0	.0%	0	.0%	3	10.7%	2	7.1%	4	14.3%
Hickleton, N=12	0	.0%	4	33.3%	0	.0%	0	.0%	1	8.3%	0	.0%	2	16.7%	3	25.0%
Marvinci, N=29	0	.0%	10	34.5%	2	6.9%	0	.0%	1	3.4%	2	6.9%	6	20.7%	13	44.8%

Table 5 Prevalence of Anomalies by Population Sample.

No cases of any infracranial congenital disorder, such as cleidocranial dysplasia, were observed among any population sample.

Relationships between anomalies

Chi-square and Fisher's exact tests of the dental anomalies and disorders are summarised in Appendix B, Section 1. Rotations are correlated to crowding among all skulls (χ^2=6.37, p=0.012). When analysed by sex, an association for males between rotations and crowding remains (Fisher's exact test, p=0.032) but is lost for females, and analysed according to geographic population and sex, supplemental teeth were associated with rotations (Fisher's exact test, p=0.043) and ectopic eruptions were associated with rotations among English males (Fisher's exact test, p=0.046).

Preliminary Craniometric Analysis

Recorded craniometrics are available in Appendix A, table 1; and summary statistics for craniometric variables are listed in Appendix B, section 2. Sex differences were significant (p<0.05) for all craniometric variables except for palatal breadth (ecm-ecm; t=1.208, p=0.23), therefore all other craniometric variable were analysed separately by sex.

Independent samples t-tests indicated that the most significantly different craniometric variables (p<0.05, see Appendix B, Section 2) were, among females, maximum cranial length (GOL; t=2.813, p=0.007), fronto-zygomatic breadth (FMT; t=2.173, p=0.035), and bicondylar breadth (BCDL; t=-2.133, p=0.040) between English and Macedonian samples. Among males, the most significant differences were upper facial height and bicondylar breadth. However, when normal skulls (no dental anomalies, no crowding) were compared, the significance dropped, although for females maximum cranial length (t=2.066, p=0.052) and for males fronto-zygomatic breath and palatal length were borderline, t=0.801, p=0.050 and t=0.676, p=0.050, respectively.

Among craniometric indices, only cranial module (CM) indicated a significant difference between the sexes (see Appendix B). Independent samples t-tests of the indices showed that the Cranial length-height index (CLHI; t=-1.992, p=0.050) and the palatal index (PI; t=-3.378, p=0.001) are the only significant differences between Macedonian and English samples, but when anomalous skulls were removed the significance was eliminated, except that palatal index remained essentially borderline (t=-1.982, p=0.054).

By far the most significant differences between Macedonian and English sample skulls are in the ratios Upper Facial Height/Total Facial Height (UHTH) and the Facial Breadth ratios. The significance is exaggerated when divided by sex, with UHTH for males reaching p=0.001 (t=-3.776) and FB2 for females, p=0.018 (t=2.517). When anomalous skulls are removed, the significance falls, but FB1 remains highly significant at t=-3.301, p=0.005, and the mandibular breadth ratio becomes significant at t=2.178, p=0.039.

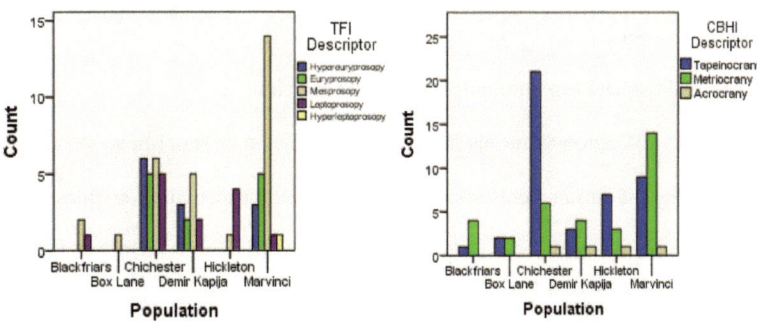

Figure 3. Bar graph illustrating relative distribution of TFI.

Figure 4. Bar graph illustrating relative distribution of CBHI.

The Macedonian and English normal sample skulls can be described using the range descriptions as interpreted by Bass (2005), summarized the bar graphs of figures 5 and 6, above. The most notable divergence between the English and Macedonian samples is in the Total Facial Index, in which the English sample is largely characterized by *leptoprosopy*, long thin faces, while the Macedonian sample is largely *mesoprosopic*, medium-faced. The samples also diverge in the Cranial Length-Height Index (CLHI) and Cranial Breadth-Height Index, both suggesting that the English sample were more characterized by "low skulls" than the Macedonian (Bass 2005:71).

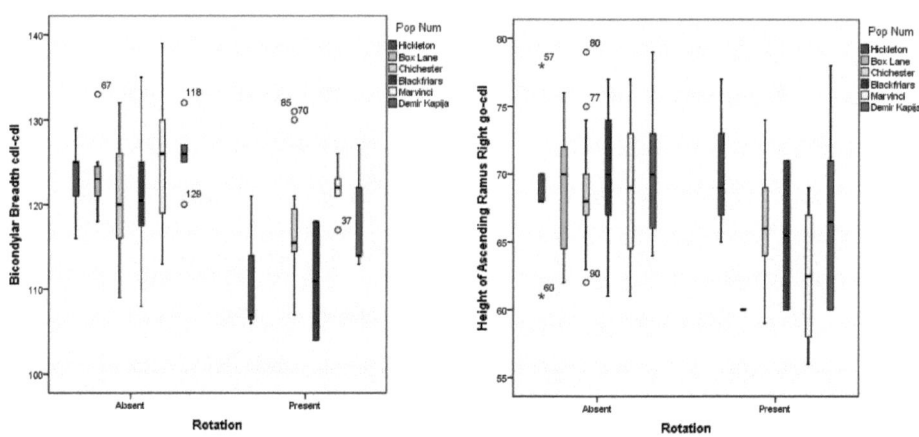

Figures 5, (left), 6 (right). Boxplots showing relative size differences in mandibular features with and without tooth rotations.

Relationships between anomalies and craniometrics

Significant differences of means from t-tests are listed in table 6, below. Among all skulls, independent sample t-tests indicated that several mandibular variables were smaller on average with rotations present: bicondylar breadth (t=3.676, p=0.000), height of ascending ramus (t=2.913, p=0.004), minimum breadth of ascending ramus (t=2.958, p=0.004), and height at mandibular symphysis (t=2.376, p=0.019). These relationships can be visualised in boxplots, figures 7 and 8, above. Rotations were also associated with smaller facial height (t=2.492, p=0.015), facial width (t=2.313, p=0.023), maximum cranial length (t=2,260, p=0.026) and cranial height (t=2.195, p=0.031).

Crowding was also shown to be associated with significantly smaller minimum ramus breadth (t=-1.993, p=0.049). Congenitally absent teeth were associated with smaller bigonial breath (t=2.357, p=0.020) while congenitally absent third molars showed a relationship with smaller facial height (t=2.407, p=0.019).

			Female			Male		
			English Mean	Macedonian Mean	All Mean	English Mean	Macedonian Mean	All Mean
Max Cranial Length	Rotation	Absent	181.00	173.72	177.36	184.04	181.86	183.04
		Present	174.71	172.10	173.18	179.10	183.17	180.63
Cranial Height	Rotation	Absent	129.38	126.55	128.08	133.67	136.00	134.60
		Present	125.00	124.80	124.91	128.60	134.00	129.85
	Congenitally Absent Teeth	Absent	128.41	126.00	127.24	132.03	134.88	133.00
		Present	124.50	.	124.50	.	148.00	148.00
	Crowding	Absent	125.41	124.45	125.04	132.52	136.50	133.66
		Present	150.00	129.40	135.29	130.00	134.43	132.38
Facial Height n-gn	Rotation	Absent	108.00	107.67	107.79	117.55	114.23	116.24
		Present	106.14	107.20	106.76	112.00	111.20	111.67
	M3 Congenitally Absent	Absent	106.92	108.24	107.69	117.12	113.39	115.56
		Present	.	100.50	100.50	103.50	.	103.50
Facial Width zy-zy	Rotation	Absent	127.20	126.79	126.96	133.61	135.00	134.26
		Present	126.00	124.50	125.17	131.25	131.80	131.46
Upper Facial Height n-pr	Ectopic, heterotopic, impaction	Absent	64.76	65.48	65.18	67.35	70.94	68.63
		Present	58.00	61.33	60.00	67.25	68.00	67.63
Maxilloalveolar Length pr-alv	Congenitally Absent Teeth	Absent	49.29	50.91	49.93	53.12	52.38	52.87
		Present	51.00	.	51.00	.	60.00	60.00
	Ectopic, heterotopic, impaction	Absent	49.24	50.91	49.89	53.29	54.18	53.57
		Present	52.00	.	52.00	51.00	48.33	49.40
Palatal Length ol-sta	Rotation	Absent	49.00	47.75	48.50	50.35	48.15	49.74
		Present	46.00	45.71	45.87	49.10	50.00	49.36
Bicondylar Breadth cdl-cdl	Rotation	Absent	119.91	122.89	121.25	122.75	127.67	124.39
		Present	111.63	119.14	115.13	119.44	121.75	120.15
Bigonial Breadth go-go	Congenitally Absent Teeth	Absent	94.62	96.57	95.64	103.32	106.21	104.44
		Present	90.00	.	90.00	75.00	103.00	89.00
Height of Ascending Ramus Right go-cdl	Rotation	Absent	67.54	67.20	67.39	70.00	70.93	70.30
		Present	65.75	63.14	64.53	67.27	70.00	67.86
Min Breadth of Ascending Ramus Right	Rotation	Absent	30.43	30.50	30.46	32.16	32.25	32.19
		Present	28.38	30.14	29.20	30.36	30.33	30.36
Height at Mandibular Symphysis gn-idi	Rotation	Absent	29.07	27.08	28.15	31.23	30.29	30.89
		Present	27.25	25.00	26.29	28.73	32.00	29.43

Table 6 Summary of mean, significant difference of craniometrics with anomalies.

When divided by sex, rotations were associated with alternate variables between the sexes: among females, smaller values for bicondylar breadth (t=2.798, p=0.009), palatal length (t=2.124, p=0.040) and height of ascending ramus (t=2.037, p=0.049), while among males cranial height and minimum breadth of ascending ramus (t=3.107, p=0.039) were significantly smaller. Females further show a significantly larger cranial height with crowding (Mann-Whitney, p=0.032), and smaller upper facial height (t=2.339, p=0.024) with ectopic eruptions. Males exhibit a strong association of ectopic eruptions with smaller maxilloalveolar length (t=2.767, p=0.009). Congenitally absent teeth were associated in males with larger cranial height (-2.412, p=0.020), maxilloalveolar length (t=-2.158, p=0.037), and bicondylar breadth (t=-2.389, p=0.021), while absence of the third molar was associated with smaller facial height (t=2.288, p=0.027).

Independent samples t-test results of anomalies with craniometric indices are listed in Appendix B. The cranial length-height index (t=-3.600, p=0.001) and cranial breadth-height index (t=-3.606, p=0.001) were significantly higher with crowding present among females while among males cranial module values were higher with other congenitally absent teeth (t=-2.490, p=0.017). The maxilloalveolar index was higher in with rotations among women (t=-3.029, p=0.005) and ectopic eruptions in males (t=-2.555, p=0.015).

Cramer's V tests to gauge associations between anomalies craniofacial indexical categories mostly indicated that anomalies are largely distributed normally across the categories (i.e., most anomalies occur within the most common type), with the exception of Total Facial Index (TFI) and Upper Facial Index (UFI). For TFI, rotations are relatively more common in English euryprosopic (wide-faced) skulls (3 of 5), and equivalent in English hypereuryprosopic (very wide-faced) skulls (3 of 6), although these were the least common facial types among the English sample. Among Macedonian skulls the converse is true: leptoprosopic (narrow-faced) skulls (2 of 3) and hyperleprosopic (very narrow-faced) skulls (1 of 1) have relatively higher rotation rates, despite being the least common skull types among the Macedonian sample. In both Macedonian and English samples, the only skulls with UFI index classified as hypereuryenic (very wide face) each contain rotations.

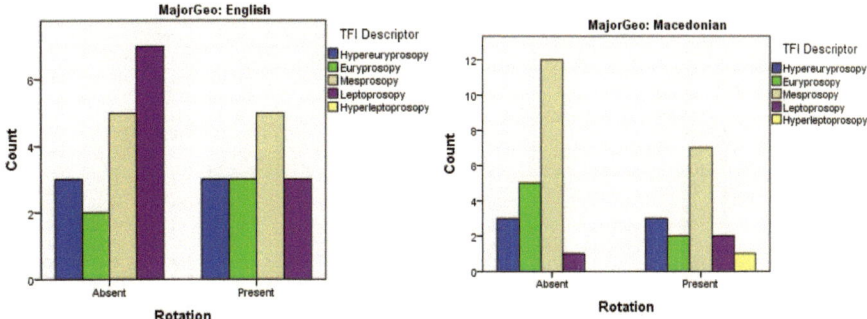

Figures 7 (left), 8 (right). Graphs showing relative frequencies of rotations among Total Facial Index categories, English and Macedonian samples.

Independent samples t-tests on anomalies with the new craniofacial ratios and indices found relationships between rotations and lower jaw breadth ratio (MAXB/BCDL; t=-2.418, p=0.019), and facial breadth (FB1, lower, t=2.529, p=0.014, and FB2, higher, t=-2.123, p=0.038). Tooth agenesis had much higher (t=-2.504, p=0.016), and ectopic eruptions, lower (t=2.170, p=0.035), upper facial index/maxilloalveolar index ratio (UFI/MAI) values among all skulls. English skulls additionally showed congenitally absent third molars related to lower (t=2.188, p=0.035), and misshapen teeth to higher (t=-2.339, p=0.025) total facial height/facial breadth (TFH/FMT) ratio values, while Macedonian skulls showed a association of crowding with higher UFH/FMT (t=-2.879, p=0.007). These results may be expected because individual paired landmark components are affected, but imply that overall dimensions and shape are affected as well.

Overall anomalies have been related to smaller size in craniometric variables, although not always statistically significant (see table 7). Crowding does not appear to have such a consistent relationship (table 8).

	Female						Male					
	English		Macedonian		All		English		Macedonian		All	
	Any Anomaly other than Crowding											
	Absent	Present	Absent	Present	Absent	Present	Absent	Present	Absent	Present	Absent	Present
	Mean	Mean	Mean	Mean	Mean	Mean	Mean	Mean	Mean	Mean	Mean	Mean
GOL	180.4	178.4	175.5	171.1	177.8	174.6	183.3	181.8	181.5	182.7	182.6	182.2
XCB	142.5	141.7	141.2	140.3	141.7	141.0	147.1	146.6	144.4	146.4	146.1	146.5
BBH	126.3	129.5	126.7	125.4	126.5	127.6	133.5	130.2	134.4	136.8	133.8	132.8
FH	108.7	106.3	111.3	106.4	110.1	106.4	119.9	111.3	116.0	111.3	118.6	111.3
ZYB	127.2	126.1	127.7	124.7	127.4	125.3	134.7	131.1	133.9	134.6	134.3	132.6
FMT	105.7	103.7	103.3	99.8	104.5	102.0	107.1	104.6	101.6	107.4	105.6	105.5
UFH	64.3	63.9	65.8	64.4	65.2	64.2	69.0	65.4	70.4	70.4	69.5	67.4
MAXL	49.3	49.5	52.8	49.3	50.6	49.4	53.4	52.7	53.9	52.0	53.5	52.4
MAXB	55.5	58.5	58.7	56.0	56.8	57.3	60.0	60.1	61.3	61.0	60.4	60.4
PL	49.5	46.9	48.6	46.1	49.2	46.5	51.0	48.6	47.8	49.3	50.2	48.9
PB	38.2	38.6	40.0	40.8	38.8	39.7	39.6	39.4	44.7	41.0	40.9	39.9
BCDL	120.0	114.8	124.4	119.8	122.0	117.1	124.2	119.1	127.7	125.3	125.0	121.6
BGO	97.6	92.6	96.3	96.7	96.9	94.7	104.4	100.3	104.5	107.4	104.4	103.5
HAR	67.9	66.2	67.0	64.9	67.5	65.6	70.6	67.6	71.0	70.6	70.7	68.6
MBAR	30.4	29.3	30.9	30.1	30.6	29.7	32.1	31.2	31.4	32.4	31.9	31.6
HMS	29.9	27.6	27.9	25.2	28.9	26.6	31.6	29.2	30.2	30.9	31.2	29.8

Table 7 Means of craniometric variables, any anomaly absent and present. Smaller values (in bold) are more common than larger values, but not always statistically significant.

	Female						Male					
	English		Macedonian		Total		English		Macedonian		Total	
	Crowding											
	Absent	Present	Absent	Present	Absent	Present	Absent	Present	Absent	Present	Absent	Present
	Mean	Mean	Mean	Mean	Mean	Mean	Mean	Mean	Mean	Mean	Mean	Mean
GOL	179.3	179.0	173.3	172.6	176.4	174.0	183.6	179.3	182.6	181.4	183.2	180.4
XCB	141.3	147.7	140.9	140.3	141.1	142.5	147.8	142.4	145.4	145.4	147.0	144.2
BBH	125.4	150.0	124.5	129.4	125.0	135.3	132.5	130.0	136.5	134.4	133.7	132.4
FH	106.8	107.5	106.6	109.2	106.7	108.8	116.5	115.0	112.1	115.4	114.9	115.2
ZYB	126.9	125.0	124.8	128.4	125.8	127.7	133.3	131.0	133.0	136.3	133.2	134.2
FMT	104.9	102.0	101.7	101.0	103.5	101.4	106.6	104.5	102.8	106.4	105.7	105.3
UFH	64.7	60.7	64.8	65.6	64.7	64.1	67.6	66.6	68.8	72.1	67.9	69.7
MAXL	49.1	51.5	50.6	51.5	49.6	51.5	53.1	53.3	52.7	53.4	53.0	53.4
MAXB	57.0	58.3	55.9	60.2	56.5	59.5	60.3	59.5	59.3	63.3	60.1	61.2
PL	48.5	45.0	48.6	48.0	47.8	46.9	50.5	48.7	48.2	49.0	50.0	48.8
PB	38.6	36.7	40.6	40.4	39.4	39.0	39.5	39.7	40.8	45.4	39.7	42.2
BCDL	116.0	118.7	121.9	120.2	118.3	119.7	121.6	122.8	124.4	128.4	122.3	125.4
BGO	94.5	93.7	98.4	92.4	96.3	92.8	103.3	100.4	106.3	105.7	104.4	103.1
HAR	67.0	66.0	65.5	65.8	66.4	65.9	69.5	68.5	69.9	72.3	69.6	69.9
MBAR	29.5	31.0	30.2	30.8	29.8	30.9	31.6	31.9	31.0	33.3	31.5	32.5
HMS	28.5	28.0	25.6	29.3	27.2	28.7	30.9	29.7	28.9	33.0	30.3	31.1

Table 8 Means of craniometric variables with crowding absent or present. Smaller values with crowding present in bold.

V. Discussion

The purpose of this investigation was to examine the relationship between dental anomalies and craniometric variation in modern humans, testing hypotheses regarding the aetiology of occlusal variation as a result of genetics or environmental and dietary modifications. Current clinical research largely posits a multifactorial origin for most dental disorders, combinations of genetic threshold traits and appropriate environmental circumstances leading to the expression of anomalous traits. A general trend in the anthropological research is that modern urbanization and agricultural changes have led to a softer diet in modern humans, resulting in smaller masticatory elements struggling to accommodate genetically-controlled tooth sizes (Lombardi 1982; Corruccini 1984; Ortner 2003). In addition to this dietary change is the increasing degree of inter-ethnic mixing, often hypothesized to introduce incongruence in the relative sizes of skeletal elements to teeth (Lombardi 1982; Mossey 1999a; Ortner 2003) due to craniometric population variation.

The first step in attempting to answer these questions is an analysis of the distribution and frequency of the dental anomalies in the sample populations, to examine differences between populations and compare with other populations and over time. A prediction of the "disease of civilization" theories would be that the premodern, mostly Mediaeval, samples would have lower rates of occlusal variation than modern populations. The second step is to examine the craniometric differences between skulls without dental anomalies and those that have dental anomalies, elucidating the relationship between morphological craniofacial variables and the expression of occlusal and dental disorders.

Palaeoepidemiology and the analysis of dental anomalies

As the study of the distribution of disease in past populations, palaeoepidemiology is burdened with the inherent problem of inferring information from often small, incomplete, and fragmented collections of specimens (Waldron 2007). Together with the limits of palaeopathology to diagnose pathologic conditions in skeletal remains, much of the interest in human diseases in the past has focused on descriptions and case studies rather than distributions and frequencies (Waldron 2007; White et al 2012). These issues limit the capability of palaeoepidemiology to describing "crude prevalence," simply the number of cases divided by the total sample number, rather than providing information that may be compared with other studies to elucidate patterns of disease distribution or predict risk (Waldron 2009:254).

Thus the modern clinical and epidemiological literature has shown significant interest in the expression and distribution of dental anomalies of shape, number, and position, but the phenomena have received little analysis within anthropology and archaeology. The relative rarity of many of the anomalies and the unlikelihood of occurrence within archaeological samples contribute to the difficulty of such palaeoepidemiological analysis (Vodanović et al 2012). There is very little likelihood of finding an anomaly such as a supernumerary or transposed tooth within the average range of skeletal remains recovered in anthropological studies; when such anomalies are found, they often yield significant results (Legoux 1974; Burnett and Weets 2001; Duncan 2009; Sholts et al 2010).

More common dental and orthodontic disorders such as crowding and rotations have more coverage within anthropology because of their frequencies but studies may still be limited because of the nature of taphonomic damage to skulls and the consequent difficulty of finding complete dentitions. Malocclusion type is difficult to infer because articulated jaws are rare, and the uncertainty of correctly matching upper and lower jaws to represent occlusion during life (Vodanović et al 2012).

With these caveats and limitations in mind, the aims of this first step of analysis will be an attempt to estimate the relative frequencies (prevalence) of the dental anomalies as they appeared in the English and Macedonian samples.

General distribution of anomalies

The overall prevalence of anomalies (exclusive of crowding) among all skulls was 48.9%. There were no statistically significant differences in prevalence between female and male skulls in the expression of anomalies in general, although crowding was more evident in males (27.6%) than females (18.2%). Including crowding, the general prevalence of all anomalies is 72.5%; 95 of 131 skulls exhibit some form of dental anomaly or occlusal disorder.

Hyperdontia

No cases of misshapen supernumeraries or mesiodens were observed. Only two cases of supplemental teeth (normally shaped supernumerary teeth) were found among the English and Macedonian samples, both in English males, Chichester 346 and Box Lane 32c. Although two occasions of supernumeraries are statistically too insignificant from which to make any inferences, the rate (1.5% among the total sample, 2.7% among English) could be expected from reported prevalence rates among modern populations (between 0.1 and 3.8% among Caucasians and more common among males than females; Rajab and Hamdam 2002). Box Lane 32c exhibited a retained deciduous mandibular first molar, impacted mandibular third molars, rotations and crowding along the anterior mandibular arch as well absent canines. Interestingly, and perhaps significantly, the maxilla had no such anomalies or crowding (although on further inspection, Box Lane 32c may be an adolescent with an unusual eruption pattern, in which the maxilla and mandible show different stages of mixed dentition). Chichester 346, conversely, while lepromatous, exhibited no crowding or other dental anomalies associated with its supplemental mandibular incisor. A supplemental fourth mandibular molar had been previously analysed from Demir Kapija by Veljanovska (2001), unfortunately the skull, DK 64, was not available for examination. Non-syndromic supernumeraries have been described to occur along with associated anomalies (the extra tooth may promote crowding and impactions) or individually (Bacetti 1998a; Rajab and Hamdam 2002). Based on this analysis of such a small sample, neither a strict hereditary aetiology nor the influence of environmental and local factors can be discounted.

Misshapen and peg-shaped teeth

Four cases of misshapen teeth were present among the samples, all of them English and male. This represents a prevalence of 3.1% among all the skulls and 5.4% among English skulls. Blackfriars 92 exhibited a peg-shaped lateral maxillary incisor, which has been associated with other dental aplasia and particularly with displacement of the maxillary canine (Brin et al 1986; Baccetti 1998a) and has an overall prevalence of between 0.3% and 8.4% (Thongudomporn and Freer 1998). Baccetti reported a frequency among Caucasians of 4.7%, and found a statistically significant association between anomalous lateral incisors and all other anomalies except for supernumerary teeth (Baccetti 1998a). Blackfrairs 92, however, has no other anomalies, and the anomalous shapes of the other specimens are among other teeth, including a peg-shaped maxillary third molar in Chichester 33 (see figure 3, Methods).

Hypodontia

The English and Macedonian samples contained a total of 4 individuals with congenitally absent teeth (excusive of M3), and 12 individuals missing the third molar, resulting in an overall prevalence of 12.2%, and 3.1% exclusive of the third molar, and 9.2% for third molar agenesis. These results are in concord with the general prevalence among modern Caucasian populations, although lower results than some premodern samples. Vodanović and colleagues (2012) found a prevalence of hypodontia at 41% among a Late Antique (3-5th century AD) and 30.1% among an Early Mediaeval Croatian sample, all of which were either the third molar or mandibular second premolars.

Congenitally absent teeth, hypodontia, is not uncommon among modern populations nor is it rare among archaeological specimens (Ortner 2003). It has been referred to as the most frequent dental anomaly in modern people (Mattheeuws et al 2004). Modern prevalence rates have been estimated as 3.5%-6.5% (Kirzioğlu et al 2005), reaching up to 39% among siblings and parents of an individual exhibiting hypodontia, suggesting a strong hereditary component to the expression of congenitally missing teeth (Vastardis 2000; Parkin et al 2009). The most common missing tooth is the third molar, reported as affecting around 20% of the general population (Vastardis 2000). According to Ortner (2003), the second most common congenitally absent teeth are the maxillary lateral incisors, followed by the second premolars. Many researchers are unsure of relative frequencies of the remaining commonly missing teeth, although Vastardis reported (2000) that some consider the mandibular second premolar is likely the second most frequent at 3.4%, compared to the lateral incisor frequency of 2.2%.

Many authors have linked hypodontia with a number of other dental and craniofacial anomalies (Mattheeuws et al 2004; Kirzioğlu et al 2005), particularly third molar agenesis with agenesis of other teeth or microdontia (Vastardis 2000; Kirzioğlu et al 2005). The sixteen specimens in this study exhibiting agenesis showed no significant associations: no individuals with absent third molars had any other missing teeth, nor was agenesis (M3 or other) statistically associated with any other anomaly. One individual, Box Lane 32c, showed a number of anomalies, but of the other 15, only three had rotations (the most common anomaly in this study), and two others had crowding (the second most common disorder).

Transpositions

No cases of transposed teeth were observed among the English and Macedonian samples. Transpositions are quite rare in modern humans, below 1% in the general population, but Chattopadhay and Srinivas (1996) reported an association between tooth agenesis and transpositions.

Rotations and reversals

Rotations were the most common dental anomaly among the analysed skulls, reaching a prevalence of 34.5% in the Marvinci sample, and an overall prevalence of 27.5%. Two Macedonian females (Marvinci) exhibited reversals. Whether or not a reversal is a fully rotated tooth, following the aetiology of rotation, or independent anomaly is unclear. Tooth rotation is apparently only rarely referred to as an independent phenomenon, usually aggregated with other symptoms characterizing crowding and general malocclusion (Harris and Smith 1980; Hillson 1996).

Although reversals were associated with crowding, the fact that rotations occur without crowding or associated disorders appears to suggest a separate cause for a specific type of rotation, perhaps unrelated to winging caused by crowding and other occlusal variables.

Ectopic eruptions and impactions

Ectopic eruptions and impactions are not normally regarded as anomalies and were recorded together to test for associations or relationships with dental anomalies or metric variables. There was a general prevalence of 12.2% among all skulls; 8 individuals in each population sample exhibited some form of impaction or heterotopic eruption. Again, the figures for the Macedonian and English samples are not out of the range of contemporary prevalence rates. Thongudomporn and Freer reported (1998) prevalence rates of 14.4% for ectopic eruptions, mostly maxillary canines, and 9.9% for impactions in their study of 111 Australian orthodontic patients.

Dental Crowding

The general prevalence of crowding among the Macedonian and English skulls was 23.7%. Importantly, the prevalence varied among the populations (although not statistically significant), from around 12% in the Blackfriars, England sample (sample size N=17) to near 45% in the Marvinci, Macedonia sample (sample size N=29).

As discussed above, crowding has had significant coverage in the anthropological research, often lending evidence to theories of the impact of modern diet and environment toward craniofacial morphology. Crowding among modern populations has been described from 40% to as high as 80% (Mockers et al 2004;

Evensen and Øgaard 2007), and the most common dental disorder among children (Melo et al 2001). Many reports have claimed little evidence of crowding (or general malocclusion) among archaeological remains or non-Western populations (Mossey 1999a; Mockers et al 2004), but Harper (1994) found more intensive crowding among a Medieval London population than modern Europeans, although he did not provide frequency. Corruccini, in his seminal work (1984) of contemporary modern populations, reported ideal occlusions in as high as 76% of non-westernised and 63% of moderately westernised populations compared to only 42% of Western, industrialized populations; significant malocclusions were present only in as low as 0.2% of the non-westernised populations compared to 16.5% of the Western populations. Further, Corruccini (1984:424) argued that crowding is the result of decreases in the sizes of the skeletal masticatory components rather than the size of the teeth, based on the lack of crowding among some populations with reduced dental attrition. In contrast, a French Copper Age site of 150 adults was described as having a 100% rate of crowding, while tooth size was congruent with modern populations (Mockers et al 2004). The Marvinci sample, which mostly consists of remains dating from the Hellenistic and Roman eras, contrasts with most data showing low crowding rates except in transitional and modern populations, and suggests, like the French Copper Age data, that the causes of dental variation are not necessarily the result of modern civilization but potentially a number of factors, genetic and environmental, that can vary among populations and times.

Relationships between dental anomalies and craniometrics

The data presented here appears to suggest that there is no significant difference between the prevalence of dental anomalies within the English and Macedonian premodern samples compared to modern Europeans (except for relatively higher rates for crowding in the Marvinci sample compared to some premodern estimates), the second step in this analysis is an examination of the differences in anomalous and nonanomalous skulls and dentitions. The null hypothesis, that there is no relationship between craniometrics and dental anomalies, can be rejected. Among all skulls, the only metric variables that showed no statistical difference between anomalous and normal skulls were maximum cranial breadth (XCB), upper facial breadth (FMT), palatal breadth (PB), and maxilloalveolar breadth (MAXB). Mandibular dimensions were most often affected but cranial dimensions in general were susceptible to variation as well. The plasticity of the craniofacial elements associated with the masticatory complex is the foundation of the field of orthodontics, but the relationship between dental anomalies and craniometrics may have significant consequences for the interpretation of phenotypic population variation and the aetiology of occlusal variation.

Heritability, population variation and dental anomalies

Craniometric variation between the English and Macedonian samples was small and not significant except for facial height and facial breadth ratios and indices. English skulls had longer, thinner faces and lower skulls than the Macedonian samples. Craniometric variation among Europeans has been described as low relative to other world populations (Strand Vidarsdóttir and O'Higgins 2003), but an analysis of intraregional populations showed that craniometric variation is significant even on a regional level, describing significant differences between Balkan subpopulations (Ross 2004). It has been argued that among modern humans regional variation is greater than global variation between populations, providing an argument against racial classifications (Howells 1989; Relethford 1994).

Estimating population distance based on craniometrics has long been a staple of physical anthropology research, and has come under close scrutiny since the advances in genetics beginning in the 1990s. Boas' influential 1912 study of Europeans and their American immigrant counterparts emphasised the plasticity of cranial shape and its relationship with the environment, but Howell's research described worldwide differences in cranial shape without distinguishing which features may be derived from genetics or influence by local environments (Howells 1989; Sparks and Jantz 2002; Gravlee et al 2003).

Progress in the field of genetics has allowed anthropologists to estimate population distances without the concern of craniometric plasticity, but many have found the data between the two largely congruent (Roseman 2004; von Cramon-Taubadel 2009a; Strauss and Hubbe 2010; von Cramon-Taubadel and Smith 2012). Some matched genetic and morphological studies argue that local variation remains higher than variation between populations (Relethford 1994; Strauss and Hubbe 2010), while others emphasize that global craniometric variation can be attributed to distance from Africa and represents earlier ideas that cranial morphology adequately recapitulates population history (Roseman 2004).

Cranial vault metrics have often been given relatively high heritability rates (h^2), so it may come as no surprise that maximum cranial breadth, XCB, showed no significant changes in skulls with dental anomalies. In their reanalysis of the Boas immigrant data, Sparks and Jantz described XCB as highly heritable, as were all of the cranial vault variables they examined, and argued against the Boasian notion of cranial plasticity (Sparks and Jantz 2002; Holloway 2002). Other studies, however, have found lower heritabilities for XCB, Martínez-Abadías et al (2009) reporting $h^2=0.36$ and Carson (2006) only $h^2=0.233$, all of the studies based on the pedigreed skulls of Halstatt, Austria. The data presented here indicates that cranial breadth shows little variation among populations or between normal skulls and skulls with anomalous dentitions, suggesting support for the claim that cranial breadth is highly heritable and relatively less sensitive to adapt to environmental or developmental stimuli.

Cranial height (BBH) was shown to be associated with larger size in female skulls with crowded dentitions and in males with congenitally absent teeth. This may be related to the angle of the cranial base, which was not measured in this analysis, often regarded as influential on the anterior displacement of the maxilla and ultimately the dimensions of the dental arch (Cendekiawan et al 2010; Cobourne and DiBiase 2010). Shorter upper facial height was related to ectopic eruptions in females and short total facial height to congenitally absent teeth in males. Facial height has been linked to 'excessive eruption' of molars (Martina et al 2005:978) and continues to grow, apparently as a result of plastic changes of the masticatory complex throughout adult life (Martina et al 2005; Cobourne and DiBiase 2010). Shorter facial height has been associated with increased jaw muscle mass and hypertrophy of dental arch structure (Forster et al 2008). It is difficult to elucidate the relationship between the anomalies presented here and facial heights, except to note that vertical facial growth is sensitive to environmental forces.

In general, heritabilities of the neurocranium have been reported as higher than the elements of the facial and masticatory functional complexes (Carson 2006; González-José et al 2005; Martínez-Abadías 2009). Although the mandible was most associated with dental anomalies in this study, the number of times that cranial vault variables (maximum cranial length, GOL, and cranial height, BBH) were associated with dental anomalies may seem surprising based on their assumed high heritabilities. This could, however, provide support for the plasticity of the cranial vault or, conversely, the heritability of neurocranial size contributing to the aetiology of the anomalies from size incongruence. As can be seen in tables 9-11, below, population samples of normal skulls (no dental anomalies) with the highest rates of tooth rotations have the smallest maximum cranial lengths, highest cranial indices, and lowest cranial breadth-height index values, while population samples with the larger cranial lengths,

Rotation Prevalence	Population					
	Chichester 36.1% Mean	Marvinci 34.5% Mean	Hickleton 33.3% Mean	Demir Kapija 21.4% Mean	Blackfriars 11.8% Mean	Box Lane 11.1% Mean
Max Cranial Length	178.50	175.14	183.80	180.00	186.33	195.33
Max Cranial Breadth	145.29	140.43	146.40	143.69	146.67	146.75
Cranial Height	129.58	130.60	129.80	130.86	134.50	140.50
Facial Height n-gn	117.50	113.75	122.33	113.83	120.00	120.50
Facial Width zy-zy	133.70	129.83	125.00	130.30	132.80	133.00
FMT Width	105.64	104.33	107.40	101.00	108.29	107.50
Upper Facial Height enm-enm	68.15	67.80	68.00	66.42	64.67	66.50
Maxilloalveolar Length pr-alv	51.75	53.00	50.80	53.50	52.67	52.50
Maxilloalveolar Breadth ect-ect	58.23	56.00	55.00	59.20	60.38	62.33
Palatal Length ol-sta	49.64	47.50	49.20	47.22	52.11	52.75
Palatal Breadth enm-enm	40.23	39.50	35.60	40.90	39.22	39.00
Bicondylar Breadth cdl-cdl	125.00	124.83	120.67	127.67	120.25	125.75
Bigonial Breadth go-go	103.75	97.17	103.67	104.56	101.25	105.75
Height of Ascending Ramus Right go-cdl	70.89	70.00	69.00	68.88	69.75	71.75
Min Breadth of Ascending Ramus Right	31.70	31.33	29.33	30.78	32.13	31.00
Height at Mandibular Symphysis gn-idi	29.44	23.67	34.67	29.45	32.13	31.25

Table 9 Means of craniometric variables by population rotation prevalence, normal skulls only.

	Population					
	Chichester	Marvinci	Hickleton	Demir Kapija	Blackfriars	Box Lane
	Mean	Mean	Mean	Mean	Mean	Mean
Cranial Index	**81.5**	**80.3**	79.7	79.8	78.2	74.1
Cranial Module	150.25	149.00	153.33	151.48	155.78	159.83
Cranial length-height Index	73.25	74.99	70.60	72.26	72.22	72.07
Cranial breadth-height Index	**89.98**	**91.76**	88.65	**91.77**	93.81	97.57
Total Facial Index	86.78	86.94	90.49	86.98	91.60	85.71
Upper Facial Index	52.27	52.30	53.12	51.75	53.93	51.88
Maxilloalveolar Index	111.37	105.56	108.94	111.26	117.50	123.46
Palatal Index	81.49	82.89	72.49	87.16	75.62	74.23

Table 10 Means of craniometric indices by population, normal skulls only.

	Population					
	Chichester	Marvinci	Hickleton	Demir Kapija	Blackfriars	Box Lane
	Mean	Mean	Mean	Mean	Mean	Mean
Palatal/max ratio	.75$_a$	.78$_a$	.67$_a$	.86$_a$	.64$_a$	.68$_a$
TFHFMT	111.08$_a$	108.04$_a$	112.85$_a$	118.94$_a$	107.14^1	111.76^1
UFHFMT	64.48$_a$	63.65$_a$	63.46$_a$	63.22$_a$	60.35$_a$	67.65^1
MAXBCDL	.48$_a$	.43$_a$	.48$_a$	.52^1	.49$_a$	.49$_a$
cdlgo	.84$_a$	.78$_a$	.86$_a$	.82$_a$	.82$_a$	.84$_a$
ZYGFMT	.80$_a$	.80$_a$	.84$_a$	.82$_a$	.83$_a$	.77^1
UHTH	.59$_a$	.60$_a$	.60$_a$	.60$_a$	.59^1	.55$_a$
FB	.93$_a$	.97$_a$	.90$_a$	.98$_a$	.93$_a$	.92^1
FB2	.85$_a$	.82$_a$	.90$_a$	.75$_a$	.90$_a$	.84$_a$

Note: Values in the same row and subtable not sharing the same subscript are significantly different at p< 0.05 in the two-sided test of equality for column means. Cells with no subscript are not included in the test. Tests assume equal variances.[2]
1. This category is not used in comparisons because the sum of case weights is less than two.
2. Tests are adjusted for all pairwise comparisons within a row of each innermost subtable using the Bonferroni correction.

Table 11 Means of new indices and ratios by population, normal skulls only.

lower cranial index, and higher cranial breadth-height index values have the lower prevalence rates of rotations (see Figure 9, below). The relationship of rotations to smaller craniometric variables, as discussed above, may suggest that the expression of rotations may be dependent on a threshold value that is more likely to arise in populations with already small skulls.

    The paired landmark variable used in this study to measure upper facial breadth, the frontomalare temporale (FMT; Buikstra and Ubelaker 1994), is not commonly one of the standard craniometrics but was used here due to the likelihood of the survivability of the element in the archaeological record, as opposed to the frequently fragmented and missing zygomatic arch. Interestingly, although an element representing the face, FMT in this study was never significantly different in anomalous versus normal skulls. FMT is one of the traits significantly correlated

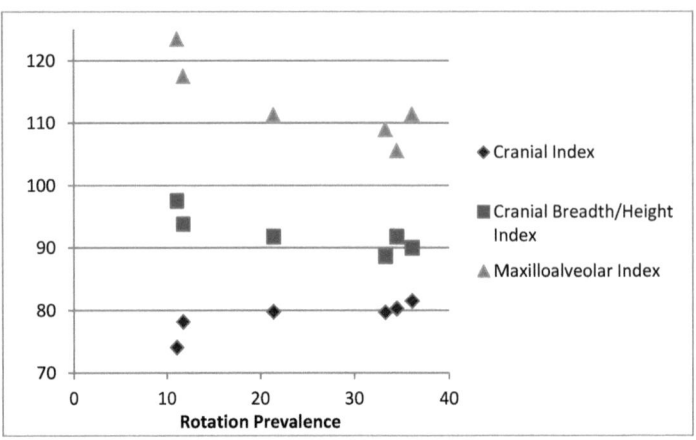

Figure 9. Scatterplot of select indices to rotation prevalence in population samples (normal skulls). Samples with higher rates of rotations cluster among high CI, and low CBHI and MAI.

with distance from Africa, suggesting a high heritability and reflection of population history rather than selection or adaptation (Betti et al 2009).

Changes in size of the mandible were especially related to dental anomalies, in particular rotations, with which the mandibular elements were reduced. While the data cannot provide insight into cause and effect, the data is congruent with theories that reduced jaw size contributes to occlusal variation. All of the populations from which these samples derived were post-transitional (that is agricultural), and we can expect a degree of malocclusion and dental disorder higher relative to prehistoric or hunter-gatherer samples.

The absence of significant size changes of palatal breadth and maxilloalveolar breadth may come as a surprise. Mandibular shape and size is often attributed to diet and environment, and the integration of the palate/maxilla with the mandible implies that the maxillary region should be as plastic. A number of studies show that maxillary features have low heritabilities along with the mandible (von Cramon-Taubadel 2011b) although as part of the facial complex, which contains a number of highly heritable components, plasticity and adaptability may be affected by modular integration (Martínez-Abadías et al 2009, 2011; von Cramon-Taubadel and Smith 2012). The data presented here does, however, indicate relationships between palatal and maxilloalveolar lengths with dental anomalies. Carson reported that in general cranial length measurements are more highly heritable than breadths, although bimaxillary breadth was estimated at $h^2=0.597$ (Carson 2006). This may suggest that the limits of the highly heritable breadth of the maxilla/palate may contribute to occlusal deviance by its inability to compensate for plastic, environmental changes to maxillary/palatal length.

Overall, the size changes among craniofacial elements examined here are congruent with most of the heritability data (variables with published high heritabilities are less affected by the presence of anomalies), the most significant of which is the variation in the size of the mandible, and slightly less significantly the overall facial dimensions. All of the measured mandibular variables associated reductions in size in skulls with rotations, and several in skulls with crowding.

Mandibular shape and size has been attributed to function rather than phylogeny since the early 20th century, believed to reflect adaptation and response to environment and diet much more than to population history (Nicholson and Harvati 2006). However, some population differences have been observed and significant differences exist between modern *Homo sapiens* and Neanderthal mandibular morphology (Nicholson and Harvati 2006). Unsurprisingly, heritability studies have shown very low h^2 estimates for mandibular variables, although Smith notes that the heritability is not significantly less than those for the whole cranium, upper face, temporal bone or cranial base measurements (Smith 2009).

Despite differences among studies of morphological and genetic congruency, few would argue that the mandible is a good estimator of genetic relationships, and von Cramon-Taubadel (2011b) found that subsistence behaviour is the determining factor in mandibular shape among modern humans (von Cramon-Taubadel 2011b). Although the maxillary-palatal complex is integrated into the masticatory complex along with the mandible, its relationship to subsistence is not as direct (von Cramon-Tabadel 2011b:19547). The mandible had become reduced in size, shorter and wider, in the transition from the hunter-gatherer lifestyle towards agriculture, supporting the masticatory stress theories of the high prevalence of occlusal disorders and dental crowding among modern, industrialized populations (von Cramon-Taubadel 2011b:19548). The data presented here, of the high degree of variability in the mandible and the relationship of smaller mandibular variables with dental anomalies, supports this theory.

Mandibular and dental arch dimensions and the aetiology of dental anomalies

Relative sizes of the dental arches have been frequently regarded as a major factor in the aetiology of malocclusion and dental anomalies (Lombardi 1982; Corruccini 1984; Forsberg 1988; Leighton 1991). In this study, the incongruence of mandibular and maxillary dimensions in the aetiology of occlusal variation seems to be supported in the involvement of maxilloalveolar breadth (MAXB) in indices in skulls with dental anomalies. While maxilloalveolar breadth itself was unaffected by the expression of anomalies, the maxilloalveolar index, lower jaw breadth ratio (MAXB/BCDL), and upper facial index/maxilloalveolar index ratio were all significantly different in skulls with rotations and ectopic eruptions. Length variables of the maxilloalveolar and palatal complexes were shown to be more

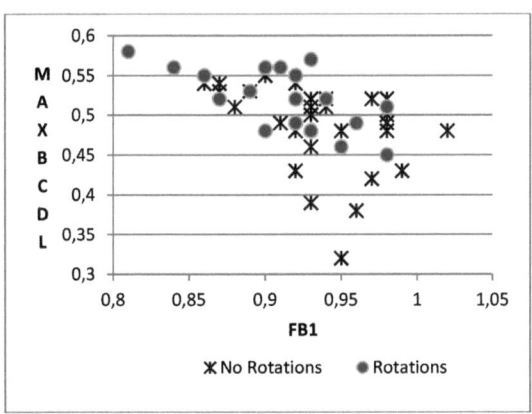

Figure 10. Scatterplot indicating skulls with rotations inclined toward higher MAX/BCDL indices and medial Facial Breadth (FB1) indices.

sensitive to change than breadths; while this may be related to the heritability of breadths, early behaviour from infants, such as suckling, may influence this growth pattern (Oyen 1996). Thus, according the data in this study, rotations, ectopic eruptions and impactions are more prevalent in skulls with relatively small mandibles and short, broad palates relative to thinner faces. See figure 10, above. Impactions and rotations have commonly been associated with small jaws (Lombardi 1982; Forsberg 1988; Leighton 1991).

Although this study found an association between crowding and rotations, it is important to note that rotations do occur without any evidence of crowding. When analysed according to population sample and by sex, crowding was only associated with rotations in males, and ecoptic eruptions only with rotations in English males. Crowding is often expected to be associated with rotations, impactions, and ectopic eruptions due to the theorized lack of space available for the teeth to grow (Barnabé and Flores-Mir 2006). For this study, the association of ectopic and impacted teeth, rotations and crowding was not consistent. Nor did crowding show any relationship with reduced masticatory elements as rotations did. Some mandibular elements, bigonial breadth and height of ascending ramus, did show some reduction in skulls with crowding, but the reduction was small, inconsistent, and not statistically significant. Upper facial breadth as measured by the frontomalare temporale showed consistent, although statistically insignificant, reduction with crowding (see results, Table 7). Baccetti (1998) has suggested a genetic contribution to the aetiology of rotations, finding an association of rotated teeth with nonadjacent tooth aplasia, although no such association was made in this analysis.

Teeth were not measured in this analysis, but many studies link the size of the teeth themselves within a dental arch that has failed to compensate for the size difference. A number of studies have described crowding as occurring when the size of the teeth exceeds the space available in the dental arches (Lombardi 1982; Howe et al 1983; Corruccini 1984; Barnabé and Flores-Mir 2006). Mossey (1990a:110) referred to this "dentoalveolar disproportion" as evidence of the genetic aetiology of crowding, and Lombardi (1982) argued that evolution has not had the time to select for teeth small enough to fit comfortably into the modern reduced jaw, causing crowding and malocclusion.

Heritability estimates for tooth dimensions are quite high, usually exceeding heritabilities of associated cranial elements. A 2001 study estimated mesiodistal lengths of at least $h^2=0.50$ and buccolingual breadths as high as $h^2=0.90$ (Dempsey and Townsend 2001). Tooth dimensions are known to vary according to geographic populations and Europeans are reported to have among the smallest teeth (Hanihara and Ishida 2005). Although dental size has been reduced over the evolution of modern humans (Lombardi 1982), because of the differences in genetic control over teeth and the masticatory apparatus, it can be expected that relatively large teeth will continue to grow into relatively small jaws. According to Mossey (1999b), the maxilla and mandible are under separate genetic control, and different regions of the mandible similarly under control of different genes. The data in this analysis supports the multifactorial and partially genetic aetiology of these occlusal variables and dental anomalies, by presenting evidence for the variation of shape and sizes of elements associated with dental anomalies. In general, most anomalies were more prevalent in elements with reduced sizes, particularly the mandible.

VI. Conclusion

This investigation studied the relationship of craniometric variation with the expression of dental anomalies of shape, size, and number. After examining a total of 131 skulls from 6 population samples from medieval England and Classical and medieval Macedonia, craniometric analyses of 16 paired landmarks found that the null hypothesis, that there is no relationship between craniometrics and dental anomalies, can be rejected. In general, dental anomalies appear to be associated in skulls with thin faces relative to short, broad palates, and particularly with reduced mandibles.

Frequencies of dental anomalies in the samples approached prevalence rates for modern Europeans, except for crowding which, although common, was not as high as many researchers have estimated for modern industrialized populations nor as low as is often expected for premodern populations. The distribution of dental anomalies varied slightly among geographic population samples, including between geographically close groups. This supports the idea of a genetic aetiology for some anomalies, but environmental and dietary influences cannot be ruled out without a clear understanding of such local variables. It is indeed interesting that two population samples close geographically but largely separated by historic periods, Marvinci and Demir Kapija, Macedonia, would have such dissimilar rates of dental anomalies.

The craniometric data presented in this study cannot establish cause and effect relationships, that is, it is not clear whether metric variation was caused by or caused the expression of dental anomalies. However, the overall higher prevalence of most anomalies in populations with generally smaller normal skulls lends evidence to theories that reduced sizes contribute to the disruption of normal tooth movement.

Dental anomalies were observed more frequently in skulls with smaller mandibles in general. Crowding, contrary to a number of studies, was not associated with consistent or significant reductions in mandible size, which is a prediction of the epidemiological transition of modern lifestyles. However, this study did not take into account size of teeth; it may be that the lower threshold of mandible size is not significant in relation to the inherited size of teeth leading to crowding.

A number of cranial vault and facial elements were also sensitive to size changes in skulls with anomalies, lending support to the plasticity of the cranium in general, although some presumed highly heritable elements were far less susceptible to size changes. Palatal (internal [maxilloalveolar] and external) lengths were far more variable than palatal breadths in the data in this study. The data presented here is generally supportive of the multifactorial, partially genetic aetiology of dental anomalies, and also supports the idea that heritable sizes of craniofacial components may contribute to incongruence between dental arch dimensions. Dental anomalies appear more likely to be expressed beyond a certain threshold of craniofacial reduction; the causes, whether these changes are largely environmental or genetic, will continue to provide interesting prospects for further research. In any case, whether from environmental or hereditary effects, the idea that the evolution of tooth size in humans is much slower than the plastic response of variable jaw and facial elements seems a reasonable theory for the aetiology of orthodontic variation.

REFERENCES

Ackermann, RR and Cheverud, JM. 2004. Detecting genetic drift versus selection in human evolution. *Proceedings of the National Academy of Sciences, USA* 101(52):17946-17951.

Aufderheide, AC; Rodriguez-Martin, C. 1998. *The Cambridge Encyclopedia of Human Paleopathology*. New York: Cambridge University Press.

Babacan, H.; Kiliç, B; Biçakçi, A. 2008. Maxillary canine-first premolar transposition in the permanent dentition. *Angle Orthodontist* 78(5):954-960.

Baccetti, T. 1998a. A controlled study of associated dental anomalies. *The Angle Orthodontist* 68(3):267-274.

Baccetti, T. 1998b. Tooth rotation associated with aplasia of nonadjacent teeth. *The Angle Orthodontist* 68(5):471-474.

Bailleul-Forestier, I; Molla, M; Verloes, A; Berdal, A 2008a. The genetic basis of inherited anomalies of the teeth: Part 1: Clinical and molecular aspects of non-syndromic dental disorders. *European Journal of Medical Genetics* 51:273-291.

Bailleul-Forestier, I; Berdal, A; Vinckier, F; de Ravel, T; Fryns, JP, Verloes, M. 2008b. The genetic basis of inherited anomalies of the teeth: Part 2: Syndromes with significant dental involvement. *European Journal of Medical Genetics* 51:383-408.

Barnabé, E; Flores-Mir, C. 2006. Dental morphology and crowding: a multivariate approach. *Angle Orthodontist* 76(1):20-25.

Basdra, EK; Kiokpasoglou, MN; Komposch, G. 2001. Congenital tooth anomalies and malocclusions: a genetic link? *European Journal of Orthodontics* 23:145-151.

Bass, WM. 2005. *Human Osteology: A Laboratory and Field Manual, 5th edition*. Springfield: Missouri Archaeological Society.

Bastir, M and Rosas, A. 2004. Facial heights: Evolutionary relevance of postnatal ontogeny for facial orientation and skull morphology in humans and chimpanzees. *Journal of Human Evolution* 47:359-381.

Bastir, M and Rosas, A. 2005. Hierarchical nature of morphological integration and modularity in the human posterior face. *American Journal of Physical Anthropology* 128:26-34.

Batra, P; Duggal, R; Parkash, H. 2005. Non-syndromic multiple supernumerary teeth transmitted as an autosomal dominant trait. *Journal of Oral Pathological Medicine* 34:621-625.

Betti, L; Balloux, F; Amos, W; Hanihara, T; Manica, A. 2009. Distance from Africa, not climate, explains within-population phenotypic diversity in humans. *Proceedings of the Royal Society B* 276:809-814.

Betti, L; Balloux, F; Hanihara, T; Manica, A. 2010. The relative role of drift and selection in shaping the human skull. *American Journal of Physical Anthropology* 141:78-82.

Bishara, SE. 2001. Chapter 5: Development of dental occlusion. In *Textbook of Orthodontics*, SE Bishara, ed. Philadelphia: WB Saunders Company.

Bogin, B. 2003. The human pattern of growth and development in palaeontological perspective. In *Patterns of Growth and Development in the Genus* Homo. Thompson, Krovitz, and Nelson, eds. Cambridge: Cambridge University Press, 15-44.

Brin, I; Becker, A; Shalhav, M. 1986. Position of the maxillary permanent canine in relation to anomalous or missing lateral incisors: a population study. *European Journal of Orthodontics* 8:12-16.

Brook, AH. 2009. Multilevel complex interactions between genetic, epigenetic and environmental factors in the aetiology of anomalies of dental development. *Archives of Oral Biology* 54(S1):S3-S17.

Buikstra, JE; Ubelaker 1994. *Standards to the data collection for recording human remains.* Arkansas Archaeological Survey Research Series 44. Fayetteville: Arkansas Archaeological Survey.

Blackburn, AC 2010. Bilateral asymmetry of the Humerus throughout growth and development. Unpublished PhD thesis, University of Manitoba, Winnipeg.

Burnett, SE and Weets, JD. 2001. Maxillary canine-first premolar transposition in two Native American skeletal samples from New Mexico. *American Journal of Physical Anthropology* 116:45-50.

Carson, EA. 2006. Maximum Likelihood estimation of human craniometric heritabilities. *American Journal of Physical Anthropology* 131:169-180.

Celikoglu, M; Bayram, M; Nur, M. 2011. Patterns of third-molar agenesis and associated dental anomalies in an orthodontic population. *American Journal of Orthodontics and Dentofacial Orthopedics* 140(6):856-860.

Cendekiawan, T; Wong, RWK; Rabie, ABM. 2010. Relations between cranial base synchondroses and craniofacial development: a review. *The Open Anatomy Journal* 2:67-75.

Chattopadhyay, A; Srinivas, K. 1996. Transposition of teeth and genetic aetiology. *The Angle Orthodontist* 66(2):147-152.

Cobourne, MT; DiBiase, AT. 2010. *Handbook of Orthodontics*. Edinburgh: Mosby Elsevier.

Corruccini RS and Beecher, RM. 1982. Occlusal variation related to soft diet in a nonhuman primate. *Science* 218:74-76.

Corruccini, RS. 1984. An epidemiological transition in dental occlusion in world populations. *American Journal of Orthodontics* 86(5):419-426.

Dempsey, PJ; Townsend, GC. 2001. Genetic and environmental contributions to variation in human tooth size. *Heredity* 86:685-693.

Doris, JM; Bernard, BW; Kuftinec, MM. 1981. A biometric study of tooth size and dental crowding. *American Journal of Orthodontics* 79(3):326-336.

Duncan, WN. 2009. Supernumerary teeth from two Mesoamerican archaeological contexts. *Dental Anthropology* 22(2):39-46.

Ely, NJ; Sherriff, M; Cobourne, MT. 2006. Dental transpositions as a disorder of genetic origin. *European Journal of Orthodontics* 28:145-151.

Enlow, DH. 1990. *Facial Growth, 3rd edition*. Philadelphia: WB Saunders Company.

Enlow, DH and Hans, MG 1996. *Essentials of Facial Growth*. Philadelphia: Saunders.

Evensen, JP; Øgaard, B. 2007. Are malocclusions more prevalent and severe now? A comparative study of medieval skulls from Norway. *American Journal of Orthodontics and Dentofacial Orthopedics* 131:710-716.

Forsberg, C-M. 1988. Tooth size, spacing, and crowding in relation to eruption or impaction of third molars. *American Journal of Orthodontics and Dentofacial Orthopedics* 94:57-62.

Forster, CM; Sunga, E; Chung, C-H. 2008. Relationship between dental arch widths and vertical facial morphology in untreated adults. *European Journal of Orthodontics* 30:288-294.

Gallucio, G; Castellano, M; La Monaca, C. 2012. Genetic basis of non-syndromic anomalies of human tooth number. *Archives of Oral Biology* 57(7):918-930.

González-José, R; Ramírez-Rozzi, F; Sardi, M; Martínez-Abadías, N; Hernández, M; Pucciarelli, HM. 2005. Functional-cranial approach to the influence of economic strategy on skull morphology. *American Journal of Physical Anthropology* 128:757-771.

Gravlee, CC; Bernard, HR; Leonard, WR. 2003. Heredity, environment, and cranial form: a reanalysis of Boas' immigrant data. *American Anthropologist* 105(1):125-138.

Hallgrímsson, B; Lieberman, DE; Liu, W.; others. 2007. Epigenetic interactions and the structure of phenotypic variation in the cranium. *Evolution and Development* 9(1):76-91.

Hanihara, T. 1996. Comparison of craniofacial features of major human groups. *American Journal of Physical Anthropology* 99:389-412.

Harper, C. 1994. A comparison of medieval and modern dentitions. *European Journal of Orthodontics* 16:163-173.

Harris, EF. 2008. Interpreting heritability estimates in the orthodontic literature. *Seminars in Orthodontics* 14(2):125-134.

Harris, EF; Smith, RJ. 1980. A study of occlusion and arch widths in families. *American Journal of Orthodontics* 78(2):155-163.

Harvati, K and Weaver, TD. 2006. Human cranial anatomy and the differential preservation of population history and climate signatures. *The Anatomical Record Part A* 282A:1225-1233.

Hillson, S. 1996. *Dental Anthropology.* Cambridge: University Press.

Holloway, RL. 2002. Head to head with Boas: did he err on the plasticity of head form? *Proceedings of the National Academy of Sciences* 99(23):14622-14623.

Howe, RP; McNamara, JA; O'Connor, KA. 1983. An examination of dental crowding and its relationship to tooth size and arch dimension. *American Journal of Orthodontics* 83(5):363-373.

Howells, WW. 1973. *Cranial Variation in Man: A Study by Multivariate Analysis of Patterns of Difference among Recent Human Populations.* Papers of the Peabody Museum 67. Cambridge: Harvard University Press.

Howells, WW. 1989. *Skull Shapes and the Map.* Papers of the Peabody Museum 79. Cambridge: Harvard University Press.

Hunt, N. 1998. Muscle function and the control of facial form. In *Clinical Oral Science.* Harris, Edgar, and Meghji eds. Oxford: Wright, 121-133.

Hunter, WS. 1990. Heredity in the craniofacial complex. In *Facial Growth, 3rd Edition*, Enlow, editor. Philadelphia: WB Saunders Company

Jacob, T; Indriati, E; Soejono, RP; Hsü, K; Frayer, DW; Eckhardt, RB; Kuperavage, AJ; Thorne, A; Hanneberg, M. 2006. Pygmoid Australomelanesian Homo sapiens skeletal remains from Liang Bua, Flores: Population affinities and pathological abnormalities. Prceedings of the National Academy of Sciences 103(36):13421-13426.

Jaenisch, R and Bird, A. 2003. Epigenetic regulation of gene expression: how the genome integrates intrinsic and environmental signals. Nature Genetics 33:245-254.

Jobling, MA; Hurles, ME; Tyler-Smith, C. 2004. *Human Evolutionary Genetics: Origins, Peoples & Disease.* Abingdon: Garland Science.

Jungers, LJ; Gingerich, PD. 1980. Supernumerary molars in Anthrpoidea, Adapidae, and *Archaeolemur*: Implications for primate homologies. *American Journal of Physical Anthropology* 52:1-5.

Killiardis, S. 1986. The relationship between masticatory function and craniofacial morhphology. III. The eruption pattern of the incisors in the growing rat fed a soft diet. *European Journal of Orthodontics* 8:71-79.

Kirzioğlu, Z; Köseler Şentut, T; Özay Ertürk, MS; Karayilmaz, H. 2005. Clinical features of hypodontia and associated dental anomalies: a retrospective study. *Oral Diseases* 11:399-404.

Konigsberg, LW. 2000. Quantitative variation and genetics. In *Human Biology: An Evolutionary and Biocultural Perspective.* Stinson, Bogin, Huss-Ashmore, and O'Rourke, eds. Wiley-Liss:135-144.

Kouskoura, T; Fragou, N; Alexiou, M; John, N; Sommer, J; Graf, D; Katsaros, C; Mitsiadis, TA. 2011. The genetic basis of craniofacial and dental abnormalities. *Schweiz Monatsschr Zahnmed* 121:636-646.

Kuroe, K; Rosas, A; Molleson, T. 2004. Variation in the cranial base orientation and facial skeleton in dry skulls from three major populations. *European Journal of Orthodontics* 26(2):201-207.

Lavelle, CLB. 1973. Variation in the secular changes in the teeth and dental charges. *The Angle Orthodontist* 43(4):412-421.

Legoux, P. 1974. Étude odontologique des restes humains périgordiens et protomagdaléniens de l'Abri-Pataud (Dordogne)(seconde partie). *Bulletins et Mémoires de la Société d'anthropologie de Paris* 13(1):45-54.

Leighton, BC. 1991. Aetiology of malocclusion of the teeth. *Archives of Disease in Childhood* 66:1011-1012.

Lieberman, DE; McBratney, BM; Krovitz, G. 2002. The evolution and development of cranial form in *Homo sapiens*. *Proceedings of the National Academy of Sciences, USA* 99(3):1134-1139.

Ling, JYK; Wong, RWK. 2010. Incisor winging in Chinese. *The Open Anthropology Journal* 3:8-11.

Lombardi, AV. 1982. The adaptive value of dental crowding: A consideration of the biologic basis of malocclusion. *American Journal of Orthodontics* 81(1):38-42.

Luac, T; Rudan, P; Rudan, I; Campbell, H. 2003. Effect of inbreeding and endogamy on occlusal traits in human isolates. *Journal of Orthodontics* 30:301-308.

Lycett, SJ and Collard, M. 2005. Do homiologies impede phylogenetic analyses of the fossil hominids? An assessment based on extant papionin craniodental morphology. *Journal of Human Evolution* 49(5):618-642.

Magilton, J; Lee, F; Boylston, A. 2008. *'Lepers outside the gate': Excavations at the cemetery of the Hospital of St James and St Mary Magdalene, Chichester, 1986-7 and 1993.* CBA Research Report 158. York: Council for British Archaeology.

Martina, R; Farella, M; Tagliaferri, R; Michelotti, A; Quaremba, G; van Eijden, TMGJ. 2005. The relationship between molar dentoalveolar and craniofacial heights. *Angle Orthodontist* 75(6):974-979.

Martínez-Abadías, N; Esparza, M; Sjøvold, T; González-José, R; Santos, M; Hernández, M. 2009. Heritability of human cranial dimensions: comparing the evolvability of different cranial regions. *Journal of Anatomy* 214:19-35.

Martínez-Abadías, N; Esparza, M; Sjøvold, T; González-José, R; Santos, M; Hernández, M; Klingenberg CP. 2012. Pervasive genetic integration directs the evolution of human skull shape. *Evolution* 66(4):1010-1023.

Mattheeuws, N; Dermaut, L; Martens, G. 2004. Has hypodontia increased in Caucasians during the 20th century? A meta-analysis. *European Journal of Orthodontics* 26:99-103.

McBratney-Owen, B and Lieberman, DE. 2003. Postnatal ontogeny of facial position in *Homo sapiens* and *Pan troglodytes*. In *Patterns of Growth and Development in the Genus* Homo. Thompson, Krovitz, and Nelson, eds. Cambridge: Cambridge University Press, 45-72.

Mishra, MB. 2011. Types of hyperdontic anomalies in permanent dentition: Report of 5 cases. *International Journal of Clinical Dental Science* 2(1):15-21.

Mockers, O; Aubrey, M; Mafart, B. 2004. Dental crowding in a prehistoric population. *European Journal of Orthodontics* 26(2):151-156.

Moss, ML. 1997a. The functional matrix hypothesis revisited. 1. The role of mechanotransduction. *American Journal of Orthodontics and Dentofacial Orthopedics* 112(1):8-11.

Moss, ML. 1997b. The functional matrix hypothesis revisited. 4. The epigenetic antithesis and the resolving synthesis. *American Journal of Orthodontics and Dentofacial Orthopedics* 112(4):410-417.

Moss, ML and Rankow, RM. 1968. The role of the functional matrix in mandibular growth. *The Angle Orthodontist* 38(2):95-103.

Moss, ML and Young, RW. 1960. A functional approach to craniology. *American Journal of Physical Anthropology* 18:281-292.

Mossey, PA. 1999a. The heritability of malocclusion: Part 1—Genetics, principles and terminology. *British Journal of Orthodontics* 26:103-113.

Mossey, PA. 1999b. The heritability of malocclusion: Part 2—The influence of genetics in malocclusion. *British oJournal of Orthodontics* 26:195-203.

Nelson, SJ; Ash, MM. 2010. *Wheeler's Dental Anatomy, Physiology, and Occlusion, Ninth Edition.* St Louis: Saunders Elsevier.

Nicholson, E; Harvati, K. 2006. Quantitative analysis of human mandibular shape using three-dimensional geometric morphometrics. *American Journal of Physical Anthropology* 131:368-383.

Normando, D; Faber, J; Guerreiro, JF; Quintão, CCA. 2011. Dental occlusion in a split Amazon indigenous population: Genetics prevails over environment. *PloS One* 6(12): e28387. doi:10.1371/journal.pone.0028387

Ortner, DJ. 2003. *Identification of Pathological Conditions in Human Skeletal Remains, 2nd Edition.* San Diego: Academic Press.

Oyen, O. 1996. Chapter 11: Masticatory function and facial growth and development. In *Essentials of Facial Growth*, Enlow and Hans, eds. Philadelphia: Saunders.

Parkin, N; Elcock, C; Smith, RN; Griffin, RC; Brook, AH. 2009. The aetiology of hypodontia: The prevalence, severity and location of hypodontia within families. *Archives of Oral Biology* 54S:S52-S56.

Paschetta, C; de Azevedo, S; Castillo, L; Martinez-Abadias, N; Hernandez, M; Lieberman, DE; Gonzalez-Jose, R. 2010. The influence of masticatory loading on craniofacial morphology: a test case across technological transitions in the Ohio Valley. *American Journal of Physical Anthropology* 141:297-314.

Papadopolous, MA; Chatzoudi, M; Karagiannis, V. 2009. Assessment of characteristic features and dental anomalies accompanying tooth transposition: A meta-analysis. *American Journal of Orthodontics and Dentofacial Orthopedics* 136(3):308.e1-308e10.

Pritchard, DJ; Korf, BR. 2011. *Medical Genetics at a Glance.* Oxford: Blackwell.

Pucciarelli, HM; Ramirez Rozzi, FV; Muñe, MC; Sardi, NL. 2006. Variation of functional cranial components in six Anthropoidea species. *Zoology* 109:231-243.

Rajab, L and Hamdam, MAM. 2002. Supernumerary teeth: review of the literature and a survey of 152 cases. *International Journal of Paediatric Dentistry* 12:244-254.

Relethford, JH. 1994. Craniometric variation among modern human populations. *American Journal of Physical Anthropology* 95:53-62.

Relethford, JH. 2004. Boas and beyond: Migration and craniometric variation. *American Journal of Human Biology* 16:379-386.

Roseman, CC. 2004. Detecting interregionally diversifying natural selection on modern human cranial form by using matched molecular and morphological data. Proceedings of the National Academy of Sciences, USA 101(35):12824-12829.

Roseman, CC and Weaver, TD. 2004. Multivariate apportionment of global human craniometric diversity. *American Journal of Physical Anthropology* 125:257-263.

Ross, AH. 2004. Regional isolation in the Balkan region: an analysis of craniofacial variation. *American Journal of Physical Anthropology* 124:73-80.

Russell, C. 2005. The Anglo-Saxon influence on Romano-Britain: Research past and present. *Durham Anthropology Journal* 13(1). Accessed online 26 May 2012 at http://www.dur.ac.uk/anthropology.journal/vol13/iss1/russell/russell.html

Sardi, ML and Ramírez Rozzi, F. 2007. Developmental connections between cranial components and the emergence of the first permanent molar in humans. *Joural of Anatomy* 210:406-417.

Scott, GR. 2008. Dental Morphology. In *Biological Anthropology of the Human Skeleton, Second Edition.* Katzenberg and Saunders, eds. Hoboken:Wiley-Liss.

Sherwood, RJ; Duren, DL; Demerath, EW; Czerwinski, SA; Siervogel, RM; Towne, B. 2008. Quantitative genetics of modern human cranial variation. *Journal of Human Evolution* 54(6):909-914.

Sholts, SB; Clement, AF; Wärmländer, SKTS. 2010. Brief communication: Additional cases of maxillary canine-first premolar transposition in several prehistoric skeletal assemblages from the Santa Barbara Channel Islands of California. *American Journal of Physical Anthropology* 143:155-160.

Smith, HF. 2009. Which cranial regions reflect molecular distances reliably in humans? Evidence from three-dimensional morphology. *American Journal of Human Biology* 21:36-47.

Sparks, CS; Jantz, RL. 2002. A reassessment of human cranial plasticity: Boas revisited. *Proceedings of the National Academy of Sciences* 99(23):14636-14639.

Sperber, G. 2006. The genetics of odontogenesis: implications in dental anthropology and palaeo-odontology. *Transactions of the Royal Society of South Africa* 61(2):121-125.

Strand Vidarsdóttir, U and O'Higgins, P. 2003. Developmental variation in the facial skeleton of anatomically modern *Homo sapiens*. In *Patterns of Growth and Development in the Genus* Homo. Thompson, Krovitz, and Nelson, eds. Cambridge: Cambridge University Press, 114-143.

Strand Vidarsdóttir, U; O'Higgins, P; Stringer, C. 2002. A geometric morphometrics study of regional differences in the ontogeny of the modern human facial skeleton. *Journal of Anatomy* 201:211-219.

Strauss, A; Hubbe, M. 2010. Craniometric similarities within and between human populations in comparison with neutral genetic data. *Human Biology* 82(3):315-330.

Stroud, G. 1984. The human bones. The human skeletal remains from Hickleton, South Yorkshire. Unpublished skeletal report held at the Biological Anthropology Resource Centre, Department of Archaeological Sciences, University of Bradford.

Swindler, DR. 2002. Fourth molars in the Anthropoidea. *Dental Anthropology* 16(1):26-28.

Thesleff, I. 2006. Research review: The genetic basis of tooth development and dental defects. *American Journal of Medical Genetics Part A* 140A:2530-2535.

Thongudomporn, U; Freer, TJ. 1998. Prevalence of dental anomalies in orthodontic patients. *Australian Dental Journal* 43(6):395-398.

Townsend, GC; Aldred, MJ; Bartold, MP. 1998. Genetic aspects of dental disorders. *American Dental Journal* 43(4):000.

Townsend, G; Hughes, T; Luciano, M; Bockmann, M; Brook, A. 2009. Genetic and environmental influences on human dental variation: A critical evaluation of studies involving twins. *Archives of Oral Biology* 54(S1):S45-S51.

Veljanovska, F. 2001[*]. *Antropoloshki Karakteristiki na Srednovekovnoto Naselenie od Crkvishte-Demir Kapija*. Skopje: Museum of Macedonia.

Veljanovska, F. 2006. *Antichkoto Naselenie od Marvinci-Valandovo*. Skopje: Museum of Macedonia.

Varella, J. 1992. Dimensional variation of craniofacial structures in relation to changing masticatory demands. *European Journal of Orthodontics* 14(1):31-36.

Vastardis, H. 2000. The genetics of human tooth agenesis: New discoveries for understanding dental anomalies. *American Journal of Orthodontics and Dentofacial Orthodpedics* 117(6):650-656.

Vodanović, M; Galić, I; Strujić, M; Peroš, K; Šlaus, M; Brkić,, H. 2012. Orthodontic anomalies and malocclusions in Late Antique and Early Mediaeval period in Croatia. *Archives of Oral Biology* 57:401-412.

von Cramon-Taubadel, N. 2009a. Congruence of individual cranial bone morphology and neutral molecular affinity patterns in modern humans. *American Journal of Physical Anthropology* 140:205-215.

---

[*] Titles published in Macedonian have been transliterated from the Cyrillic by the author.

von Cramon-Taubadel, N. 2009b. Revisiting the homoiology hypothesis: the impact of phenotypic plasticity on the reconstruction of human population history from craniometric data. *Journal of Human Evolution* 57:179-190.

von Cramon-Taubadel, N. 2011a. The relative efficacy of functional and developmental cranial modules for reconstructing global human population history. *American Journal of Physical Anthropology* 146:83-93.

von Cramon-Taubadel, N. 2011b. Global human mandibular variation reflects differences in agricultural and hunter-gatherer subsistence strategies. *Proceedings of the National Academy of Sciences* 108(49):19546-19551.

von Cramon-Taubadel, N; Smith, HF. 2012. The relative congruence of cranial and genetic estimates of hominoid taxon relationships: Implications for the reconstruction of hominin phylogeny. *Journal of Human Evolution* 62:640-653.

Waldron, T. 2007. *Palaeoepidemiology: The Measure of Disease in the Human Past*. Walnut Creek: Left Coast Press.

Waldron, T. 2009. *Palaeopathology. Cambridge Manuals in Archaeology.* Cambridge: University Press.

Watnick, SS. 1972. Inheritance of craniofacial morphology. *The Angle Orthodontist* 42(4):339-351.

White, TD; Black, MT; Folkens, PA. *Human Osteology, Third Edition.* Burlington: Elsevier.

White, TD; Folkens, PA. 2005. *The Human Bone Manual*. Burlington: Elsevier.

Appendices

Appendix A 1 Craniometrics and data recorded, all skulls 85
Appendix A 2 93
Section 1. Frequencies and Distributions of Anomalies. 93
Section 2. Craniometric Means and Variances. 105
        Part 1. General Craniometrics. 105
        Part 2. Craniometrics and Dental anomalies 110
Section 3. Independent T-Tests Results. 118
        Part 3. General Craniometrics 118
        Part 4. Craniometrics with anomalies Independent Samples T-tests.... 127

Appendix A 1 Craniometrics and data recorded, all skulls

Table 1. Craniometrics, All skulls

	Sex	Skeleton	GOL	XCB	BBH	NGN	ZYB	FMT	NPH	MAXL	MAXB	PL	PB	BCDL	BGB	HARR	MBAR	HMS
Blackfriars	F	103	185	147	-	-	145	112	-	-	62	50	47	135	115	72	28	35
Blackfriars	F	107	-	-	-	-	-	-	-	45	59	51	38	115	93	66	33	33
Blackfriars	F	122	186	-	130	-	125	109	-	-	60	48	40	123	93	67	31	26
Blackfriars	M	134	-	-	-	-	-	-	-	-	60	45	41	121	104	70	31	33
Blackfriars	F	167	181	142	133	-	123	105	66	-	55	47	30	108	92	61	27	27
Blackfriars	F	200	180	137	-	-	-	103	-	52	55	48	38	-	-	92	-	33	29
Blackfriars	M	233	-	-	-	-	-	108	-	-	-	55	-	-	120	109	74	34	31
Blackfriars	F	281	177	145	-	-	-	102	-	-	60	49	40	120	86	66	30	28
Blackfriars	M	287	-	-	-	-	-	-	-	-	58	47	32	118	103	71	29	32
Blackfriars	M	302	192	150	139	120	131	112	71	61	67	58	42	-	106	74	39	36
Blackfriars	M	311	-	-	-	-	-	-	-	-	62	58	39	-	117	76	34	38
Blackfriars	M	317	-	141	133	-	134	106	-	-	52	50	32	-	108	67	36	33
Blackfriars	M	411	-	151	-	-	-	104	57	52	58	49	38	-	94	70	34	30
Blackfriars	M	414	186	143	136	-	140	110	-	-	60	49	40	-	-	-	-	-
Blackfriars	F	420	188	147	-	-	-	106	-	-	-	59	39	-	100	72	31	32
Blackfriars	M	92	190	151	138	118	136	102	66	-	59	47	41	127	111	77	34	30
Blackfriars	F	98	160	125	-	98	114	96	61	46	58	45	-	104	88	60	29	26
Box Lane	M	16	-	153	-	-	-	113	-	-	58	63	53	43	133	110	72	31	31
Box Lane	M	32c	177	126	-	-	-	98	66	-	62	50	40	-	-	75	60	30	28
Box Lane	F	35 1/2	192	131	-	-	-	109	-	-	-	-	-	-	125	99	71	30	28
Box Lane	M	42	-	-	-	-	-	105	-	-	56	47	36	123	98	62	29	30
Box Lane	M	48	193	146	142	127	-	-	64	-	-	56	33	124	109	76	29	31
Box Lane	M	49a	192	156	140	106	-	-	62	50	-	52	42	119	109	69	29	29
Box Lane	M	63	196	146	-	-	-	-	-	47	65	51	43	123	104	67	32	30
Box Lane	M	67	197	142	139	114	133	102	69	-	59	51	37	123	100	72	32	33
Box Lane	F	73	176	142	119	-	-	106	-	-	-	56	-	118	91	62	29	30
Chichester	M	021	164	135	122	120	-	100	60	-	62	47	40	120	103	63	30	33
Chichester	M	033	-	-	126	122	-	102	69	-	46	39	109	91	67	32	30
Chichester	F	039	160	144	120	109	127	100	63	49	60	44	36	107	93	64	29	29
Chichester	M	065	180	140	121	106	118	96	63	51	55	42	35	113	97	67	28	26
Chichester	M	100	182	147	-	-	127	103	66	49	61	44	42	120	92	65	32	30
Chichester	M	109	182	190	131	-	-	102	61	52	56	48	36	114	99	63	27	26
Chichester	M	142	175	143	113	109	128	112	67	53	64	49	42	115	94	59	27	26
Chichester	M	149	184	150	140	115	135	107	72	52	62	52	38	-	-	70	34	32
Chichester	F	150	187	145	125	102	130	101	63	49	48	43	42	-	99	67	27	29
Chichester	F	174	172	140	117	116	132	107	70	55	63	53	41	123	100	74	32	27
Chichester	M	19	178	150	136	113	139	107	60	-	68	-	45	130	111	65	39	26
Chichester	F	190	180	140	129	107	127	107	63	52	60	49	39	111	99	68	32	27
Chichester	F	208	165	140	123	102	123	101	62	-	54	48	34	121	90	70	32	28
Chichester	M	216	184	138	-	100	122	105	65	55	61	47	41	118	91	62	30	30
Chichester	F	238	169	143	127	-	128	105	63	50	57	46	42	-	-	-	-	-
Chichester	F	252	187	146	129	96	128	110	63	50	55	46	39	115	100	63	27	23
Chichester	F	257	172	136	129	108	125	104	65	54	60	53	38	116	89	64	34	30
Chichester	M	267	179	147	134	-	132	109	73	51	-	48	-	-	-	33	29
Chichester	F	279	183	152	134	105	136	112	67	50	61	48	41	118	92	69	27	30
Chichester	M	295	-	140	129	107	131	111	64	53	62	52	43	116	107	66	31	29
Chichester	F	311	181	138	131	-	-	103	66	52	45	51	32	-	-	-	-	-

Site	Sex	ID															
Chichester	M	315	175	147	129	106 -		104	65 -		55	49	41 -		98	67	31	26
Chichester	M	328	177	152	124	112	143	106	69	58	64	52	44	131	115	66	31	29
Chichester	M	335	179	157 -		113	142	106	69	54	52	53	42	132	112	75	33	32
Chichester	M	337	170	152	131	132	143	110	78	58	57	51	41	132	109	79	35	35
Chichester	M	342	179	145	125 -		132	104	72	50	59	46	41 -	-	-	-	-
Chichester	M	345	-	-	-	-	-	106	61	50	64	48	41 -	-	-	-	-
Chichester	M	346	188	146 -		106	135	110	63	53	62	50	40	118	104	69	34	28
Chichester	M	354	179	150	137	122	130	105	68 -		61	51	41 -		72	30	33
Chichester	M	371	181	145	126	125	137	109	73	56	61	53	40	125	92	70	38	35
Chichester	M	372	180	136	138 -	-		109 -			58	52	38	117	91	74	31	32
Chichester	M	373	182	148	134 -			106 -		48	62	47	43	126	90	68	33	28
Chichester	M	57	187	135	132	122	132	107	71 -		62	58	37	114	106	69	31	20
Chichester	M	58	171	151	137 -												
Chichester	M	81a	195	148 -		120	131	108	68	52	64	52	43	128	111	73	29 -
Chichester	F	92	-	156 -		125	100	64	49	60	44	40	115	96	66	30	28
Demir Kapija	F	1	176	144 -		100	122	91	62	51	58	47	39 -		91	74	29	29
Demir Kapija	F	115	168	138 -		86	121	99	62 -		50	46	40 -		97	60	24	14
Demir Kapija	M	142	189	144 -		112	131	108 -		-		57 -		114	111	63	27	34
Demir Kapija	M	157	184	147 -		-		104	74	52	60	43	51	127	112	78	33	33
Demir Kapija	F	162	185	142 -		-		98	73 -		65	52	44 -		-	-	-	-
Demir Kapija	F	17a	173	145 -		110	122	111	73 -		65	47	44	114	94	71	31 -
Demir Kapija	M	205a	185	140 -		-	-		73 -		66	51	39 -		112 -		31	36
Demir Kapija	M	205b	-	148 -		-	130	101 -		58	67 -		47 -		-	-	-	34
Demir Kapija	M	205c	190	144	135	119	131	106	73	53	65	48	40 -		110	64	33	29
Demir Kapija	M	205d	186	149	138 -		130	106	66	55	66	52	41 -		-	-	-	-
Demir Kapija	M	205e*	182	143	137 -		132 -		68 -		-		-		-	-	-	-	-
Demir Kapija	F	205g*	177	137	136 -		130	102	72	54	61	54	40 -		82 -		32	30
Demir Kapija	F	205i	180	143 -			129	104	71	55	60	51	38 -		98 -		-	-
Demir Kapija	F	205lj	175	142	116 -		-		99	65 -		53	45	33 -		-	-	26
Demir Kapija	M	232*	167	152 -		116 -		66 -		-		-		-	132	105	75	30	34
Demir Kapija	F	237	167	139 -		-		102	52	46	47	40	37 -		-	-	-	-
Demir Kapija	F	250a	181	144 -		112	128	102	67 -		56	49	36	122	110	70	35	31
Demir Kapija	F	264*	170	145 -		95	122 -		53 -		54	40	40	113	90	60	27	25
Demir Kapija	F	286a*	170	137	123 -		-		97 -		-		-		-	-	66	27	29
Demir Kapija	M	30*	195	145 -		115	134 -		67 -		52	54	37 -		103	71	31	28
Demir Kapija	M	37a	171	160 -		-	-		-		-	-	-		-	102	70	33	25
Demir Kapija	M	407a	183	142 -		95	135	109	61	46	63	44	42	120	109	66	29	26
Demir Kapija	F	466*	180	150 -		114	128	107	64	55 -		-		126	102	67	31	28
Demir Kapija	F	52	183	140	136	112	128	114	67 -		65	48	44	125	108	66	35	31
Demir Kapija	F	55a	182	141 -		-	130	108	63 -		-	-	-		101 -		30	29
Demir Kapija	M	74	177	141 -		-	-	-		53 -		-	-		108	72	30	28
Demir Kapija	M	82b	181	143	131	107	131	105	68	53	52	35	48 -		106	70	30	28
Demir Kapija	M	99a	198 -		143 -		-	-		-		-	-		127	102	79	36	30
Hickleton	M	10	181	148	135	129 -		120	74	54	49	52	29	125	102	78	29	35
Hickleton	M	103a	182	147	126 -		130	100	68 -		-	-	-		-	-	-	-
Hickleton	M	12	181	139	131	115	131	105	69	53	59	48	36	121	107	77	31	29
Hickleton	F	20	186	151	171	107 -		102	53 -		55	38	32	125	96	68	29	26
Hickleton	F	34	173	135	124	115	124	103	70	46	59	45	40	107	84	69	27	26
Hickleton	F	36	195	146	120	118	131	100	69	50	61	48	42	106	90	65	26	28
Hickleton	M	46	186	150	130	117	130	102	69	58	61	50	41	121	108	61	29	37
Hickleton	M	50	189	147	139	121	133	104	76	53	63	51	39	116	101	68	30	32

Population	Sex	Skeleton																
Hickleton	M	52*	183	-	-	118	-	108	69	-	58	47	42	129	113	70	30	30
Hickleton	F	7	183	136	126	-	-	104	68	51	62	48	42	-	-	-	-	-
Hickleton	F	8	181	145	120	-	125	102	62	48	53	48	37	-	-	-	-	-
Hickleton	F	9	182	142	125	-	112	109	59	41	49	45	32	-	-	-	-	-
Marvinci	F	213	174	142	134	108	124	98	65	54	60	50	44	126	97	73	28	27
Marvinci	M	215*	181	146	135	116	135	-	69	-	-	-	-	123	110	-	-	-
Marvinci	M	220a*	182	157	140	110	147	-	70	-	-	-	-	134	120	-	-	-
Marvinci	F	220b*	170	143	127	115	128	-	72	-	-	-	-	-	100	-	-	-
Marvinci	M	237e*	170	145	135	-	-	-	-	-	-	-	-	-	102	-	-	-
Marvinci	M	240	183	145	129	113	128	116	71	49	63	48	42	115	113	65	29	30
Marvinci	M	246a*	180	139	134	104	130	105	66	52	60	49	43	-	102	69	31	29
Marvinci	F	249*	163	146	118	-	130	-	-	-	-	-	-	125	90	-	-	-
Marvinci	M	250a*	177	144	134	111	133	104	70	50	63	48	41	131	103	68	35	28
Marvinci	F	254	173	138	-	111	125	107	64	-	-	-	-	120	92	63	33	23
Marvinci	F	260/I*	169	139	118	121	124	101	66	44	62	43	39	121	108	60	31	22
Marvinci	F	260/II*	168	135	118	95	122	99	59	-	37	44	58	116	97	61	29	20
Marvinci*	F	269	171	136	123	114	127	98	68	52	64	50	41	117	92	65	33	32
Marvinci	M	286a	180	146	139	119	143	108	70	52	52	45	35	137	102	74	33	21
Marvinci	F	286b	173	139	130	116	132	105	66	46	61	45	40	126	91	69	32	30
Marvinci	F	287*	171	140	130	113	128	-	66	-	-	-	-	121	96	-	-	-
Marvinci	M	288	184	145	126	118	138	112	76	-	68	49	47	127	109	73	30	30
Marvinci	F	289*	185	147	-	105	135	-	68	-	-	-	-	126	102	-	-	-
Marvinci	M	290*	176	142	133	114	138	-	69	-	-	-	-	123	102	-	-	-
Marvinci	M	292	180	141	131	117	137	106	73	-	67	50	45	129	109	69	36	36
Marvinci	F	293	161	138	128	112	125	99	66	54	61	51	41	118	94	69	30	-
Marvinci	M	294	183	133	-	-	-	-	-	-	-	-	-	113	93	-	-	-
Marvinci	M	298*	180	140	138	117	132	-	72	-	-	-	-	128	109	-	-	-
Marvinci	M	299	192	158	148	128	144	110	80	60	59	53	35	139	103	77	40	38
Marvinci	M	300	175	152	-	-	135	104	71	53	63	49	62	-	95	-	30	34
Marvinci	F	316*	163	134	126	101	110	93	59	-	51	45	36	-	91	56	30	26
Marvinci	F	317	167	138	129	101	125	100	59	49	53	46	36	124	98	64	30	23
Marvinci	F	318a*	173	138	124	-	125	-	68	-	-	-	-	-	-	-	-	-
Marvinci	F	bb1	189	140	-	110	125	103	71	55	54	51	35	-	-	-	-	-

Table 2. All skulls, anomalies and conditions.

Population	Sex	Skeleton	Pathology	SL	MD	Rotation	Reversal	Mis	Absent	M3	Ectopic	Crowding
Blackfriars	F	103	Path Max/cloaca	0	0	0	0	0	0	0	0	0
Blackfriars	F	107	-	0	0	0	0	0	0	0	0	0
Blackfriars	F	122	-	0	0	0	0	0	0	0	0	0
Blackfriars	M	134	-	0	0	0	0	0	0	0	0	1
Blackfriars	F	167	-	0	0	0	0	0	0	0	0	0
Blackfriars	F	200	-	0	0	0	0	0	0	1	0	0
Blackfriars	M	233	-	0	0	0	0	0	0	0	0	1
Blackfriars	F	281	Poss SUP?	0	0	0	0	0	0	0	1	0
Blackfriars	M	287	-	0	0	1	0	0	0	0	0	0
Blackfriars	M	302	-	0	0	0	0	0	0	0	0	0
Blackfriars	M	311	-	0	0	0	0	0	0	0	0	0
Blackfriars	M	317	-	0	0	0	0	0	0	1	0	0
Blackfriars	M	411	-	0	0	0	0	0	0	0	0	0
Blackfriars	M	414	-	0	0	0	0	0	0	0	0	0

* some metric data provided by Dr Veljanovska (Veljanovska 2001, 2006), as current condition of skull prevented measurement

Site	Sex	ID	Notes									
Blackfriars	F	420	-	0	0	0	0	0	0	0	0	0
Blackfriars	M	92	-	0	0	0	0	1	0	0	0	0
Blackfriars	F	98	-	0	0	1	0	0	0	0	0	0
Box Lane	M	16	Gingivitis	0	0	0	0	0	0	0	0	0
Box Lane	M	32c	retained decid M1	1	0	1	0	0	1	0	1	1
Box Lane	F	35 1/2	-	0	0	0	0	0	0	1	0	0
Box Lane	M	42	-	0	0	0	0	0	0	0	0	1
Box Lane	M	48	-	0	0	0	0	0	0	0	0	0
Box Lane	M	49a	dental	0	0	0	0	1	0	0	0	0
Box Lane	M	63	palatal porosity	0	0	0	0	0	0	0	0	0
Box Lane	M	67	-	0	0	0	0	0	0	0	0	0
Box Lane	F	73	diastema, ?M3??	0	0	0	0	0	0	1	1	0
Chichester	M	021	-	0	0	0	0	0	0	0	0	0
Chichester	M	033	leprosy	0	0	0	0	1	0	0	0	0
Chichester	F	039	-	0	0	1	0	0	0	0	0	0
Chichester	M	065	-	0	0	1	0	0	0	0	0	1
Chichester	M	100	-	0	0	0	0	0	0	0	1	0
Chichester	M	109	Occribra orbitalia	0	0	1	0	0	0	1	0	0
Chichester	M	142	leprosy	0	0	1	0	0	0	0	0	0
Chichester	M	149	Trauma left jaw/tm	0	0	0	0	0	0	0	0	0
Chichester	F	150	-	0	0	0	0	0	0	0	0	0
Chichester	F	174	-	0	0	0	0	0	0	0	0	0
Chichester	M	19	-	0	0	1	0	0	0	0	0	1
Chichester	F	190	-	0	0	0	0	0	0	0	1	0
Chichester	F	208	diastema	0	0	1	0	0	1	0	0	0
Chichester	M	216	-	0	0	0	0	0	0	1	0	0
Chichester	F	238	-	0	0	0	0	0	0	0	0	0
Chichester	F	252	partly edent	0	0	1	0	0	0	0	0	0
Chichester	F	257	-	0	0	0	0	0	0	0	0	1
Chichester	M	267	-	0	0	0	0	0	0	0	0	0
Chichester	F	279	-	0	0	1	0	0	0	0	0	0
Chichester	M	295	-	0	0	1	0	0	0	1	0	0
Chichester	F	311	-	0	0	0	0	0	0	0	0	0
Chichester	M	315	-	0	0	0	0	0	0	0	0	1
Chichester	M	328	diastema, space	0	0	1	0	0	0	0	0	0
Chichester	M	335	mostly edentulous	0	0	0	0	0	0	0	0	0
Chichester	M	337	-	0	0	0	0	0	0	0	0	0
Chichester	M	342	-	0	0	0	0	0	0	0	0	0
Chichester	M	345	-	0	0	0	0	0	0	0	0	0
Chichester	M	346	-	1	0	0	0	0	0	0	0	0
Chichester	M	354	C(13)erupt?	0	0	1	0	1	0	0	1	1
Chichester	M	371	-	0	0	0	0	0	0	0	0	1
Chichester	M	372	max inc diastema	0	0	1	0	0	0	0	0	0
Chichester	M	373	-	0	0	0	0	0	0	0	0	0
Chichester	M	57	alv. porosity etc	0	0	0	0	0	0	0	0	0
Chichester	M	58	leprosy	0	0	0	0	0	0	0	0	0
Chichester	M	81a	-	0	0	0	0	0	0	0	0	0
Chichester	F	92	-	0	0	1	0	0	0	0	0	1
Demir Kapija	F	1	-	0	0	0	0	0	0	1	0	0
Demir Kapija	F	115	edentulous mand	0	0	1	0	0	0	0	0	0
Demir Kapija	M	142	-	0	0	1	0	0	0	0	0	0

Site	Sex	ID	Notes									
Demir Kapija	M	157	-	0	0	1	0	0	0	0	0	1
Demir Kapija	F	162	-	0	0	0	0	0	0	0	0	0
Demir Kapija	F	17a	-	0	0	1	0	0	0	0	0	0
Demir Kapija	M	205a	-	0	0	0	0	0	0	1	0	1
Demir Kapija	M	205b	-	0	0	0	0	0	0	0	0	0
Demir Kapija	M	205c	-	0	0	0	0	0	0	0	0	0
Demir Kapija	M	205d	-	0	0	0	0	0	0	0	0	0
Demir Kapija	M	205e	-	0	0	0	0	0	0	0	0	0
Demir Kapija	F	205g	-	0	0	0	0	0	0	0	0	1
Demir Kapija	F	205i	rudimentray M3s	0	0	0	0	0	0	0	0	0
Demir Kapija	F	205lj	-	0	0	0	0	0	0	0	0	0
Demir Kapija	M	232	-	0	0	0	0	0	0	0	0	0
Demir Kapija	F	237	edentulous	0	0	0	0	0	0	0	0	0
Demir Kapija	F	250a	diastema	0	0	1	0	0	0	0	0	0
Demir Kapija	F	264	-	0	0	1	0	0	0	0	0	1
Demir Kapija	F	286a	-	0	0	0	0	0	0	0	0	0
Demir Kapija	M	30	-	0	0	0	0	0	0	0	0	0
Demir Kapija	M	37a	only mand m3 hypo	0	0	0	0	0	0	1	0	0
Demir Kapija	M	407a	-	0	0	0	0	0	0	0	1	0
Demir Kapija	F	466	-	0	0	0	0	0	0	0	0	0
Demir Kapija	F	52	-	0	0	0	0	0	0	0	0	0
Demir Kapija	F	55a	-	0	0	0	0	0	0	0	0	0
Demir Kapija	M	74	edentulous maxilla	0	0	0	0	0	0	0	0	0
Demir Kapija	M	82b	-	0	0	0	0	0	0	0	0	0
Demir Kapija	M	99a	-	0	0	0	0	0	0	0	1	0
Hickleton	M	10	-	0	0	0	0	0	0	0	0	0
Hickleton	M	103a	-	0	0	1	0	0	0	0	0	0
Hickleton	M	12	-	0	0	1	0	0	0	0	1	1
Hickleton	F	20	cranial dep. frac.	0	0	0	0	0	0	0	1	1
Hickleton	F	34	-	0	0	1	0	0	0	0	0	0
Hickleton	F	36	-	0	0	1	0	0	0	0	0	0
Hickleton	M	46	-	0	0	0	0	0	0	0	0	0
Hickleton	M	50	-	0	0	0	0	0	0	0	0	0
Hickleton	M	52	-	0	0	0	0	0	0	0	0	1
Hickleton	F	7	-	0	0	0	0	0	1	0	0	0
Hickleton	F	8	-	0	0	0	0	0	0	0	0	0
Hickleton	F	9	-	0	0	0	0	0	0	0	0	0
Marvinci	F	213	-	0	0	0	0	0	0	0	0	0
Marvinci	M	215	-	0	0	1	0	0	0	0	0	1
Marvinci	M	220a	M3; c4-c7 trauma?	0	0	0	0	0	0	0	1	0
Marvinci	F	220b	-	0	0	1	0	0	0	0	0	0
Marvinci	M	237e	-	0	0	0	0	0	0	1	0	0
Marvinci	M	240	-	0	0	0	0	0	0	0	1	0
Marvinci	M	246a	-	0	0	1	0	0	0	0	0	1
Marvinci	F	249	-	0	0	0	0	0	0	0	0	0
Marvinci	M	250a	molar crowding	0	0	0	0	0	0	0	1	1
Marvinci	F	254	-	0	0	0	0	0	0	0	0	0
Marvinci	F	260/I	-	0	0	1	0	0	0	0	0	0
Marvinci	F	260/II	M1 5-cusp pattern	0	0	0	0	0	0	0	1	0
Marvinci	F	269	-	0	0	1	0	0	0	0	0	1
Marvinci	M	286a	-	0	0	0	0	0	0	0	0	0

Population	Sex	Skeleton	Notes											
Marvinci	F	286b	LI REVERSAL(42)	0	0	0	1	0	0	0	0	1		
Marvinci	F	287	-	0	0	1	0	0	0	0	1	1		
Marvinci	M	288	-	0	0	0	0	0	0	0	0	1		
Marvinci	F	289	-	0	0	1	0	0	0	0	0	1		
Marvinci	M	290	-	0	0	1	0	0	0	0	0	1		
Marvinci	M	292	-	0	0	0	0	0	0	0	0	1		
Marvinci	F	293	Void, REVERSAL	0	0	0	1	0	0	0	0	1		
Marvinci	M	294	-	0	0	0	0	0	0	0	0	0		
Marvinci	M	298	-	0	0	0	0	0	0	0	0	0		
Marvinci	M	299	I3 absent AM?	0	0	0	0	0	1	0	0	1		
Marvinci	M	300	-	0	0	0	0	0	0	0	0	1		
Marvinci	F	316	-	0	0	1	0	0	0	0	1	0		
Marvinci	F	317	-	0	0	0	0	0	0	1	0	0		
Marvinci	F	318a	-	0	0	0	0	0	0	0	0	0		
Marvinci	M	bb1	-	0	0	1	0	0	0	0	0	0		

Table 3. All skull, craniometric indices and ratios

Population	Skeleton	CI	CM	CLHI	CBHI	TFI	UFI	MAI	PI	PMR	TFHFMT	UFHFMT	MAXBCDL	cdlgo	ZYGFMT	UHTH	FB	FB2	UFIMAI
Blackfriars	103	79.5	-	-	-	-	-	-	94.00	-	-	-	-	0.46	0.85	0.77	-	0.93	0.83	-
Blackfriars	107	-	-	-	-	-	-	131.11	74.51	0.57	-	-	-	0.51	0.81	-	-	-	-	-
Blackfriars	122	-	-	69.89	-	-	-	-	83.33	-	-	-	-	0.49	0.76	0.87	-	0.98	0.89	-
Blackfriars	134	-	-	-	-	-	-	-	91.11	-	-	-	-	0.50	0.86	-	-	-	-	-
Blackfriars	167	78.5	152.00	73.48	93.66	-	53.66	-	63.83	-	-	-	62.86	0.51	0.85	0.85	-	0.88	0.97	-
Blackfriars	200	76.1	-	-	-	-	-	105.77	79.17	0.75	-	-	-	-	-	-	-	-	-	-
Blackfriars	233	-	-	-	-	-	-	-	-	-	-	-	-	-	0.91	-	-	-	0.90	-
Blackfriars	281	81.9	-	-	-	-	-	-	81.63	-	-	-	-	0.50	0.72	-	-	-	0.85	-
Blackfriars	287	-	-	-	-	-	-	-	68.09	-	-	-	-	0.49	0.87	-	-	-	-	-
Blackfriars	302	78.1	160.33	72.40	92.67	91.60	54.20	109.84	72.41	0.66	107.14	63.39	-	-	0.85	0.59	-	-	0.49
Blackfriars	311	-	-	-	-	-	-	-	67.24	-	-	-	-	-	-	-	-	-	-	-
Blackfriars	317	-	-	-	94.33	-	-	-	64.00	-	-	-	-	-	-	0.79	-	-	-	-
Blackfriars	411	-	-	-	-	-	-	111.54	77.55	0.70	-	-	54.81	-	-	-	-	-	-	-
Blackfriars	414	76.9	155.00	73.12	95.10	-	-	-	81.63	-	-	-	-	-	-	0.79	-	-	-	-
Blackfriars	420	78.2	-	-	-	-	-	-	66.10	-	-	-	-	-	-	-	-	-	-	-
Blackfriars	92	79.5	159.67	72.63	91.39	86.76	48.53	-	87.23	-	115.69	64.71	0.46	0.87	0.75	0.56	0.93	0.80	-
Blackfriars	98	78.1	-	-	-	85.96	53.51	126.09	-	-	102.08	63.54	0.56	0.85	0.84	0.62	0.91	0.92	0.42
Box Lane	16	-	-	-	-	-	-	108.62	81.13	0.75	-	-	-	0.47	0.83	-	-	-	0.85	-
Box Lane	32c	71.2	-	-	-	-	-	-	80.00	-	-	67.35	-	-	-	-	-	-	-	-
Box Lane	35 1/2	68.2	-	-	-	-	-	-	-	-	-	-	-	0.79	-	-	-	0.87	-
Box Lane	42	-	-	-	-	-	-	-	76.60	-	-	-	-	0.46	0.80	-	-	-	0.85	-
Box Lane	48	75.6	160.33	73.58	97.26	-	-	-	58.93	-	-	-	-	-	0.88	-	0.50	-	-	-
Box Lane	49a	81.3	162.67	72.92	89.74	-	-	-	80.77	-	-	-	-	-	0.92	-	0.58	-	-	-
Box Lane	63	74.5	-	-	-	-	-	138.30	84.31	0.61	-	-	-	0.53	0.85	-	-	-	-	-
Box Lane	67	72.1	159.33	70.56	97.89	85.71	51.88	-	72.55	-	111.76	67.65	0.48	0.81	0.77	0.61	0.92	0.83	-
Box Lane	73	80.7	145.67	67.61	83.80	-	-	-	-	-	-	-	-	-	0.77	-	-	-	0.90	-
Chichester	021	82.3	140.33	74.39	90.37	-	-	-	85.11	-	120.00	60.00	0.52	0.86	-	0.50	-	0.83	-
Chichester	033	-	-	-	-	-	-	-	84.78	-	119.61	67.65	-	0.83	-	0.57	-	0.94	-
Chichester	039	90.0	141.33	75.00	83.33	85.85	49.61	122.45	81.82	0.67	109.00	63.00	0.56	0.87	0.79	0.58	0.84	0.93	0.41
Chichester	065	77.8	147.00	67.22	86.43	89.83	53.39	107.84	83.33	0.77	110.42	65.63	0.49	0.86	0.81	0.59	0.96	0.85	0.50
Chichester	100	80.8	-	-	-	-	51.97	124.49	95.45	0.77	-	64.08	0.51	0.77	0.81	-	0.94	0.86	0.42
Chichester	109	104.4	167.67	71.98	68.95	-	-	107.69	75.00	0.70	-	59.80	0.49	0.87	-	-	-	0.89	-
Chichester	142	81.7	143.67	64.57	79.02	85.16	52.34	120.75	85.71	0.71	97.32	59.82	0.56	0.82	0.88	0.61	0.90	0.97	0.43
Chichester	149	81.5	158.00	76.09	93.33	85.19	53.33	119.23	73.08	0.61	107.48	67.29	-	-	0.79	0.63	-	-	0.45

Site	ID															
Chichester	150	77.5	152.33	66.84	86.21	78.46	48.46	97.96	97.67	1.00	100.99	62.38	-	-	0.78	0.62 - -	0.49
Chichester	174	81.4	143.00	68.02	83.57	87.88	53.03	114.55	77.36	0.68	108.41	65.42	0.51 0.81	0.81	0.60 0.93 0.87	0.46
Chichester	19	84.3	154.67	76.40	90.67	81.29	43.17 -	-	-		105.61	56.07	0.52 0.85	0.77	0.53 0.94 0.82 -	
Chichester	190	77.8	149.67	71.67	92.14	84.25	49.61	115.38	79.59	0.69	100.00	58.88	0.54 0.89	0.84	0.59 0.87 0.96	0.43
Chichester	208	84.8	142.67	74.55	87.86	82.93	50.41 -		70.83 -		100.99	61.39	0.45 0.74	0.82	0.61 0.98 0.83 -	
Chichester	216	75.0 -	-	-		81.97	53.28	110.91	87.23	0.79	95.24	61.90	0.52 0.77	0.86	0.65 0.97 0.89	0.48
Chichester	238	84.6	146.33	75.15	88.81 -		49.22	114.00	91.30	0.80 -		60.00 -	-	0.82 -	- - -	0.43
Chichester	252	78.1	154.00	68.98	88.36	75.00	49.22	110.00	84.78	0.77	87.27	57.27	0.48 0.87	0.86	0.66 0.90 0.96	0.45
Chichester	257	79.1	145.67	75.00	94.85	86.40	52.00	111.11	71.70	0.65	103.85	62.50	0.52 0.77	0.83	0.60 0.93 0.90	0.47
Chichester	267	82.1	153.33	74.86	91.16 -			55.30 -				66.97 -			0.83 -		
Chichester	279	83.1	156.33	73.22	88.16	77.21	49.26	122.00	85.42	0.70	93.75	59.82	0.52 0.78	0.82	0.64 0.87 0.95	0.40
Chichester	295	-	-	-	92.14	81.68	48.85	116.98	82.69	0.71	96.40	57.66	0.53 0.92	0.85	0.60 0.89 0.96	0.42
Chichester	311	76.2	150.00	72.38	94.93 -			86.54	62.75	0.73 -		64.08 -			-		
Chichester	315	84.0	150.33	73.71	87.76 -	-			83.67 -		101.92	62.50 -			0.61 -		
Chichester	328	85.9	151.00	70.06	81.58	78.32	48.25	110.34	84.62	0.77	105.66	65.09	0.49 0.88	0.74	0.62 0.92 0.81	0.44
Chichester	335	87.7 -			79.58	48.59	96.30	79.25	0.82		106.60	65.09	0.39 0.85	0.75	0.61 0.93 0.80	0.50
Chichester	337	89.4	151.00	77.06	86.18	92.31	54.55	98.28	80.39	0.82	120.00	70.91	0.43 0.83	0.77	0.59 0.92 0.83	0.56
Chichester	342	81.0	149.67	69.83	86.21 -		54.55	118.00	89.13	0.76 -		69.23 -			0.79 -	-	0.46
Chichester	345	-	-	-			128.00	85.42	0.67 -			57.55 -			-	-	
Chichester	346	77.7 -	-	-		78.52	46.67	116.98	80.00	0.68	96.36	57.27	0.53 0.88	0.81	0.59 0.87 0.93	0.40
Chichester	354	83.8	155.33	76.54	91.33	93.85	52.31 -		80.39 -		116.19	64.76 -			0.81	0.56 -	
Chichester	371	80.1	150.67	69.61	86.90	91.24	53.28	108.93	75.47	0.69	114.68	66.97	0.49 0.74	0.80	0.58 0.91 0.87	0.49
Chichester	372	75.6	151.33	76.67	101.47 -	-			73.08 -		-			0.50 0.78 -	-	- 0.93 -	
Chichester	373	81.3	154.67	73.63	90.54 -			129.17	91.49	0.71 -		-		0.49 0.71 -	-	- 0.84 -	
Chichester	57	72.2	151.33	70.59	97.78	92.42	53.79 -		63.79 -		114.02	66.36	0.54 0.93	0.81	0.58 0.86 0.94 -	
Chichester	58	88.3	153.00	80.12	90.73 -	-	-	-	-		-						
Chichester	81a	75.9 -	-	-		91.60	51.91	123.08	82.69	0.67	111.11	62.96	0.50 0.87	0.82	0.57 0.98 0.84	0.42
Chichester	92	-	-	-	-	51.20	122.45	90.91	0.74 -			64.00	0.52 0.83	0.80 -		0.92 0.87	0.42
Demir Kapija	1	81.8 -	-	-		81.97	50.82	113.73	82.98	0.73	109.89	68.13 -			0.75	0.62 - -	0.45
Demir Kapija	115	82.1 -	-	-		71.07	51.24 -		86.96 -		86.87	62.63 -			0.82	0.72 - -	
Demir Kapija	142	76.2 -	-	-		85.50 -			-		103.70 -			0.97	0.82 -	- 0.87 0.95 -	
Demir Kapija	157	79.9 -	-	-	-		115.38	118.60	1.03 -			71.15	0.47 0.88 -		-	- 0.82 -	
Demir Kapija	162	76.8 -	-	-	-			84.62 -				74.49 -			-	-	
Demir Kapija	17a	83.8 -	-	-		90.16	59.84 -		93.62 -		99.10	65.77	0.57 0.82	0.91	0.66 0.93 0.97 -	
Demir Kapija	205a	75.7 -	-	-	-	-		76.47 -		-							
Demir Kapija	205b	-	-	-	-	-	115.52 -		-		-			0.78 -			
Demir Kapija	205c	75.8	156.33	71.05	93.75	90.84	55.73	122.64	83.33	0.68	112.26	68.87 -			0.81	0.61 - -	0.45
Demir Kapija	205d	80.1	157.67	74.19	92.62 -		50.77	120.00	78.85	0.66 -		62.26 -			0.82 -	- -	0.42
Demir Kapija	205e	78.6	154.00	75.27	95.80 -		51.52 -		-			-					
Demir Kapija	205g	77.4	150.00	76.84	99.27 -		55.38	112.96	74.07	0.66 -		70.59 -			0.78 -	- -	0.49
Demir Kapija	205i	79.4 -	-	-		55.04	109.09	74.51	0.68 -			68.27 -			0.81 -	- -	0.50
Demir Kapija	205lj	81.1	144.33	66.29	81.69 -	-	-		73.33 -		-		65.66 -			-		
Demir Kapija	232	91.0 -	-	-	-	-			175.76 -			-		0.80 -		- 0.50 -	
Demir Kapija	237	83.2 -	-	-	-		102.17	92.50	0.91 -			50.98 -			-		
Demir Kapija	250a	79.6 -	-	-		87.50	52.34 -		73.47 -		109.80	65.69	0.46 0.90	0.80	0.60 0.95 0.84 -	
Demir Kapija	264	85.3 -	-	-		62.30	43.44 -		100.00 -		-		0.48 0.80 -			0.56 0.93 -	
Demir Kapija	286a	80.6	143.33	72.35	89.78 -	-	-	-	-		-						
Demir Kapija	30	74.4 -	-	-		85.82	50.00 -		68.52 -		-	-				0.58 - - -	
Demir Kapija	37a	93.6 -	-	-	-	-	-	-	-		-						
Demir Kapija	407a	77.6 -	-	-		70.37	45.19	136.96	95.45	0.70	87.16	55.96	0.53 0.91	0.81	0.64 0.89 0.91	0.33
Demir Kapija	466	83.3 -	-	-		89.06	50.00 -	-	-		106.54	59.81 -		0.81	0.84	0.56 0.98 0.85 -	

Site	No.																
Demir Kapija	52	76.5	153.00	74.32	97.14	87.50	52.34	-	91.67	-	98.25	58.77	0.52	0.86	0.89	0.60 0.98	0.91 -
Demir Kapija	55a	77.5 -	-	-	-	48.46	-	-	-	-	-	58.33	-	-	0.83 -	- -	-
Demir Kapija	74	79.7 -	-	-	-	-	-	-	-	-	-	-	-	-	-	-	-
Demir Kapija	82b	79.0	151.67	72.38	91.61	81.68	51.91	98.11	137.14	1.40	101.90	64.76 -		-	0.80	0.64 -	-	0.53
Demir Kapija	99a	-	-	72.22 -		-	-	-	-	-	-	-	0.80 -		-	- -	-
Hickleton	10	81.8	154.67	74.59	91.22 -		-	90.74	55.77	0.61	107.50	61.67	0.39	0.82 -		0.57 -	0.96 -
Hickleton	103a	80.8	151.67	69.23	85.71 -		52.31 -		-	-	-	68.00 -		-	0.77 -	- -	-
Hickleton	12	76.8	150.33	72.38	94.24	87.79	52.67	111.32	75.00	0.67	109.52	65.71	0.49	0.88	0.80	0.60 0.92	0.87	0.47
Hickleton	20	81.2	169.33	91.94	113.25 -		-	84.21 -		-	104.90	51.96	0.44	0.77 -		0.50 -	0.82 -
Hickleton	34	78.0	144.00	71.68	91.85	92.74	56.45	128.26	88.89	0.69	111.65	67.96	0.55	0.79	0.83	0.61 0.86	0.96	0.44
Hickleton	36	74.9	153.67	61.54	82.19	90.08	52.67	122.00	87.50	0.72	118.00	69.00	0.58	0.85	0.76	0.58 0.81	0.94	0.43
Hickleton	46	80.6	155.33	69.89	86.67	90.00	53.08	105.17	82.00	0.78	114.71	67.65	0.50	0.89	0.78	0.59 0.93	0.84	0.50
Hickleton	50	77.8	158.33	73.54	94.56	90.98	57.14	118.87	76.47	0.64	116.35	73.08	0.54	0.87	0.78	0.63 0.87	0.90	0.48
Hickleton	52	-	-	-	-	-	-	-	89.36 -		109.26	63.89	0.45	0.88 -		0.58 -	0.84 -
Hickleton	7	74.3	148.33	68.85	92.65 -		-	121.57	87.50	0.72 -		65.38 -		-	-	- -	-
Hickleton	8	80.1	148.67	66.30	82.76 -		49.60	110.42	77.08	0.70 -		60.78 -		-	0.82 -	- -	0.45
Hickleton	9	78.0	149.67	68.68	88.03 -		52.68	119.51	71.11	0.60 -		54.13 -		-	0.97 -	- -	0.44
Marvinci	213	81.6	150.00	77.01	94.37	87.10	52.42	111.11	88.00	0.79	110.20	66.33	0.48	0.77	0.79	0.60 1.02	0.78	0.47
Marvinci	215	80.7	154.00	74.59	92.47	85.93	51.11 -		-	-	-	-	-	0.89 -		0.59 0.91	- -
Marvinci	220a	86.3	159.67	76.92	89.17	74.83	47.62 -		-	-	-	-	-	0.90 -		0.64 0.91	- -
Marvinci	220b	84.1	146.67	74.71	88.81	89.84	56.25 -		-	-	-	-	-	-	-	0.63 -	- -
Marvinci	237e	85.3	150.00	79.41	93.10 -		-	-	-	-	-	-	-	-	-	-	-
Marvinci	240	79.2	152.33	70.49	88.97	88.28	55.47	128.57	87.50	0.68	97.41	61.21	0.55	0.98	0.91	0.63 0.90	1.01	0.43
Marvinci	246a	77.2	151.00	74.44	96.40	80.00	50.77	115.38	87.76	0.76	99.05	62.86 -		-	0.81	0.63 -	-	0.44
Marvinci	249	89.6	142.33	72.39	80.82 -		-	-	-	-	-	-	-	0.72 -		0.96 -	- -
Marvinci	250a	81.4	151.67	75.71	93.06	83.46	52.63	126.00	85.42	0.68	106.73	67.31	0.48	0.79	0.78	0.63 0.98	0.79	0.42
Marvinci	254	79.8 -		-	-	88.80	51.20 -		-	-	103.74	59.81 -		0.77	0.86	0.58 0.96	0.89 -
Marvinci	260/I	82.2	142.00	69.82	84.89	97.58	53.23	140.91	90.70	0.64	119.80	65.35	0.51	0.89	0.81	0.55 0.98	0.83	0.38
Marvinci	260/II	80.4	140.33	70.24	87.41	77.87	48.36 -		131.82 -		95.96	59.60	0.32	0.84	0.81	0.62 0.95	0.85 -
Marvinci	269	79.5	143.33	71.93	90.44	89.76	53.54	123.08	82.00	0.67	116.33	69.39	0.55	0.79	0.77	0.60 0.92	0.84	0.44
Marvinci	286a	81.1	155.00	77.22	95.21	83.22	48.95	100.00	77.78	0.78	110.19	64.81	0.38	0.74	0.76	0.59 0.96	0.79	0.49
Marvinci	286b	80.3	147.33	75.14	93.53	87.88	50.00	132.61	88.89	0.67	110.48	62.86	0.48	0.72	0.80	0.57 0.95	0.83	0.38
Marvinci	287	81.9	147.00	76.02	92.86	88.28	51.56 -		-	-	-	-	-	0.79 -		0.58 0.95	- -
Marvinci	288	78.8	151.67	68.48	86.90	85.51	55.07 -		95.92 -		105.36	67.86	0.54	0.86	0.81	0.64 0.92	0.88 -
Marvinci	289	79.5 -		-	-	77.78	50.37 -		-	-	-	-	-	0.81 -		0.65 0.93	- -
Marvinci	290	80.7	150.33	75.57	93.66	82.61	50.00 -		-	-	-	-	-	0.83 -		0.61 0.89	- -
Marvinci	292	78.3	150.67	72.78	92.91	85.40	53.28 -		90.00 -		110.38	68.87	0.52	0.84	0.77	0.62 0.94	0.82 -
Marvinci	293	85.7	142.33	79.50	92.75	89.60	52.80	112.96	80.39	0.71	113.13	66.67	0.52	0.80	0.79	0.59 0.94	0.84	0.47
Marvinci	294	72.7 -		-	-	-	-	-	-	-	-	-	-	0.82 -		- -	- -
Marvinci	298	77.8	152.67	76.37	98.57	88.64	54.55 -		-	-	-	-	-	0.85 -		0.62 0.97	- -
Marvinci	299	82.3	166.00	77.08	93.67	88.89	55.56	98.33	66.04	0.67	116.36	72.73	0.42	0.74	0.76	0.63 0.97	0.79	0.56
Marvinci	300	86.9 -		-	-	-	52.59	118.87	126.53	1.06 -		68.27 -		-	-	0.77 -	- -	0.44
Marvinci	316	82.2	141.00	77.30	94.03	91.82	53.64 -		80.00 -		108.60	63.44 -		-	0.85	0.58 -	- -
Marvinci	317	82.6	144.67	77.25	93.48	80.80	47.20	108.16	78.26	0.72	101.00	59.00	0.43	0.79	0.80	0.58 0.99	0.81	0.44
Marvinci	318a	79.8	145.00	71.68	89.86 -		54.40 -		-	-	-	-	-	-	-	- -	- -
Marvinci	bb1	74.1 -		-	-	88.00	56.80	98.18	68.63	0.70	106.80	68.93 -		-	0.82	0.65 -	-	0.58

Appendix A 2

Section 1. Frequencies and Distributions of Anomalies.

Supplemental Teeth * Rotation

Chi-Square Tests

Sex	MajorGeo		Value	df	Asymp. Sig. (2-sided)	Exact Sig. (2-sided)	Exact Sig. (1-sided)
Female	English	Pearson Chi-Square	.[a]				
		N of Valid Cases	27				
	Macedonian	Pearson Chi-Square	.[a]				
		N of Valid Cases	28				
Male	English	Pearson Chi-Square	.658[b]	1	.417		
		Continuity Correction[c]	.000	1	1.000		
		Likelihood Ratio	.576	1	.448		
		Fisher's Exact Test				.450	.450
		Linear-by-Linear Association	.644	1	.422		
		N of Valid Cases	47				
	Macedonian	Pearson Chi-Square	.[a]				
		N of Valid Cases	29				

a. No statistics are computed because Supplemental Teeth is a constant.
b. 2 cells (50.0%) have expected count less than 5. The minimum expected count is .51.
c. Computed only for a 2x2 table

Supplemental Teeth * Reversal

Chi-Square Tests

Sex	MajorGeo		Value
Female	English	Pearson Chi-Square	.[a]
		N of Valid Cases	27
	Macedonian	Pearson Chi-Square	.[b]
		N of Valid Cases	28
Male	English	Pearson Chi-Square	.[c]
		N of Valid Cases	47
	Macedonian	Pearson Chi-Square	.[a]
		N of Valid Cases	29

a. No statistics are computed because Supplemental Teeth and Reversal are constants.
b. No statistics are computed because Supplemental Teeth is a constant.
c. No statistics are computed because Reversal is a constant.

Supplemental Teeth * Peg, Misshapen

Chi-Square Tests

Sex	MajorGeo		Value	df	Asymp. Sig. (2-sided)	Exact Sig. (2-sided)	Exact Sig. (1-sided)
Female	English	Pearson Chi-Square	.[a]				
		N of Valid Cases	27				
	Macedonian	Pearson Chi-Square	.[a]				
		N of Valid Cases	28				
Male	English	Pearson Chi-Square	.194[b]	1	.659		
		Continuity Correction[c]	.000	1	1.000		
		Likelihood Ratio	.364	1	.546		
		Fisher's Exact Test				1.000	.835
		Linear-by-Linear Association	.190	1	.663		
		N of Valid Cases	47				
	Macedonian	Pearson Chi-Square	.[a]				
		N of Valid Cases	29				

a. No statistics are computed because Supplemental Teeth and Peg, Misshapen are constants.
b. 3 cells (75.0%) have expected count less than 5. The minimum expected count is .17.
c. Computed only for a 2x2 table

Supplemental Teeth * Congenitally Absent Teeth

Chi-Square Tests

Sex	MajorGeo		Value	df	Asymp. Sig. (2-sided)	Exact Sig. (2-sided)	Exact Sig. (1-sided)
Female	English	Pearson Chi-Square	.ᵃ				
		N of Valid Cases	27				
	Macedonian	Pearson Chi-Square	.ᵇ				
		N of Valid Cases	28				
Male	English	Pearson Chi-Square	22.989ᶜ	1	.000		
		Continuity Correctionᵈ	5.248	1	.022		
		Likelihood Ratio	6.906	1	.009		
		Fisher's Exact Test				.043	.043
		Linear-by-Linear Association	22.500	1	.000		
		N of Valid Cases	47				
	Macedonian	Pearson Chi-Square	.ᵃ				
		N of Valid Cases	29				

a. No statistics are computed because Supplemental Teeth is a constant.
b. No statistics are computed because Supplemental Teeth and Congenitally Absent Teeth are constants.
c. 3 cells (75.0%) have expected count less than 5. The minimum expected count is .04.
d. Computed only for a 2x2 table

M3 Congenitally Absent * Rotation

Chi-Square Tests

Sex	MajorGeo		Value	df	Asymp. Sig. (2-sided)	Exact Sig. (2-sided)	Exact Sig. (1-sided)
Female	English	Pearson Chi-Square	1.421ᵃ	1	.233		
		Continuity Correctionᵇ	.272	1	.602		
		Likelihood Ratio	2.263	1	.133		
		Fisher's Exact Test				.532	.331
		Linear-by-Linear Association	1.368	1	.242		
		N of Valid Cases	27				
	Macedonian	Pearson Chi-Square	1.197ᶜ	1	.274		
		Continuity Correctionᵇ	.108	1	.743		
		Likelihood Ratio	1.852	1	.174		
		Fisher's Exact Test				.524	.405
		Linear-by-Linear Association	1.154	1	.283		
		N of Valid Cases	28				
Male	English	Pearson Chi-Square	1.377ᵈ	1	.241		
		Continuity Correctionᵇ	.329	1	.566		
		Likelihood Ratio	1.215	1	.270		
		Fisher's Exact Test				.266	.266
		Linear-by-Linear Association	1.347	1	.246		
		N of Valid Cases	47				
	Macedonian	Pearson Chi-Square	.873ᵉ	1	.350		
		Continuity Correctionᵇ	.033	1	.856		
		Likelihood Ratio	1.479	1	.224		
		Fisher's Exact Test				1.000	.485
		Linear-by-Linear Association	.843	1	.359		
		N of Valid Cases	29				

a. 2 cells (50.0%) have expected count less than 5. The minimum expected count is .89.
b. Computed only for a 2x2 table
c. 2 cells (50.0%) have expected count less than 5. The minimum expected count is .71.
d. 2 cells (50.0%) have expected count less than 5. The minimum expected count is 1.02.
e. 2 cells (50.0%) have expected count less than 5. The minimum expected count is .62.

M3 Congenitally Absent * Reversal

Chi-Square Tests

Sex	MajorGeo		Value	df	Asymp. Sig. (2-sided)	Exact Sig. (2-sided)	Exact Sig. (1-sided)
Female	English	Pearson Chi-Square	.[a]				
		N of Valid Cases	27				
	Macedonian	Pearson Chi-Square	.166[b]	1	.684		
		Continuity Correction[c]	.000	1	1.000		
		Likelihood Ratio	.308	1	.579		
		Fisher's Exact Test				1.000	.860
		Linear-by-Linear Association	.160	1	.689		
		N of Valid Cases	28				
Male	English	Pearson Chi-Square	.[a]				
		N of Valid Cases	47				
	Macedonian	Pearson Chi-Square	.[a]				
		N of Valid Cases	29				

a. No statistics are computed because Reversal is a constant.
b. 3 cells (75.0%) have expected count less than 5. The minimum expected count is .14.
c. Computed only for a 2x2 table

M3 Congenitally Absent * Peg, Misshapen

Chi-Square Tests

Sex	MajorGeo		Value	df	Asymp. Sig. (2-sided)	Exact Sig. (2-sided)	Exact Sig. (1-sided)
Female	English	Pearson Chi-Square	.[a]				
		N of Valid Cases	27				
	Macedonian	Pearson Chi-Square	.[a]				
		N of Valid Cases	28				
Male	English	Pearson Chi-Square	.407[b]	1	.524		
		Continuity Correction[c]	.000	1	1.000		
		Likelihood Ratio	.745	1	.388		
		Fisher's Exact Test				1.000	.692
		Linear-by-Linear Association	.398	1	.528		
		N of Valid Cases	47				
	Macedonian	Pearson Chi-Square	.[a]				
		N of Valid Cases	29				

a. No statistics are computed because Peg, Misshapen is a constant.
b. 3 cells (75.0%) have expected count less than 5. The minimum expected count is .34.
c. Computed only for a 2x2 table

M3 Congenitally Absent * Congenitally Absent Teeth

Chi-Square Tests

Sex	MajorGeo		Value	df	Asymp. Sig. (2-sided)	Exact Sig. (2-sided)	Exact Sig. (1-sided)
Female	English	Pearson Chi-Square	.270[a]	1	.603		
		Continuity Correction[b]	.000	1	1.000		
		Likelihood Ratio	.491	1	.484		
		Fisher's Exact Test				1.000	.786
		Linear-by-Linear Association	.260	1	.610		
		N of Valid Cases	27				
	Macedonian	Pearson Chi-Square	.[c]				
		N of Valid Cases	28				
Male	English	Pearson Chi-Square	.095[d]	1	.758		
		Continuity Correction[b]	.000	1	1.000		
		Likelihood Ratio	.180	1	.671		
		Fisher's Exact Test				1.000	.915
		Linear-by-Linear Association	.093	1	.760		
		N of Valid Cases	47				

Sex	MajorGeo		Value	df	Asymp. Sig. (2-sided)	Exact Sig. (2-sided)	Exact Sig. (1-sided)
	Macedonian	Pearson Chi-Square	.120^e	1	.730		
		Continuity Correction^b	.000	1	1.000		
		Likelihood Ratio	.222	1	.637		
		Fisher's Exact Test				1.000	.897
		Linear-by-Linear Association	.115	1	.734		
		N of Valid Cases	29				

a. 3 cells (75.0%) have expected count less than 5. The minimum expected count is .22.
b. Computed only for a 2x2 table
c. No statistics are computed because Congenitally Absent Teeth is a constant.
d. 3 cells (75.0%) have expected count less than 5. The minimum expected count is .09.
e. 3 cells (75.0%) have expected count less than 5. The minimum expected count is .10.

Ectopic, heterotopic, impaction * Rotation

Chi-Square Tests

Sex	MajorGeo		Value	df	Asymp. Sig. (2-sided)	Exact Sig. (2-sided)	Exact Sig. (1-sided)
Female	English	Pearson Chi-Square	1.977^a	1	.160		
		Continuity Correction^b	.661	1	.416		
		Likelihood Ratio	3.095	1	.079		
		Fisher's Exact Test				.285	.221
		Linear-by-Linear Association	1.904	1	.168		
		N of Valid Cases	27				
	Macedonian	Pearson Chi-Square	1.402^c	1	.236		
		Continuity Correction^b	.299	1	.585		
		Likelihood Ratio	1.336	1	.248		
		Fisher's Exact Test				.284	.284
		Linear-by-Linear Association	1.352	1	.245		
		N of Valid Cases	28				
Male	English	Pearson Chi-Square	5.627^d	1	.018		
		Continuity Correction^b	3.143	1	.076		
		Likelihood Ratio	4.782	1	.029		
		Fisher's Exact Test				.046	.046
		Linear-by-Linear Association	5.507	1	.019		
		N of Valid Cases	47				
	Macedonian	Pearson Chi-Square	1.576^e	1	.209		
		Continuity Correction^b	.421	1	.517		
		Likelihood Ratio	2.577	1	.108		
		Fisher's Exact Test				.553	.283
		Linear-by-Linear Association	1.522	1	.217		
		N of Valid Cases	29				

a. 2 cells (50.0%) have expected count less than 5. The minimum expected count is 1.19.
b. Computed only for a 2x2 table
c. 2 cells (50.0%) have expected count less than 5. The minimum expected count is 1.07.
d. 2 cells (50.0%) have expected count less than 5. The minimum expected count is 1.02.
e. 3 cells (75.0%) have expected count less than 5. The minimum expected count is 1.03.

Ectopic, heterotopic, impaction * Reversal

Chi-Square Tests

Sex	MajorGeo		Value	df	Asymp. Sig. (2-sided)	Exact Sig. (2-sided)	Exact Sig. (1-sided)
Female	English	Pearson Chi-Square	.^{a}				
		N of Valid Cases	27				
	Macedonian	Pearson Chi-Square	.258^b	1	.611		
		Continuity Correction^c	.000	1	1.000		
		Likelihood Ratio	.471	1	.492		
		Fisher's Exact Test				1.000	.794
		Linear-by-Linear Association	.249	1	.618		

		N of Valid Cases	28				
Male	English	Pearson Chi-Square	.[a]				
		N of Valid Cases	47				
	Macedonian	Pearson Chi-Square	.[a]				
		N of Valid Cases	29				

a. No statistics are computed because Reversal is a constant.
b. 3 cells (75.0%) have expected count less than 5. The minimum expected count is .21.
c. Computed only for a 2x2 table

Ectopic, heterotopic, impaction * Peg, Misshapen
Chi-Square Tests

Sex	MajorGeo		Value	df	Asymp. Sig. (2-sided)	Exact Sig. (2-sided)	Exact Sig. (1-sided)
Female	English	Pearson Chi-Square	.[a]				
		N of Valid Cases	27				
	Macedonian	Pearson Chi-Square	.[a]				
		N of Valid Cases	28				
Male	English	Pearson Chi-Square	1.527[b]	1	.217		
		Continuity Correction[c]	.089	1	.765		
		Likelihood Ratio	1.100	1	.294		
		Fisher's Exact Test				.308	.308
		Linear-by-Linear Association	1.494	1	.222		
		N of Valid Cases	47				
	Macedonian	Pearson Chi-Square	.[a]				
		N of Valid Cases	29				

a. No statistics are computed because Peg, Misshapen is a constant.
b. 3 cells (75.0%) have expected count less than 5. The minimum expected count is .34.
c. Computed only for a 2x2 table

Ectopic, heterotopic, impaction * Congenitally Absent Teeth
Chi-Square Tests

Sex	MajorGeo		Value	df	Asymp. Sig. (2-sided)	Exact Sig. (2-sided)	Exact Sig. (1-sided)
Female	English	Pearson Chi-Square	.376[a]	1	.540		
		Continuity Correction[b]	.000	1	1.000		
		Likelihood Ratio	.669	1	.414		
		Fisher's Exact Test				1.000	.721
		Linear-by-Linear Association	.362	1	.548		
		N of Valid Cases	27				
	Macedonian	Pearson Chi-Square	.[c]				
		N of Valid Cases	28				
Male	English	Pearson Chi-Square	10.984[d]	1	.001		
		Continuity Correction[b]	2.259	1	.133		
		Likelihood Ratio	5.180	1	.023		
		Fisher's Exact Test				.085	.085
		Linear-by-Linear Association	10.750	1	.001		
		N of Valid Cases	47				
	Macedonian	Pearson Chi-Square	.216[e]	1	.642		
		Continuity Correction[b]	.000	1	1.000		
		Likelihood Ratio	.386	1	.534		
		Fisher's Exact Test				1.000	.828
		Linear-by-Linear Association	.208	1	.648		
		N of Valid Cases	29				

a. 3 cells (75.0%) have expected count less than 5. The minimum expected count is .30.
b. Computed only for a 2x2 table
c. No statistics are computed because Congenitally Absent Teeth is a constant.
d. 3 cells (75.0%) have expected count less than 5. The minimum expected count is .09.
e. 3 cells (75.0%) have expected count less than 5. The minimum expected count is .17.

Crowding * Rotation

Chi-Square Tests

Sex	MajorGeo		Value	df	Asymp. Sig. (2-sided)	Exact Sig. (2-sided)	Exact Sig. (1-sided)
Female	English	Pearson Chi-Square	.022[a]	1	.882		
		Continuity Correction[b]	.000	1	1.000		
		Likelihood Ratio	.022	1	.883		
		Fisher's Exact Test				1.000	.669
		Linear-by-Linear Association	.021	1	.884		
		N of Valid Cases	27				
	Macedonian	Pearson Chi-Square	1.867[c]	1	.172		
		Continuity Correction[b]	.830	1	.362		
		Likelihood Ratio	1.810	1	.178		
		Fisher's Exact Test				.207	.181
		Linear-by-Linear Association	1.800	1	.180		
		N of Valid Cases	28				
Male	English	Pearson Chi-Square	2.998[d]	1	.083		
		Continuity Correction[b]	1.786	1	.181		
		Likelihood Ratio	2.776	1	.096		
		Fisher's Exact Test				.118	.094
		Linear-by-Linear Association	2.934	1	.087		
		N of Valid Cases	47				
	Macedonian	Pearson Chi-Square	3.468[e]	1	.063		
		Continuity Correction[b]	1.905	1	.168		
		Likelihood Ratio	3.322	1	.068		
		Fisher's Exact Test				.143	.086
		Linear-by-Linear Association	3.349	1	.067		
		N of Valid Cases	29				

a. 2 cells (50.0%) have expected count less than 5. The minimum expected count is .89.
b. Computed only for a 2x2 table
c. 2 cells (50.0%) have expected count less than 5. The minimum expected count is 2.50.
d. 1 cells (25.0%) have expected count less than 5. The minimum expected count is 2.81.
e. 2 cells (50.0%) have expected count less than 5. The minimum expected count is 2.07.

Crowding * Reversal

Chi-Square Tests

Sex	MajorGeo		Value	df	Asymp. Sig. (2-sided)	Exact Sig. (2-sided)	Exact Sig. (1-sided)
Female	English	Pearson Chi-Square	.[a]				
		N of Valid Cases	27				
	Macedonian	Pearson Chi-Square	6.462[b]	1	.011		
		Continuity Correction[c]	2.872	1	.090		
		Likelihood Ratio	6.034	1	.014		
		Fisher's Exact Test				.056	.056
		Linear-by-Linear Association	6.231	1	.013		
		N of Valid Cases	28				
Male	English	Pearson Chi-Square	.[a]				
		N of Valid Cases	47				
	Macedonian	Pearson Chi-Square	.[a]				
		N of Valid Cases	29				

a. No statistics are computed because Reversal is a constant.
b. 2 cells (50.0%) have expected count less than 5. The minimum expected count is .50.
c. Computed only for a 2x2 table

Crowding * Peg, Misshapen

Chi-Square Tests

Sex	MajorGeo		Value	df	Asymp. Sig. (2-sided)	Exact Sig. (2-sided)	Exact Sig. (1-sided)
Female	English	Pearson Chi-Square	.[a]				
		N of Valid Cases	27				
	Macedonian	Pearson Chi-Square	.[a]				
		N of Valid Cases	28				
Male	English	Pearson Chi-Square	.006[b]	1	.937		
		Continuity Correction[c]	.000	1	1.000		
		Likelihood Ratio	.006	1	.938		
		Fisher's Exact Test				1.000	.670
		Linear-by-Linear Association	.006	1	.938		
		N of Valid Cases	47				
	Macedonian	Pearson Chi-Square	.[a]				
		N of Valid Cases	29				

a. No statistics are computed because Peg, Misshapen is a constant.
b. 2 cells (50.0%) have expected count less than 5. The minimum expected count is .94.
c. Computed only for a 2x2 table

Crowding * Congenitally Absent Teeth

Chi-Square Tests

Sex	MajorGeo		Value	df	Asymp. Sig. (2-sided)	Exact Sig. (2-sided)	Exact Sig. (1-sided)
Female	English	Pearson Chi-Square	.270[a]	1	.603		
		Continuity Correction[b]	.000	1	1.000		
		Likelihood Ratio	.491	1	.484		
		Fisher's Exact Test				1.000	.786
		Linear-by-Linear Association	.260	1	.610		
		N of Valid Cases	27				
	Macedonian	Pearson Chi-Square	.[c]				
		N of Valid Cases	28				
Male	English	Pearson Chi-Square	3.344[d]	1	.067		
		Continuity Correction[b]	.403	1	.525		
		Likelihood Ratio	2.977	1	.084		
		Fisher's Exact Test				.234	.234
		Linear-by-Linear Association	3.273	1	.070		
		N of Valid Cases	47				
	Macedonian	Pearson Chi-Square	1.968[e]	1	.161		
		Continuity Correction[b]	.110	1	.740		
		Likelihood Ratio	2.198	1	.138		
		Fisher's Exact Test				.345	.345
		Linear-by-Linear Association	1.900	1	.168		
		N of Valid Cases	29				

a. 3 cells (75.0%) have expected count less than 5. The minimum expected count is .22.
b. Computed only for a 2x2 table
c. No statistics are computed because Congenitally Absent Teeth is a constant.
d. 2 cells (50.0%) have expected count less than 5. The minimum expected count is .23.
e. 2 cells (50.0%) have expected count less than 5. The minimum expected count is .34.

Rotation * Peg, Misshapen

Chi-Square Tests

Sex	MajorGeo		Value	df	Asymp. Sig. (2-sided)	Exact Sig. (2-sided)	Exact Sig. (1-sided)
Female	English	Pearson Chi-Square	.[a]				
		N of Valid Cases	27				
	Macedonian	Pearson Chi-Square	.[a]				
		N of Valid Cases	28				
Male	English	Pearson Chi-Square	.001[b]	1	.980		

			Continuity Correction[c]	.000	1	1.000		
			Likelihood Ratio	.001	1	.980		
			Fisher's Exact Test				1.000	.734
			Linear-by-Linear Association	.001	1	.980		
			N of Valid Cases	47				
		Macedonian	Pearson Chi-Square	.[a]				
			N of Valid Cases	29				

a. No statistics are computed because Peg, Misshapen is a constant.
b. 2 cells (50.0%) have expected count less than 5. The minimum expected count is 1.02.
c. Computed only for a 2x2 table

Rotation * Congenitally Absent Teeth

Chi-Square Tests

Sex	MajorGeo		Value	df	Asymp. Sig. (2-sided)	Exact Sig. (2-sided)	Exact Sig. (1-sided)
Female	English	Pearson Chi-Square	.430[a]	1	.512		
		Continuity Correction[b]	.000	1	1.000		
		Likelihood Ratio	.395	1	.530		
		Fisher's Exact Test				.513	.513
		Linear-by-Linear Association	.414	1	.520		
		N of Valid Cases	27				
	Macedonian	Pearson Chi-Square	.[c]				
		N of Valid Cases	28				
Male	English	Pearson Chi-Square	2.980[d]	1	.084		
		Continuity Correction[b]	.322	1	.571		
		Likelihood Ratio	2.795	1	.095		
		Fisher's Exact Test				.255	.255
		Linear-by-Linear Association	2.917	1	.088		
		N of Valid Cases	47				
	Macedonian	Pearson Chi-Square	.270[e]	1	.603		
		Continuity Correction[b]	.000	1	1.000		
		Likelihood Ratio	.473	1	.492		
		Fisher's Exact Test				1.000	.793
		Linear-by-Linear Association	.261	1	.610		
		N of Valid Cases	29				

a. 2 cells (50.0%) have expected count less than 5. The minimum expected count is .59.
b. Computed only for a 2x2 table
c. No statistics are computed because Congenitally Absent Teeth is a constant.
d. 2 cells (50.0%) have expected count less than 5. The minimum expected count is .26.
e. 2 cells (50.0%) have expected count less than 5. The minimum expected count is .21.

Reversal * Peg, Misshapen

Chi-Square Tests

Sex	MajorGeo		Value
Female	English	Pearson Chi-Square	.[a]
		N of Valid Cases	27
	Macedonian	Pearson Chi-Square	.[b]
		N of Valid Cases	28
Male	English	Pearson Chi-Square	.[c]
		N of Valid Cases	47
	Macedonian	Pearson Chi-Square	.[a]
		N of Valid Cases	29

a. No statistics are computed because Reversal and Peg, Misshapen are constants.
b. No statistics are computed because Peg, Misshapen is a constant.
c. No statistics are computed because Reversal is a constant.

Reversal * Congenitally Absent Teeth

Chi-Square Tests

Sex	MajorGeo		Value
Female	English	Pearson Chi-Square	.[a]
		N of Valid Cases	27
	Macedonian	Pearson Chi-Square	.[b]
		N of Valid Cases	28
Male	English	Pearson Chi-Square	.[a]
		N of Valid Cases	47
	Macedonian	Pearson Chi-Square	.[a]
		N of Valid Cases	29

a. No statistics are computed because Reversal is a constant.
b. No statistics are computed because Congenitally Absent Teeth is a constant.

Supplemental Teeth * M3 Congenitally Absent

Chi-Square Tests

Sex	MajorGeo		Value	df	Asymp. Sig. (2-sided)	Exact Sig. (2-sided)	Exact Sig. (1-sided)
Female	English	Pearson Chi-Square	.[a]				
		N of Valid Cases	27				
	Macedonian	Pearson Chi-Square	.[a]				
		N of Valid Cases	28				
Male	English	Pearson Chi-Square	.194[b]	1	.659		
		Continuity Correction[c]	.000	1	1.000		
		Likelihood Ratio	.364	1	.546		
		Fisher's Exact Test				1.000	.835
		Linear-by-Linear Association	.190	1	.663		
		N of Valid Cases	47				
	Macedonian	Pearson Chi-Square	.[a]				
		N of Valid Cases	29				

a. No statistics are computed because Supplemental Teeth is a constant.
b. 3 cells (75.0%) have expected count less than 5. The minimum expected count is .17.
c. Computed only for a 2x2 table

Supplemental Teeth * Ectopic, heterotopic, impaction

Chi-Square Tests

Sex	MajorGeo		Value	df	Asymp. Sig. (2-sided)	Exact Sig. (2-sided)	Exact Sig. (1-sided)
Female	English	Pearson Chi-Square	.[a]				
		N of Valid Cases	27				
	Macedonian	Pearson Chi-Square	.[a]				
		N of Valid Cases	28				
Male	English	Pearson Chi-Square	4.618[b]	1	.032		
		Continuity Correction[c]	.729	1	.393		
		Likelihood Ratio	2.544	1	.111		
		Fisher's Exact Test				.165	.165
		Linear-by-Linear Association	4.520	1	.034		
		N of Valid Cases	47				
	Macedonian	Pearson Chi-Square	.[a]				
		N of Valid Cases	29				

a. No statistics are computed because Supplemental Teeth is a constant.
b. 3 cells (75.0%) have expected count less than 5. The minimum expected count is .17.
c. Computed only for a 2x2 table

Supplemental Teeth * Crowding

Chi-Square Tests

Sex	MajorGeo		Value	df	Asymp. Sig. (2-sided)	Exact Sig. (2-sided)	Exact Sig. (1-sided)
Female	English	Pearson Chi-Square	.ᵃ				
		N of Valid Cases	27				
	Macedonian	Pearson Chi-Square	.ᵃ				
		N of Valid Cases	28				
Male	English	Pearson Chi-Square	.824ᵇ	1	.364		
		Continuity Correctionᶜ	.003	1	.957		
		Likelihood Ratio	.701	1	.403		
		Fisher's Exact Test				.417	.417
		Linear-by-Linear Association	.807	1	.369		
		N of Valid Cases	47				
	Macedonian	Pearson Chi-Square	.ᵃ				
		N of Valid Cases	29				

a. No statistics are computed because Supplemental Teeth is a constant.
b. 2 cells (50.0%) have expected count less than 5. The minimum expected count is .47.
c. Computed only for a 2x2 table

Supplemental Teeth * M3 Congenitally Absent

Chi-Square Tests

	Value	df	Asymp. Sig. (2-sided)	Exact Sig. (2-sided)	Exact Sig. (1-sided)
Pearson Chi-Square	.205ᵃ	1	.651		
Continuity Correctionᵇ	.000	1	1.000		
Likelihood Ratio	.387	1	.534		
Fisher's Exact Test				1.000	.825
Linear-by-Linear Association	.203	1	.652		
N of Valid Cases	131				

a. 2 cells (50.0%) have expected count less than 5. The minimum expected count is .18.
b. Computed only for a 2x2 table

Supplemental Teeth * Ectopic, heterotopic, impaction

Chi-Square Tests

	Value	df	Asymp. Sig. (2-sided)	Exact Sig. (2-sided)	Exact Sig. (1-sided)
Pearson Chi-Square	2.705ᵃ	1	.100		
Continuity Correctionᵇ	.310	1	.578		
Likelihood Ratio	1.735	1	.188		
Fisher's Exact Test				.230	.230
Linear-by-Linear Association	2.684	1	.101		
N of Valid Cases	131				

a. 2 cells (50.0%) have expected count less than 5. The minimum expected count is .24.
b. Computed only for a 2x2 table

Supplemental Teeth * Crowding

Chi-Square Tests

	Value	df	Asymp. Sig. (2-sided)	Exact Sig. (2-sided)	Exact Sig. (1-sided)
Pearson Chi-Square	.780ᵃ	1	.377		
Continuity Correctionᵇ	.002	1	.964		
Likelihood Ratio	.662	1	.416		
Fisher's Exact Test				.419	.419
Linear-by-Linear Association	.774	1	.379		
N of Valid Cases	131				

a. 2 cells (50.0%) have expected count less than 5. The minimum expected count is .47.
b. Computed only for a 2x2 table

Rotation * M3 Congenitally Absent

Chi-Square Tests

	Value	df	Asymp. Sig. (2-sided)	Exact Sig. (2-sided)	Exact Sig. (1-sided)
Pearson Chi-Square	.775[a]	1	.379		
Continuity Correction[b]	.293	1	.588		
Likelihood Ratio	.850	1	.357		
Fisher's Exact Test				.510	.306
Linear-by-Linear Association	.769	1	.380		
N of Valid Cases	131				

a. 1 cells (25.0%) have expected count less than 5. The minimum expected count is 3.30.
b. Computed only for a 2x2 table

Rotation * Ectopic, heterotopic, impaction

Chi-Square Tests

	Value	df	Asymp. Sig. (2-sided)	Exact Sig. (2-sided)	Exact Sig. (1-sided)
Pearson Chi-Square	.130[a]	1	.719		
Continuity Correction[b]	.004	1	.951		
Likelihood Ratio	.127	1	.722		
Fisher's Exact Test				.767	.462
Linear-by-Linear Association	.129	1	.720		
N of Valid Cases	131				

a. 1 cells (25.0%) have expected count less than 5. The minimum expected count is 4.40.
b. Computed only for a 2x2 table

Rotation * Crowding

Chi-Square Tests

	Value	df	Asymp. Sig. (2-sided)	Exact Sig. (2-sided)	Exact Sig. (1-sided)
Pearson Chi-Square	6.370[a]	1	.012		
Continuity Correction[b]	5.261	1	.022		
Likelihood Ratio	5.986	1	.014		
Fisher's Exact Test				.020	.013
Linear-by-Linear Association	6.321	1	.012		
N of Valid Cases	131				

a. 0 cells (.0%) have expected count less than 5. The minimum expected count is 8.52.
b. Computed only for a 2x2 table

Reversal * M3 Congenitally Absent

Chi-Square Tests

	Value	df	Asymp. Sig. (2-sided)	Exact Sig. (2-sided)	Exact Sig. (1-sided)
Pearson Chi-Square	.205[a]	1	.651		
Continuity Correction[b]	.000	1	1.000		
Likelihood Ratio	.387	1	.534		
Fisher's Exact Test				1.000	.825
Linear-by-Linear Association	.203	1	.652		
N of Valid Cases	131				

a. 2 cells (50.0%) have expected count less than 5. The minimum expected count is .18.
b. Computed only for a 2x2 table

Reversal * Ectopic, heterotopic, impaction

Chi-Square Tests

	Value	df	Asymp. Sig. (2-sided)	Exact Sig. (2-sided)	Exact Sig. (1-sided)
Pearson Chi-Square	.283[a]	1	.595		
Continuity Correction[b]	.000	1	1.000		
Likelihood Ratio	.525	1	.469		
Fisher's Exact Test				1.000	.770
Linear-by-Linear Association	.280	1	.596		
N of Valid Cases	131				

a. 2 cells (50.0%) have expected count less than 5. The minimum expected count is .24.
b. Computed only for a 2x2 table

Reversal * Crowding

Chi-Square Tests

	Value	df	Asymp. Sig. (2-sided)	Exact Sig. (2-sided)	Exact Sig. (1-sided)
Pearson Chi-Square	6.552[a]	1	.010		
Continuity Correction[b]	2.963	1	.085		
Likelihood Ratio	5.866	1	.015		
Fisher's Exact Test				.055	.055
Linear-by-Linear Association	6.502	1	.011		
N of Valid Cases	131				

a. 2 cells (50.0%) have expected count less than 5. The minimum expected count is .47.
b. Computed only for a 2x2 table

Supplemental Teeth * Rotation

Chi-Square Tests

	Value	df	Asymp. Sig. (2-sided)	Exact Sig. (2-sided)	Exact Sig. (1-sided)
Pearson Chi-Square	.517[a]	1	.472		
Continuity Correction[b]	.000	1	1.000		
Likelihood Ratio	.461	1	.497		
Fisher's Exact Test				.476	.476
Linear-by-Linear Association	.513	1	.474		
N of Valid Cases	131				

a. 2 cells (50.0%) have expected count less than 5. The minimum expected count is .55.
b. Computed only for a 2x2 table

Appendix B

Section 2. Craniometric Means and Variances.

Part 1. General Craniometrics.

Table 1. Craniometric landmarks, all skulls, Macedonian versus English.

	MajorGeo	N	Mean	Std. Deviation	Std. Error Mean
Max Cranial Length	English	61	181.26	8.236	1.054
	Macedonian	56	177.64	8.176	1.093
Max Cranial Breadth	English	64	144.98	8.764	1.096
	Macedonian	56	143.05	5.538	.740
Cranial Height	English	50	130.50	8.979	1.270
	Macedonian	33	130.97	7.573	1.318
Facial Height n-gn	English	39	113.28	8.693	1.392
	Macedonian	37	110.32	8.489	1.396
Facial Width zy-zy	English	44	130.34	7.104	1.071
	Macedonian	45	129.76	6.634	.989
FMT Width	English	66	105.47	4.330	.533
	Macedonian	39	102.74	8.071	1.292
Upper Facial Height n-pr	English	54	66.19	4.798	.653
	Macedonian	47	67.40	5.511	.804
Maxilloalveolar Length pr-alv	English	44	51.59	3.842	.579
	Macedonian	25	52.04	3.802	.760
Maxilloalveolar Breadth ect-ect	English	64	58.97	4.468	.559
	Macedonian	36	58.97	6.797	1.133
Palatal Length ol-sta	English	70	49.33	3.937	.471
	Macedonian	36	47.75	4.423	.737
Palatal Breadth enm-enm	English	67	39.10	3.701	.452
	Macedonian	36	41.67	6.090	1.015
Bicondylar Breadth cdl-cdl	English	52	119.87	7.319	1.015
	Macedonian	32	123.72	6.764	1.196
Bigonial Breadth go-go	English	61	99.64	8.905	1.140
	Macedonian	48	101.52	7.850	1.133
Height of Ascending Ramus Right go-cdl	English	62	68.45	4.824	.613
	Macedonian	34	68.15	5.560	.954
Min Breadth of Ascending Ramus Right	English	64	31.00	2.862	.358
	Macedonian	38	31.16	3.009	.488
Height at Mandibular Symphysis gn-idi	English	63	29.81	3.330	.420
	Macedonian	38	28.58	4.847	.786

Table 2. Craniometric landmarks, normal skulls, Macedonian versus English

	MajorGeo	N	Mean	Std. Deviation	Std. Error Mean
Max Cranial Length	English	28	182.93	8.326	1.574
	Macedonian	22	178.45	7.732	1.648
Max Cranial Breadth	English	29	145.97	5.109	.949
	Macedonian	23	142.70	4.487	.936
Cranial Height	English	23	131.43	6.788	1.415
	Macedonian	12	130.75	8.281	2.390
Facial Height n-gn	English	14	119.14	7.482	2.000
	Macedonian	10	113.80	4.237	1.340
Facial Width zy-zy	English	20	131.70	7.498	1.677
	Macedonian	16	130.13	4.395	1.099
FMT Width	English	28	106.75	4.300	.813
	Macedonian	16	101.63	10.557	2.639
Upper Facial Height enm-enm	English	23	67.52	5.648	1.178
	Macedonian	17	66.82	4.953	1.201
Maxilloalveolar Length pr-alv	English	22	51.73	4.651	.992
	Macedonian	10	53.40	3.098	.980
Maxilloalveolar Breadth ect-ect	English	29	58.69	5.613	1.042
	Macedonian	12	58.67	7.062	2.039
Palatal Length ol-sta	English	32	50.66	3.981	.704
	Macedonian	11	47.27	5.711	1.722
Palatal Breadth enm-enm	English	31	39.03	4.151	.746
	Macedonian	12	40.67	4.793	1.384
Bicondylar Breadth cdl-cdl	English	18	123.39	7.171	1.690
	Macedonian	9	125.78	6.778	2.259
Bigonial Breadth go-go	English	23	103.22	7.592	1.583
	Macedonian	15	101.60	6.412	1.656
Height of Ascending Ramus Right go-cdl	English	24	70.42	4.925	1.005
	Macedonian	11	69.18	4.167	1.256
Min Breadth of Ascending Ramus Right	English	25	31.44	2.740	.548
	Macedonian	12	30.92	2.275	.657
Height at Mandibular Symphysis gn-idi	English	24	31.29	4.005	.818
	Macedonian	14	28.21	3.534	.944

Table 3. Macedonian v. Englsih craniometrics, all skulls by sex.

Sex		MajorGeo	N	Mean	Std. Deviation	Std. Error Mean
Female	Max Cranial Length	English	25	179.24	9.098	1.820
		Macedonian	28	173.14	6.604	1.248
	Max Cranial Breadth	English	25	142.04	6.693	1.339
		Macedonian	28	140.71	3.857	.729
	Cranial Height	English	19	128.00	11.508	2.640
		Macedonian	16	126.00	6.450	1.612
	Facial Height n-gn	English	12	106.92	6.921	1.998
		Macedonian	19	107.42	8.903	2.042
	Facial Width zy-zy	English	18	126.67	7.300	1.721
		Macedonian	24	125.83	4.896	.999
	FMT Width	English	26	104.54	4.022	.789
		Macedonian	22	101.55	5.501	1.173
	Upper Facial Height n-pr	English	19	64.05	4.075	.935
		Macedonian	26	65.00	5.463	1.071
	Maxilloalveolar Length pr-alv	English	18	49.39	3.363	.793
		Macedonian	11	50.91	4.036	1.217
	Maxilloalveolar Breadth ect-ect	English	24	57.13	4.712	.962
		Macedonian	19	57.00	7.303	1.675
	Palatal Length ol-sta	English	26	48.08	4.251	.834
		Macedonian	19	47.00	3.844	.882
	Palatal Breadth enm-enm	English	24	38.38	4.020	.821
		Macedonian	19	40.53	5.253	1.205
	Bicondylar Breadth cdl-cdl	English	19	116.42	8.044	1.845
		Macedonian	16	121.25	4.509	1.127
	Bigonial Breadth go-go	English	22	94.41	6.580	1.403
		Macedonian	23	96.57	6.687	1.394
	Height of Ascending Ramus Right go-cdl	English	21	66.86	3.772	.823
		Macedonian	17	65.53	5.100	1.237
	Min Breadth of Ascending Ramus Right	English	22	29.68	2.338	.498
		Macedonian	19	30.37	2.753	.632
	Height at Mandibular Symphysis gn-idi	English	22	28.41	2.631	.561
		Macedonian	18	26.39	4.616	1.088
Male	Max Cranial Length	English	36	182.67	7.387	1.231
		Macedonian	28	182.14	7.111	1.344
	Max Cranial Breadth	English	39	146.87	9.471	1.517
		Macedonian	28	145.39	6.021	1.138
	Cranial Height	English	31	132.03	6.770	1.216
		Macedonian	17	135.65	5.267	1.277
	Facial Height n-gn	English	27	116.11	7.949	1.530
		Macedonian	18	113.39	7.022	1.655
	Facial Width zy-zy	English	26	132.88	5.840	1.145
		Macedonian	21	134.24	5.449	1.189
	FMT Width	English	40	106.08	4.463	.706
		Macedonian	17	104.29	10.510	2.549
	Upper Facial Height n-pr	English	35	67.34	4.814	.814
		Macedonian	21	70.38	3.968	.866
	Maxilloalveolar Length pr-alv	English	26	53.12	3.433	.673
		Macedonian	14	52.93	3.496	.934
	Maxilloalveolar Breadth ect-ect	English	40	60.08	3.977	.629
		Macedonian	17	61.18	5.593	1.356
	Palatal Length ol-sta	English	44	50.07	3.585	.541
		Macedonian	17	48.59	4.976	1.207
	Palatal Breadth enm-enm	English	43	39.51	3.494	.533
		Macedonian	17	42.94	6.842	1.659
	Bicondylar Breadth cdl-cdl	English	33	121.85	6.155	1.071
		Macedonian	16	126.19	7.825	1.956
	Bigonial Breadth go-go	English	39	102.59	8.747	1.401
		Macedonian	25	106.08	5.873	1.175
	Height of Ascending Ramus Right go-cdl	English	41	69.27	5.133	.802
		Macedonian	17	70.76	4.816	1.168
	Min Breadth of Ascending Ramus Right	English	42	31.69	2.892	.446
		Macedonian	19	31.95	3.118	.715
	Height at Mandibular Symphysis gn-idi	English	41	30.56	3.450	.539
		Macedonian	20	30.55	4.249	.950

Table 4. Macedonian v. English Indices and Ratios, all skulls.

	MajorGeo	N	Mean	Std. Deviation	Std. Error Mean
Cranial Index	English	59	79.999	5.4007	.7031
	Macedonian	55	80.760	4.0144	.5413
Cranial Module	English	46	152.2464	6.34110	.93494
	Macedonian	32	149.6042	5.92815	1.04796
Cranial length-height Index	English	47	72.3177	4.61867	.67370
	Macedonian	33	74.1595	3.11882	.54292
Cranial breadth-height Index	English	48	89.9942	6.56627	.94776
	Macedonian	32	91.8432	4.25828	.75276
Total Facial Index	English	31	85.8882	5.29110	.95031
	Macedonian	36	84.6010	6.86265	1.14378
Upper Facial Index	English	40	51.6479	2.76939	.43788
	Macedonian	42	51.9853	3.18502	.49146
Maxilloalveolar Index	English	42	114.5840	10.83095	1.67125
	Macedonian	23	115.6842	12.18048	2.53981
Palatal Index	English	66	79.6506	8.93554	1.09989
	Macedonian	35	88.3347	16.95302	2.86558
Palatal/max ratio	English	41	.7126	.07565	.01181
	Macedonian	22	.7715	.18103	.03860
TFHFMT	English	37	107.3362	8.04718	1.32295
	Macedonian	28	107.9553	15.48025	2.92549
UFHFMT	English	52	63.2273	4.41083	.61167
	Macedonian	35	64.7828	5.00687	.84632
MAXBCDL	English	46	.4988	.04036	.00595
	Macedonian	19	.4840	.06236	.01431
cdlgo	English	52	.8328	.05356	.00743
	Macedonian	32	.8279	.06505	.01150
ZYGFMT	English	44	.8108	.04228	.00637
	Macedonian	33	.8099	.03879	.00675
UHTH	English	39	.5902	.03636	.00582
	Macedonian	35	.6112	.03436	.00581
FB	English	32	.9123	.04126	.00729
	Macedonian	28	.9443	.03447	.00651
FB2	English	46	.8845	.05201	.00767
	Macedonian	22	.8412	.09783	.02086
UFIMAI	English	31	.4536	.03658	.00657
	Macedonian	20	.4554	.06070	.01357

Table 5. Macedonian v. English indices and ratios, by sex

Sex		MajorGeo	N	Mean	Std. Deviation	Std. Error Mean
Female	Cranial Index	English	24	79.181	4.1951	.8563
		Macedonian	28	81.347	2.8825	.5447
	Cranial Module	English	18	149.5926	6.50546	1.53335
		Macedonian	16	145.1667	3.58598	.89650
	Cranial length-height Index	English	19	71.6201	6.10627	1.40088
		Macedonian	16	73.9241	3.47208	.86802
	Cranial breadth-height Index	English	18	89.8003	7.21046	1.69952
		Macedonian	16	90.6952	5.11583	1.27896
	Total Facial Index	English	11	84.2486	5.47463	1.65066
		Macedonian	19	85.0880	8.18120	1.87690
	Upper Facial Index	English	16	51.2864	2.22923	.55731
		Macedonian	23	51.9078	3.36308	.70125
	Maxilloalveolar Index	English	18	115.6201	11.04014	2.60219
		Macedonian	10	116.6785	11.97044	3.78539
	Palatal Index	English	24	80.5417	9.45814	1.93063
		Macedonian	19	86.7252	13.33151	3.05846
	Palatal/max ratio	English	17	.7150	.09295	.02254
		Macedonian	10	.7181	.07913	.02502
	TFHFMT	English	12	103.4080	8.08071	2.33270
		Macedonian	15	105.9793	8.56506	2.21149
	UFHFMT	English	19	61.8080	4.25081	.97520
		Macedonian	21	63.8832	5.25566	1.14688
	MAXBCDL	English	17	.5111	.03965	.00962
		Macedonian	11	.4827	.06762	.02039
	cdlgo	English	19	.8087	.04924	.01130
		Macedonian	16	.8050	.05132	.01283
	ZYGFMT	English	18	.8276	.04727	.01114
		Macedonian	18	.8164	.04038	.00952
	UHTH	English	12	.6003	.03975	.01148
		Macedonian	19	.6024	.04150	.00952
	FB	English	14	.9017	.04998	.01336
		Macedonian	16	.9581	.02566	.00641
	FB2	English	18	.9016	.05087	.01199
		Macedonian	12	.8537	.05118	.01477

107

Male	UFIMAI	English	14	.4391	.02469	.00660
		Macedonian	9	.4452	.04491	.01497
	Cranial Index	English	35	80.561	6.0873	1.0289
		Macedonian	27	80.151	4.9078	.9445
	Cranial Module	English	28	153.9524	5.71455	1.07995
		Macedonian	16	154.0417	4.21439	1.05360
	Cranial length-height Index	English	28	72.7910	3.30320	.62425
		Macedonian	17	74.3811	2.83630	.68790
	Cranial breadth-height Index	English	30	90.1106	6.27398	1.14547
		Macedonian	16	92.9912	2.91400	.72850
	Total Facial Index	English	20	86.7899	5.10068	1.14055
		Macedonian	17	84.0566	5.20839	1.26322
	Upper Facial Index	English	24	51.8889	3.10039	.63286
		Macedonian	19	52.0792	3.04399	.69834
	Maxilloalveolar Index	English	24	113.8069	10.84242	2.21320
		Macedonian	13	114.9194	12.77007	3.54178
	Palatal Index	English	42	79.1415	8.69876	1.34225
		Macedonian	16	90.2459	20.76051	5.19013
	Palatal/max ratio	English	24	.7109	.06273	.01281
		Macedonian	12	.8159	.22957	.06627
	TFHFMT	English	25	109.2217	7.46919	1.49384
		Macedonian	13	110.2352	21.04963	5.83812
	UFHFMT	English	33	64.0445	4.35410	.75795
		Macedonian	14	66.1322	4.44980	1.18926
	MAXBCDL	English	29	.4917	.03969	.00737
		Macedonian	8	.4856	.05883	.02080
	cdlgo	English	33	.8467	.05162	.00899
		Macedonian	16	.8509	.07062	.01766
	ZYGFMT	English	26	.7992	.03481	.00683
		Macedonian	15	.8020	.03656	.00944
	UHTH	English	27	.5858	.03460	.00666
		Macedonian	16	.6216	.01990	.00498
	FB	English	18	.9206	.03208	.00756
		Macedonian	12	.9260	.03707	.01070
	FB2	English	28	.8736	.05061	.00957
		Macedonian	10	.8260	.13663	.04321
	UFIMAI	English	17	.4654	.04101	.00995
		Macedonian	11	.4637	.07224	.02178

Table 6. Macedonian v. English indices and ratios, normal skulls.

Sex		MajorGeo	N	Mean	Std. Deviation	Std. Error Mean
Female	Max Cranial Length	English	10	181.20	6.250	1.977
		Macedonian	12	175.42	6.762	1.952
	Max Cranial Breadth	English	9	143.22	3.073	1.024
		Macedonian	12	141.50	3.680	1.062
	Cranial Height	English	8	126.00	5.477	1.936
		Macedonian	6	125.17	8.208	3.351
	Facial Height n-gn	English	2	109.00	9.899	7.000
		Macedonian	4	111.25	2.500	1.250
	Facial Width zy-zy	English	8	127.50	9.304	3.290
		Macedonian	8	127.38	2.387	.844
	FMT Width	English	10	105.90	3.446	1.090
		Macedonian	10	103.40	5.582	1.765
	Upper Facial Height enm-enm	English	7	64.14	3.532	1.335
		Macedonian	10	65.20	5.653	1.788
	Maxilloalveolar Length pr-alv	English	7	48.57	4.577	1.730
		Macedonian	4	52.50	4.359	2.179
	Maxilloalveolar Breadth ect-ect	English	10	55.10	6.208	1.963
		Macedonian	6	58.33	7.090	2.894
	Palatal Length ol-sta	English	11	49.18	4.378	1.320
		Macedonian	6	47.67	4.502	1.838
	Palatal Breadth enm-enm	English	11	38.18	5.135	1.548
		Macedonian	6	40.00	4.690	1.915
	Bicondylar Breadth cdl-cdl	English	5	120.80	10.109	4.521
		Macedonian	5	124.40	2.510	1.122
	Bigonial Breadth go-go	English	7	98.86	7.946	3.003
		Macedonian	7	98.29	6.130	2.317
	Height of Ascending Ramus Right go-cdl	English	7	68.43	4.504	1.702
		Macedonian	5	67.00	3.674	1.643
	Min Breadth of Ascending Ramus Right	English	7	29.86	2.478	.937
		Macedonian	6	30.67	3.011	1.229
	Height at Mandibular Symphysis gn-idi	English	7	29.86	3.485	1.317
		Macedonian	7	27.57	2.573	.972
Male	Max Cranial Length	English	18	183.89	9.311	2.195
		Macedonian	10	182.10	7.520	2.378
	Max Cranial Breadth	English	20	147.20	5.415	1.211
		Macedonian	11	144.00	5.079	1.531
	Cranial Height	English	15	134.33	5.615	1.450
		Macedonian	6	136.33	2.944	1.202
	Facial Height n-gn	English	12	120.83	5.952	1.718
		Macedonian	6	115.50	4.461	1.821
	Facial Width zy-zy	English	12	134.50	4.543	1.311
		Macedonian	8	132.88	4.291	1.517
	FMT Width	English	18	107.22	4.735	1.116
		Macedonian	6	98.67	16.170	6.601
	Upper Facial Height enm-enm	English	16	69.00	5.842	1.461
		Macedonian	7	69.14	2.610	.986
	Maxilloalveolar Length pr-alv	English	15	53.20	4.021	1.038
		Macedonian	6	54.00	2.191	.894
	Maxilloalveolar Breadth ect-ect	English	19	60.58	4.337	.995
		Macedonian	6	59.00	7.694	3.141
	Palatal Length ol-sta	English	21	51.43	3.627	.792
		Macedonian	5	46.80	7.463	3.338
	Palatal Breadth enm-enm	English	20	39.50	3.561	.796
		Macedonian	6	41.33	5.241	2.140
	Bicondylar Breadth cdl-cdl	English	13	124.38	5.910	1.639
		Macedonian	4	127.50	10.344	5.172
	Bigonial Breadth go-go	English	16	105.13	6.820	1.705
		Macedonian	8	104.50	5.425	1.918
	Height of Ascending Ramus Right go-cdl	English	17	71.24	4.982	1.208
		Macedonian	6	71.00	3.899	1.592
	Min Breadth of Ascending Ramus Right	English	18	32.06	2.645	.623
		Macedonian	6	31.17	1.472	.601
	Height at Mandibular Symphysis gn-idi	English	17	31.88	4.152	1.007
		Macedonian	7	28.86	4.413	1.668

Part 2. Craniometrics and Dental anomalies

Table 7. Means, Craniometrics and Rotations, Reversals.

			Female				Male				All			
			Rotation		Reversal		Rotation		Reversal		Rotation		Reversal	
			Absent Mean	Present Mean	Absent Mean	Present Mean	Absent Mean	Present Mean	Absent Mean	Present Mean	Absent Mean	Present Mean	Absent Mean	Present Mean
MajorGeo	English	Max Cranial Length	181.00	174.71	179.24	.	184.04	179.10	182.67	.	182.80	177.29	181.26	.
		Max Cranial Breadth	141.59	143.00	142.04	.	146.96	146.64	146.87	.	144.93	145.11	144.98	.
		Cranial Height	129.38	125.00	128.00	.	133.67	128.60	132.03	.	132.03	127.25	130.50	.
		Facial Height n-gn	108.00	106.14	106.92	.	117.55	112.00	116.11	.	115.64	109.07	113.28	.
		Facial Width zy-zy	127.20	126.00	126.67	.	133.61	131.25	132.88	.	131.32	128.63	130.34	.
		FMT Width	105.33	102.75	104.54	.	106.62	104.64	106.08	.	106.13	103.84	105.47	.
		Upper Facial Height	63.45	64.88	64.05	.	68.08	65.50	67.34	.	66.67	65.22	66.19	.
		MAXL	49.91	48.57	49.39	.	53.05	53.33	53.12	.	51.94	50.77	51.59	.
		MAXB	56.44	58.50	57.13	.	59.86	60.64	60.08	.	58.64	59.74	58.97	.
		Palatal Length	49.00	46.00	48.08	.	50.35	49.10	50.07	.	49.88	47.72	49.33	.
		Palatal Breadth	38.18	38.86	38.38	.	39.59	39.27	39.51	.	39.10	39.11	39.10	.
		Bicondylar Breadth	119.91	111.63	116.42	.	122.75	119.44	121.85	.	121.86	115.76	119.87	.
		Bigonial Breadth	96.00	91.63	94.41	.	103.52	99.90	102.59	.	101.07	96.22	99.64	.
		HAR	67.54	65.75	66.86	.	70.00	67.27	69.27	.	69.26	66.63	68.45	.
		MBAR	30.43	28.38	29.68	.	32.16	30.36	31.69	.	31.62	29.53	31.00	.
		HMS	29.07	27.25	28.41	.	31.23	28.73	30.56	.	30.55	28.11	29.81	.
	Macedonian	Max Cranial Length	173.72	172.10	173.62	167.00	181.86	183.17	182.14	.	178.20	176.25	178.04	167.00
		Max Cranial Breadth	140.50	141.10	140.88	138.50	146.05	143.00	145.39	.	143.55	141.81	143.22	138.50
		Cranial Height	126.55	124.80	125.57	129.00	136.00	134.00	135.65	.	131.84	128.25	131.10	129.00
		Facial Height n-gn	107.67	107.20	106.65	114.00	114.23	111.20	113.39	.	111.55	108.53	110.11	114.00
		Facial Width zy-zy	126.79	124.50	125.59	128.50	135.00	131.80	134.24	.	131.17	126.93	129.81	128.50
		FMT Width	101.88	100.67	101.50	102.00	104.08	105.00	104.29	.	102.86	102.40	102.78	102.00
		Upper Facial Height	64.75	65.40	64.92	66.00	70.56	69.80	70.38	.	67.66	66.87	67.47	66.00
		MAXL	51.56	48.00	51.11	50.00	52.91	53.00	52.93	.	52.30	51.00	52.22	50.00
		MAXB	56.75	57.43	56.53	61.00	61.86	58.00	61.18	.	59.50	57.60	58.85	61.00
		Palatal Length	47.75	45.71	46.88	48.00	48.15	50.00	48.59	.	47.96	47.27	47.74	48.00
		Palatal Breadth	41.17	39.43	40.53	40.50	42.93	43.00	42.94	.	42.12	40.50	41.74	40.50
		Bicondylar Breadth	122.89	119.14	121.14	122.00	127.67	121.75	126.19	.	125.62	120.09	123.83	122.00
		Bigonial Breadth	95.46	98.00	96.95	92.50	105.75	107.40	106.08	.	101.70	101.13	101.91	92.50
		HAR	67.20	63.14	65.07	69.00	70.93	70.00	70.76	.	69.38	65.20	68.09	69.00
		MBAR	30.50	30.14	30.29	31.00	32.25	30.33	31.95	.	31.50	30.20	31.17	31.00
		HMS	27.08	25.00	26.18	30.00	30.29	32.00	30.55	.	28.97	27.33	28.54	30.00
	All	Max Cranial Length	177.36	173.18	176.37	167.00	183.04	180.63	182.44	.	180.61	176.79	179.75	167.00
		Max Cranial Breadth	141.03	141.94	141.45	138.50	146.56	145.35	146.25	.	144.28	143.60	144.18	138.50
		Cranial Height	128.08	124.91	126.97	129.00	134.60	129.85	133.31	.	131.95	127.58	130.73	129.00
		Facial Height n-gn	107.79	106.76	106.76	114.00	116.24	111.67	115.02	.	113.72	108.79	111.78	114.00
		Facial Width zy-zy	126.96	125.17	126.08	128.50	134.26	131.46	133.49	.	131.24	127.81	130.08	128.50
		FMT Width	103.71	101.86	103.22	102.00	105.83	104.73	105.54	.	104.88	103.34	104.50	102.00
		Upper Facial Height	64.22	65.17	64.53	66.00	69.05	66.93	68.48	.	67.13	65.97	66.77	66.00
		MAXL	50.65	48.44	49.96	50.00	53.00	53.22	53.05	.	52.08	50.83	51.81	50.00
		MAXB	56.57	58.00	56.88	61.00	60.51	60.07	60.40	.	58.96	59.00	58.93	61.00
		Palatal Length	48.50	45.87	47.60	48.00	49.74	49.36	49.66	.	49.26	47.55	48.81	48.00
		Palatal Breadth	39.41	39.14	39.27	40.50	40.67	40.07	40.48	.	40.15	39.61	39.99	40.50
		Bicondylar Breadth	121.25	115.13	118.42	122.00	124.39	120.15	123.27	.	123.27	117.46	121.32	122.00
		Bigonial Breadth	95.74	95.17	95.65	92.50	104.43	102.40	103.95	.	101.34	98.45	100.62	92.50
		HAR	67.39	64.53	66.11	69.00	70.30	67.86	69.71	.	69.30	66.14	68.33	69.00
		MBAR	30.46	29.20	29.95	31.00	32.19	30.36	31.77	.	31.58	29.76	31.06	31.00
		HMS	28.15	26.29	27.44	30.00	30.89	29.43	30.56	.	29.92	27.86	29.34	30.00

Table 8. Means, craniometrics and supplemental (supernumerary) teeth and misshapen teeth.

			Female				Male				All			
			Supplemental Teeth		Peg, Misshapen		Supplemental Teeth		Peg, Misshapen		Supplemental Teeth		Peg, Misshapen	
			Absent Mean	Present Mean	Absent Mean	Present Mean	Absent Mean	Present Mean	Absent Mean	Present Mean	Absent Mean	Present Mean	Absent Mean	Present Mean
MajorGeo	English	Max Cranial Length	179.24	.	179.24	.	182.68	182.50	182.27	187.00	181.22	182.50	180.97	187.00
		Max Cranial Breadth	142.04	.	142.04	.	147.46	136.00	146.42	152.33	145.27	136.00	144.62	152.33
		Cranial Height	128.00	.	128.00	.	132.03	.	131.56	135.25	130.50	.	130.09	135.25
		Facial Height n-gn	106.92	.	106.92	.	116.50	106.00	115.96	117.00	113.47	106.00	112.86	117.00
		Facial Width zy-zy	126.67	.	126.67	.	132.80	135.00	132.88	133.00	130.23	135.00	130.21	133.00
		FMT Width	104.54	.	104.54	.	106.18	104.00	106.32	103.00	105.52	104.00	105.59	103.00
		Upper Facial Height	64.05	.	64.05	.	67.52	64.50	67.48	66.25	66.25	64.50	66.18	66.25
		MAXL	49.39	.	49.39	.	53.12	53.00	53.24	50.00	51.56	53.00	51.63	50.00
		MAXB	57.13	.	57.13	.	59.97	62.00	60.08	60.00	58.87	62.00	58.94	60.00
		Palatal Length	48.08	.	48.08	.	50.07	50.00	50.18	49.00	49.31	50.00	49.35	49.00
		Palatal Breadth	38.38	.	38.38	.	39.49	40.00	39.38	40.75	39.08	40.00	39.00	40.75
		Bicondylar Breadth	116.42	.	116.42	.	121.97	118.00	122.20	118.33	119.90	118.00	119.96	118.33
		Bigonial Breadth	94.41	.	94.41	.	103.30	89.50	102.50	103.67	99.98	89.50	99.43	103.67
		HAR	66.86	.	66.86	.	69.51	64.50	69.05	71.25	68.58	64.50	68.26	71.25
		MBAR	29.68	.	29.68	.	31.68	32.00	31.74	31.25	30.97	32.00	30.91	31.25
		HMS	28.41	.	28.41	.	30.69	28.00	30.57	30.50	29.87	28.00	29.76	30.50
	Macedonian	Max Cranial Length	173.14	.	173.14	.	182.14	.	182.14	.	177.64	.	177.64	.
		Max Cranial Breadth	140.71	.	140.71	.	145.39	.	145.39	.	143.05	.	143.05	.
		Cranial Height	126.00	.	126.00	.	135.65	.	135.65	.	130.97	.	130.97	.
		Facial Height n-gn	107.42	.	107.42	.	113.39	.	113.39	.	110.32	.	110.32	.
		Facial Width	125.83	.	125.83	.	134.24	.	134.24	.	129.76	.	129.76	.
		FMT Width	101.55	.	101.55	.	104.29	.	104.29	.	102.74	.	102.74	.
		UFH	65.00	.	65.00	.	70.38	.	70.38	.	67.40	.	67.40	.
		MAXL	50.91	.	50.91	.	52.93	.	52.93	.	52.04	.	52.04	.
		MAXB	57.00	.	57.00	.	61.18	.	61.18	.	58.97	.	58.97	.
		Palatal Length	47.00	.	47.00	.	48.59	.	48.59	.	47.75	.	47.75	.
		Palatal Breadth	40.53	.	40.53	.	42.94	.	42.94	.	41.67	.	41.67	.
		Bicondylar Breadth	121.25	.	121.25	.	126.19	.	126.19	.	123.72	.	123.72	.
		Bigonial Breadth	96.57	.	96.57	.	106.08	.	106.08	.	101.52	.	101.52	.
		HAR	65.53	.	65.53	.	70.76	.	70.76	.	68.15	.	68.15	.
		MBAR	30.37	.	30.37	.	31.95	.	31.95	.	31.16	.	31.16	.
		HMS	26.39	.	26.39	.	30.55	.	30.55	.	28.58	.	28.58	.
	All	Max Cranial Length	176.02	.	176.02	.	182.44	182.50	182.21	187.00	179.48	182.50	179.33	187.00
		Max Cranial Breadth	141.34	.	141.34	.	146.57	136.00	145.97	152.33	144.22	136.00	143.87	152.33
		Cranial Height	127.09	.	127.09	.	133.31	.	133.14	135.25	130.69	.	130.46	135.25
		Facial Height n-gn	107.23	.	107.23	.	115.23	106.00	114.83	117.00	111.92	106.00	111.56	117.00
		Facial Width zy-zy	126.19	.	126.19	.	133.46	135.00	133.51	133.00	129.99	135.00	129.98	133.00
		FMT Width	103.17	.	103.17	.	105.60	104.00	105.69	103.00	104.47	104.00	104.50	103.00
		Upper Facial Height	64.60	.	64.60	.	68.63	64.50	68.65	66.25	66.80	64.50	66.77	66.25
		MAXL	49.97	.	49.97	.	53.05	53.00	53.13	50.00	51.74	53.00	51.78	50.00
		MAXB	57.07	.	57.07	.	60.35	62.00	60.42	60.00	58.91	62.00	58.95	60.00
		Palatal Length	47.62	.	47.62	.	49.64	50.00	49.70	49.00	48.77	50.00	48.78	49.00
		Palatal Breadth	39.33	.	39.33	.	40.50	40.00	40.46	40.75	40.00	40.00	39.97	40.75
		Bicondylar Breadth	118.63	.	118.63	.	123.38	118.00	123.59	118.33	121.37	118.00	121.44	118.33
		Bigonial Breadth	95.51	.	95.51	.	104.42	89.50	103.97	103.67	100.67	89.50	100.38	103.67
		HAR	66.26	.	66.26	.	69.89	64.50	69.59	71.25	68.43	64.50	68.22	71.25
		MBAR	30.00	.	30.00	.	31.76	32.00	31.81	31.25	31.04	32.00	31.05	31.25
		HMS	27.50	.	27.50	.	30.64	28.00	30.56	30.50	29.37	28.00	29.30	30.50

Table 9. Means, congenitally missing teeth and missing M3.

			Female				Male				All			
			Congenitally Absent Teeth		M3 Congenitally Absent		Congenitally Absent Teeth		M3 Congenitally Absent		Congenitally Absent Teeth		M3 Congenitally Absent	
			Absent Mean	Present Mean	Absent Mean	Present Mean	Absent Mean	Present Mean	Absent Mean	Present Mean	Absent Mean	Present Mean	Absent Mean	Present Mean
MajorGeo	English	Max Cranial Length	179.70	174.00	178.77	182.67	182.83	177.00	182.65	183.00	181.59	175.00	181.13	182.80
		Max Cranial Breadth	142.39	138.00	142.77	136.67	147.42	126.00	146.26	152.25	145.52	134.00	144.91	145.57
		Cranial Height	128.41	124.50	128.50	119.00	132.03	.	132.14	131.00	130.75	124.50	130.72	128.00
		Facial Height n-gn	107.36	102.00	106.92	.	116.11	.	117.12	103.50	113.58	102.00	113.81	103.50
		Facial Width zy-zy	126.88	123.00	126.67	.	132.88	.	133.39	129.00	130.51	123.00	130.44	129.00
		FMT Width	104.71	102.50	104.35	106.00	106.28	98.00	106.08	106.00	105.68	101.00	105.41	106.00
		Upper Facial Height	63.94	65.00	64.05	.	67.38	66.00	67.72	63.33	66.24	65.33	66.35	63.33
		MAXL	49.29	51.00	49.24	52.00	53.12	.	53.09	53.33	51.60	51.00	51.45	53.00
		MAXB	57.05	58.00	57.22	55.00	60.03	62.00	60.33	57.75	58.95	59.33	59.12	57.20
		Palatal Length	48.08	48.00	47.75	52.00	50.07	50.00	50.15	49.25	49.36	48.67	49.25	50.17
		Palatal Breadth	38.41	38.00	38.39	38.00	39.50	40.00	39.67	38.00	39.13	38.67	39.19	38.00
		Bicondylar Breadth	116.17	121.00	115.82	121.50	121.85	.	122.43	116.00	119.84	121.00	120.04	118.20
		Bigonial Breadth	94.62	90.00	94.47	94.00	103.32	75.00	102.74	101.25	100.22	82.50	99.83	98.14
		HAR	66.70	70.00	66.89	66.50	69.50	60.00	69.78	64.50	68.57	65.00	68.80	65.17
		MBAR	29.57	32.00	29.53	30.67	31.73	30.00	31.76	31.00	31.00	31.00	31.02	30.86
		HMS	28.43	28.00	28.32	29.00	30.63	28.00	30.68	29.50	29.87	28.00	29.88	29.29
	Macedonian	Max Cranial Length	173.14	.	173.27	171.50	181.78	192.00	182.96	175.33	177.38	192.00	178.02	173.80
		Max Cranial Breadth	140.71	.	140.69	141.00	144.93	158.00	145.04	148.33	142.78	158.00	142.82	145.40
		Cranial Height	126.00	.	125.80	129.00	134.88	148.00	135.69	135.00	130.44	148.00	130.90	132.00
		Facial Height n-gn	107.42	.	108.24	100.50	112.53	128.00	113.39	.	109.83	128.00	110.89	100.50
		Facial Width zy-zy	125.83	.	126.05	123.50	133.75	144.00	134.24	.	129.43	144.00	130.05	123.50
		FMT Width	101.55	.	102.15	95.50	103.94	110.00	104.29	.	102.55	110.00	103.14	95.50
		Upper Facial Height	65.00	.	65.38	60.50	69.90	80.00	70.25	73.00	67.13	80.00	67.59	64.67
		MAXL	50.91	.	51.11	50.00	52.38	60.00	52.93	.	51.71	60.00	52.22	50.00
		MAXB	57.00	.	57.18	55.50	61.31	59.00	60.88	66.00	58.97	59.00	58.97	59.00
		Palatal Length	47.00	.	47.06	46.50	48.31	53.00	48.44	51.00	47.60	53.00	47.73	48.00
		Palatal Breadth	40.53	.	40.88	37.50	43.44	35.00	43.19	39.00	41.86	35.00	42.00	38.00
		Bicondylar Breadth	121.25	.	121.07	124.00	125.33	139.00	126.19	.	123.23	139.00	123.71	124.00
		Bigonial Breadth	96.57	.	96.76	94.50	106.21	103.00	106.18	105.33	101.49	103.00	101.58	101.00
		HAR	65.53	.	65.07	69.00	70.38	77.00	70.81	70.00	67.88	77.00	68.03	69.33
		MBAR	30.37	.	30.47	29.50	31.50	40.00	31.94	32.00	30.92	40.00	31.21	30.75
		HMS	26.39	.	26.44	26.00	30.16	38.00	30.56	30.50	28.32	38.00	28.62	28.25
	All	Max Cranial Length	176.10	174.00	175.79	178.20	182.37	184.50	182.78	178.40	179.54	179.25	179.64	178.30
		Max Cranial Breadth	141.47	138.00	141.65	138.40	146.38	142.00	145.75	150.57	144.22	140.00	143.93	145.50
		Cranial Height	127.24	124.50	127.27	124.00	133.00	148.00	133.43	132.00	130.63	132.33	130.79	129.33
		Facial Height n-gn	107.40	102.00	107.69	100.50	114.73	128.00	115.56	103.50	111.76	115.00	112.39	102.00
		Facial Width zy-zy	126.27	123.00	126.33	123.50	133.26	144.00	133.80	129.00	129.97	133.50	130.24	126.80
		FMT Width	103.20	102.50	103.33	101.80	105.60	104.00	105.51	106.00	104.50	103.25	104.53	103.67
		Upper Facial Height	64.58	65.00	64.79	60.50	68.31	73.00	68.69	65.75	66.66	69.00	66.93	64.00
		MAXL	49.93	51.00	49.88	50.67	52.87	60.00	53.03	53.33	51.64	55.50	51.73	52.00
		MAXB	57.02	58.00	57.20	55.33	60.40	60.50	60.50	59.40	58.96	59.25	59.07	57.88
		Palatal Length	47.60	48.00	47.46	49.25	49.59	51.50	49.66	49.60	48.75	49.75	48.73	49.44
		Palatal Breadth	39.39	38.00	39.45	37.67	40.59	37.50	40.69	38.20	40.09	37.75	40.17	38.00
		Bicondylar Breadth	118.56	121.00	118.28	122.33	122.94	139.00	123.74	116.00	121.12	130.00	121.50	119.17
		Bigonial Breadth	95.64	90.00	95.68	94.20	104.44	89.00	104.07	103.00	100.78	89.33	100.61	99.33
		HAR	66.16	70.00	66.09	67.75	69.75	68.50	70.09	65.60	68.32	69.00	68.53	66.56
		MBAR	29.95	32.00	29.97	30.20	31.66	35.00	31.82	31.33	30.97	34.00	31.09	30.82
		HMS	27.49	28.00	27.46	27.80	30.47	33.00	30.64	29.83	29.29	31.33	29.40	28.91

112

Table 10. Means, ectopic and impacted teeth and crowding.

			Female				Male				All			
			Ectopic, heterotopic, impaction		Crowding		Ectopic, heterotopic, impaction		Crowding		Ectopic, heterotopic, impaction		Crowding	
			Absent Mean	Present Mean	Absent Mean	Present Mean	Absent Mean	Present Mean	Absent Mean	Present Mean	Absent Mean	Present Mean	Absent Mean	Present Mean
Major Geo	English	Max Cranial Length	179.14	179.75	179.26	179.00	183.03	179.75	183.64	179.25	181.49	179.75	181.67	179.20
		Max Cranial Breadth	141.57	144.50	141.27	147.67	147.60	140.50	147.84	142.43	145.34	142.50	145.17	144.00
		Cranial Height	125.81	139.67	125.41	150.00	131.90	134.00	132.52	130.00	129.73	137.40	129.64	135.00
		Facial Height n-gn	106.90	107.00	106.80	107.50	115.92	118.50	116.50	115.00	113.34	112.75	113.27	113.33
		Facial Width zy-zy	126.65	127.00	126.88	125.00	133.35	129.33	133.33	131.00	130.50	128.75	130.54	129.29
		FMT Width	104.59	104.25	104.87	102.00	106.44	102.75	106.60	104.50	105.74	103.50	105.85	103.92
		Upper Facial Height	64.76	58.00	64.69	60.67	67.35	67.25	67.56	66.63	66.44	64.17	66.49	65.00
		MAXL	49.24	52.00	49.13	51.50	53.29	51.00	53.09	53.33	51.61	51.33	51.46	52.60
		MAXB	56.95	58.33	56.95	58.33	60.00	60.75	60.27	59.50	58.88	59.71	58.90	59.23
		Palatal Length	48.09	48.00	48.48	45.00	50.25	48.25	50.47	48.70	49.48	48.13	49.67	47.85
		Palatal Breadth	38.57	37.00	38.62	36.67	39.49	39.75	39.45	39.70	39.17	38.57	39.13	39.00
		Bicondylar Breadth	115.87	118.50	116.00	118.67	121.94	120.50	121.56	122.75	119.96	119.17	119.39	121.64
		Bigonial Breadth	94.72	93.00	94.53	93.67	103.53	91.33	103.34	100.40	100.59	92.29	99.85	98.85
		HAR	67.06	66.00	67.00	66.00	69.35	68.50	69.53	68.55	68.63	67.25	68.58	68.00
		MBAR	29.61	30.00	29.47	31.00	31.79	30.75	31.61	31.91	31.09	30.38	30.80	31.71
		HMS	28.56	27.75	28.47	28.00	30.62	30.00	30.87	29.73	29.95	28.88	29.94	29.36
	Macedonian	Max Cranial Length	173.84	167.33	173.33	172.57	181.61	184.60	182.56	181.40	177.56	178.13	177.59	177.76
		Max Cranial Breadth	141.24	136.33	140.86	140.29	145.13	147.00	145.39	145.40	143.14	142.43	142.95	143.29
		Cranial Height	126.31	124.67	124.45	129.40	135.38	136.50	136.50	134.43	130.85	131.43	130.19	132.33
		Facial Height n-gn	108.25	103.00	106.62	109.17	115.14	107.25	112.09	115.43	111.47	105.43	109.13	112.54
		Facial Width zy-zy	126.67	120.00	124.76	128.43	133.88	135.75	133.00	136.25	129.89	129.00	128.33	132.60
		FMT Width	102.10	96.00	101.67	101.00	103.14	109.67	102.80	106.43	102.53	104.20	102.07	104.45
		Upper Facial Height	65.48	61.33	64.79	65.57	70.94	68.00	68.82	72.10	67.80	65.14	66.27	69.41
		MAXL	50.91	.	50.57	51.50	54.18	48.33	52.67	53.40	52.55	48.33	51.75	52.56
		MAXB	58.53	44.00	55.86	60.20	60.79	63.00	59.33	63.25	59.55	55.40	57.22	62.08
		Palatal Length	47.29	44.50	46.64	48.00	49.00	46.67	48.22	49.00	48.06	45.80	47.26	48.62
		Palatal Breadth	39.76	47.00	40.57	40.40	43.21	41.67	40.78	45.38	41.32	43.80	40.65	43.46
		Bicondylar Breadth	121.64	118.50	121.90	120.17	126.55	125.40	124.44	128.43	123.80	123.43	123.11	124.62
		Bigonial Breadth	96.85	94.67	98.38	92.43	105.25	109.40	106.33	105.70	101.05	103.88	102.23	100.24
		HAR	66.47	58.50	65.46	65.75	71.15	69.50	69.91	72.33	68.64	65.83	67.50	69.70
		MBAR	30.47	29.50	30.21	30.80	31.87	32.25	31.00	33.25	31.13	31.33	30.56	32.31
		HMS	26.81	23.00	25.57	29.25	31.06	28.50	28.92	33.00	28.74	26.67	27.12	31.75
	All	Max Cranial Length	176.26	174.43	176.43	174.00	182.44	182.44	183.22	180.44	179.62	178.94	179.90	178.30
		Max Cranial Breadth	141.39	141.00	141.07	142.50	146.59	143.75	146.96	144.18	144.31	142.47	144.24	143.56
		Cranial Height	126.03	132.17	125.04	135.29	132.98	135.67	133.66	132.38	130.14	133.92	129.83	133.40
		Facial Height n-gn	107.73	104.60	106.70	108.75	115.64	111.00	114.94	115.21	112.48	108.09	111.43	112.86
		Facial Width zy-zy	126.66	121.75	125.79	127.67	133.58	133.00	133.21	134.23	130.21	128.91	129.55	131.55
		FMT Width	103.40	101.50	103.46	101.43	105.52	105.71	105.65	105.29	104.55	103.77	104.54	104.37
		Upper Facial Height	65.18	60.00	64.74	64.10	68.63	67.63	67.92	69.67	67.06	64.69	66.40	67.68
		MAXL	49.89	52.00	49.57	51.50	53.57	49.40	52.97	53.38	51.94	49.83	51.55	52.57
		MAXB	57.66	52.60	56.51	59.50	60.22	61.71	60.05	61.17	59.11	57.92	58.38	60.65
		Palatal Length	47.74	46.83	47.78	46.88	49.93	47.57	50.00	48.83	49.01	47.23	48.98	48.23
		Palatal Breadth	39.11	41.00	39.40	40.57	40.47	40.75	39.74	42.22	39.90	40.75	39.58	41.23
		Bicondylar Breadth	118.66	118.50	118.27	119.67	123.14	124.00	122.32	125.40	121.31	121.46	120.57	123.25
		Bigonial Breadth	95.84	93.71	96.29	92.80	104.14	102.63	104.36	103.05	100.79	98.47	100.78	99.63
		HAR	66.78	63.50	66.35	65.86	69.82	69.00	69.63	69.88	68.63	66.64	68.22	68.71
		MBAR	30.03	29.83	29.79	30.88	31.81	31.50	31.45	32.47	31.10	30.79	30.72	32.00
		HMS	27.74	26.17	27.24	28.71	30.75	29.25	30.31	31.29	29.57	27.93	28.96	30.46

Table 11. Index and ratio means, rotations and reversals.

			Female				Male				Total			
			Rotation		Reversal		Rotation		Reversal		Rotation		Reversal	
			Absent Mean	Present Mean	Absent Mean	Present Mean	Absent Mean	Present Mean	Absent Mean	Present Mean	Absent Mean	Present Mean	Absent Mean	Present Mean
MajorGeo	English	Cranial Index	78.4	81.0	79.2	.	79.9	82.2	80.6	.	79.3	81.7	80.0	.
		Cranial Module	150.06	148.67	149.59	.	154.63	152.52	153.95	.	152.86	150.98	152.25	.
		Cranial length-height Index	71.99	70.83	71.62	.	73.32	71.67	72.79	.	72.78	71.33	72.32	.
		Cranial breadth-height Index	91.22	86.96	89.80	.	91.59	87.15	90.11	.	91.45	87.08	89.99	.
		Total Facial Index	84.25	84.25	84.25	.	87.53	85.42	86.79	.	86.76	84.83	85.89	.
		Upper Facial Index	51.03	51.54	51.29	.	52.63	50.41	51.89	.	52.10	50.98	51.65	.
		Maxilloalveolar Index	111.63	121.89	115.62	.	114.25	112.49	113.81	.	113.25	117.55	114.58	.
		Palatal Index	78.99	84.31	80.54	.	79.25	78.79	79.14	.	79.16	81.06	79.65	.
		Palatal/max ratio	.71	.72	.71	.	.71	.72	.71	.	.71	.72	.71	.
		TFHFMT	103.63	103.25	103.41	.	110.52	105.87	109.22	.	109.03	104.56	107.34	.
		UFHFMT	60.76	63.25	61.81	.	64.50	62.99	64.04	.	63.29	63.10	63.23	.
		MAXBCDL	.50	.53	.51	.	.49	.51	.49	.	.49	.52	.50	.
		cdlgo	.80	.82	.81	.	.84	.86	.85	.	.83	.84	.83	.
		ZYGFMT	.84	.82	.83	.	.80	.80	.80	.	.81	.81	.81	.
		UHTH	.58	.61	.60	.	.59	.59	.59	.	.58	.60	.59	.
		FB	.92	.89	.90	.	.92	.92	.92	.	.92	.90	.91	.
		FB2	.89	.92	.90	.	.87	.89	.87	.	.87	.91	.88	.
		UFIMAI	.45	.42	.44	.	.47	.45	.47	.	.46	.44	.45	.
	Macedonian	Cranial Index	81.0	82.0	81.2	83.0	80.7	78.1	80.2	.	80.8	80.6	80.7	83.0
		Cranial Module	145.70	144.00	145.21	144.83	154.56	151.78	154.04	.	150.50	146.92	149.92	144.83
		Cranial length-height Index	73.91	73.96	73.44	77.32	74.28	74.87	74.38	.	74.12	74.30	73.96	77.32
		Cranial breadth-height Index	90.92	90.21	90.35	93.14	92.72	94.18	92.99	.	91.89	91.70	91.76	93.14
		Total Facial Index	85.62	84.61	84.66	88.74	83.91	84.41	84.06	.	84.64	84.54	84.36	88.74
		Upper Facial Index	51.42	52.55	51.96	51.40	52.05	52.17	52.08	.	51.76	52.44	52.01	51.40
		Maxilloalveolar Index	112.85	131.99	115.15	122.79	116.50	109.65	114.92	.	114.88	118.59	115.01	122.79
		Palatal Index	86.75	86.68	86.97	84.64	89.92	91.66	90.25	.	88.40	88.17	88.56	84.64
		Palatal/max ratio	.73	.65	.72	.69	.81	.83	.82	.	.77	.76	.78	.69
		TFHFMT	105.47	106.75	105.08	111.80	112.35	103.18	110.24	.	109.09	105.56	107.66	111.80
		UFHFMT	63.29	65.38	63.79	64.76	65.72	67.65	66.11	.	64.32	66.13	64.78	64.76
		MAXBCDL	.46	.51	.48	.50	.49	.47	.49	.	.47	.51	.48	.50
		cdlgo	.79	.83	.81	.76	.84	.89	.85	.	.81	.85	.83	.76
		ZYGFMT	.81	.83	.82	.79	.80	.82	.80	.	.80	.82	.81	.79
		UHTH	.59	.61	.61	.58	.62	.62	.62	.	.61	.61	.61	.58
		FB	.97	.94	.96	.95	.94	.89	.93	.	.95	.93	.94	.95
		FB2	.85	.87	.86	.84	.81	.88	.83	.	.83	.87	.84	.84
		UFIMAI	.46	.41	.45	.42	.45	.51	.46	.	.45	.46	.46	.42
	Total	Cranial Index	79.7	81.6	80.2	83.0	80.3	80.7	80.4	.	80.0	81.2	80.3	83.0
		Cranial Module	147.97	146.55	147.68	144.83	154.60	152.33	153.98	.	151.83	149.57	151.33	144.83
		Cranial length-height Index	72.87	72.25	72.39	77.32	73.73	72.47	73.39	.	73.36	72.36	72.97	77.32
		Cranial breadth-height Index	91.08	88.43	90.04	93.14	92.03	88.78	91.11	.	91.64	88.62	90.67	93.14
		Total Facial Index	85.20	84.46	84.50	88.74	85.79	85.00	85.53	.	85.59	84.68	85.09	88.74
		Upper Facial Index	51.27	52.10	51.67	51.40	52.35	51.00	51.97	.	51.91	51.66	51.83	51.40
		Maxilloalveolar Index	112.14	124.14	115.48	122.79	115.05	111.54	114.20	.	113.88	117.84	114.73	122.79
		Palatal Index	82.20	85.49	83.21	84.64	82.33	81.76	82.20	.	82.28	83.70	82.62	84.64
		Palatal/max ratio	.72	.70	.72	.69	.74	.76	.75	.	.73	.73	.73	.69
		TFHFMT	104.81	104.87	104.28	111.80	111.18	105.07	109.57	.	109.05	104.95	107.47	111.80
		UFHFMT	62.22	64.16	62.80	64.76	64.90	64.06	64.67	.	63.74	64.11	63.83	64.76
		MAXBCDL	.48	.52	.50	.50	.49	.50	.49	.	.48	.51	.49	.50
		cdlgo	.79	.83	.81	.76	.84	.87	.85	.	.82	.85	.83	.76
		ZYGFMT	.82	.82	.82	.79	.80	.81	.80	.	.81	.81	.81	.79
		UHTH	.59	.61	.60	.58	.60	.60	.60	.	.60	.61	.60	.58
		FB	.95	.91	.93	.95	.93	.91	.92	.	.94	.91	.93	.95
		FB2	.87	.90	.89	.84	.85	.89	.86	.	.86	.90	.87	.84
		UFIMAI	.46	.42	.44	.42	.46	.47	.46	.	.46	.44	.46	.42

Table 12. Index and ratio means, supplemental and misshapen teeth.

			Female				Male				Total				
			Supplemental Teeth		Peg, Misshapen		Supplemental Teeth		Peg, Misshapen		Supplemental Teeth		Peg, Misshapen		
			Absent Mean	Present Mean	Absent Mean	Present Mean	Absent Mean	Present Mean	Absent Mean	Present Mean	Absent Mean	Present Mean	Absent Mean	Present Mean
MajorGeo	English	Cranial Index	79.2	.	79.2	.	80.9	74.4	80.5	81.5	80.2	74.4	79.9	81.5
		Cranial Module	149.59	.	149.59	.	153.95	.	153.32	159.22	152.25	.	151.76	159.22
		CLHI	71.62	.	71.62	.	72.79	.	72.64	74.03	72.32	.	72.20	74.03
		CBHI	89.80	.	89.80	.	90.11	.	90.03	90.82	89.99	.	89.94	90.82
		Total Facial Index	84.25	.	84.25	.	87.23	78.52	86.40	90.31	86.13	78.52	85.58	90.31
		Upper Facial Index	51.29	.	51.29	.	52.12	46.67	52.02	50.42	51.78	46.67	51.71	50.42
		MAI	115.62	.	115.62	.	113.67	116.98	113.81	.	114.53	116.98	114.58	.
		Palatal Index	80.54	.	80.54	.	79.10	80.00	78.70	83.29	79.64	80.00	79.42	83.29
		Palatal/max ratio	.71	.	.71	.	.71	.68	.71	.	.71	.68	.71	.
		TFHFMT	103.41	.	103.41	.	109.76	96.36	108.14	117.16	107.64	96.36	106.47	117.16
		UFHFMT	61.81	.	61.81	.	64.16	62.31	63.88	65.70	63.26	62.31	63.08	65.70
		MAXBCDL	.51	.	.51	.	.49	.53	.49	.46	.50	.53	.50	.46
		cdlgo	.81	.	.81	.	.85	.88	.84	.87	.83	.88	.83	.87
		ZYGFMT	.83	.	.83	.	.80	.81	.80	.78	.81	.81	.81	.78
		UHTH	.60	.	.60	.	.59	.59	.59	.57	.59	.59	.59	.57
		FB	.90	.	.90	.	.92	.87	.92	.93	.91	.87	.91	.93
		FB2	.90	.	.90	.	.87	.93	.87	.87	.88	.93	.89	.87
		UFIMAI	.44	.	.44	.	.47	.40	.47	.	.46	.40	.45	.
	Macedonian	Cranial Index	81.3	.	81.3	.	80.2	.	80.2	.	80.8	.	80.8	.
		Cranial Module	145.17	.	145.17	.	154.04	.	154.04	.	149.60	.	149.60	.
		CLHI	73.92	.	73.92	.	74.38	.	74.38	.	74.16	.	74.16	.
		CBHI	90.70	.	90.70	.	92.99	.	92.99	.	91.84	.	91.84	.
		Total Facial Index	85.09	.	85.09	.	84.06	.	84.06	.	84.60	.	84.60	.
		Upper Facial Index	51.91	.	51.91	.	52.08	.	52.08	.	51.99	.	51.99	.
		MAI	116.68	.	116.68	.	114.92	.	114.92	.	115.68	.	115.68	.
		Palatal Index	86.73	.	86.73	.	90.25	.	90.25	.	88.33	.	88.33	.
		Palatal/max ratio	.72	.	.72	.	.82	.	.82	.	.77	.	.77	.
		TFHFMT	105.98	.	105.98	.	110.24	.	110.24	.	107.96	.	107.96	.
		UFHFMT	63.88	.	63.88	.	66.13	.	66.13	.	64.78	.	64.78	.
		MAXBCDL	.48	.	.48	.	.49	.	.49	.	.48	.	.48	.
		cdlgo	.80	.	.80	.	.85	.	.85	.	.83	.	.83	.
		ZYGFMT	.82	.	.82	.	.80	.	.80	.	.81	.	.81	.
		UHTH	.60	.	.60	.	.62	.	.62	.	.61	.	.61	.
		FB	.96	.	.96	.	.93	.	.93	.	.94	.	.94	.
		FB2	.85	.	.85	.	.83	.	.83	.	.84	.	.84	.
		UFIMAI	.45	.	.45	.	.46	.	.46	.	.46	.	.46	.
	Total	Cranial Index	80.3	.	80.3	.	80.6	74.4	80.3	81.5	80.5	74.4	80.3	81.5
		Cranial Module	147.51	.	147.51	.	153.98	.	153.60	159.22	151.16	.	150.84	159.22
		CLHI	72.67	.	72.67	.	73.39	.	73.35	74.03	73.08	.	73.04	74.03
		CBHI	90.22	.	90.22	.	91.11	.	91.13	90.82	90.73	.	90.73	90.82
		Total Facial Index	84.78	.	84.78	.	85.73	78.52	85.26	90.31	85.30	78.52	85.04	90.31
		Upper Facial Index	51.65	.	51.65	.	52.10	46.67	52.05	50.42	51.88	46.67	51.86	50.42
		MAI	116.00	.	116.00	.	114.12	116.98	114.20	.	114.94	116.98	114.97	.
		Palatal Index	83.27	.	83.27	.	82.28	80.00	82.12	83.29	82.71	80.00	82.63	83.29
		Palatal/max ratio	.72	.	.72	.	.75	.68	.75	.	.73	.68	.73	.
		TFHFMT	104.84	.	104.84	.	109.93	96.36	108.92	117.16	107.78	96.36	107.14	117.16
		UFHFMT	62.90	.	62.90	.	64.77	62.31	64.60	65.70	63.89	62.31	63.79	65.70
		MAXBCDL	.50	.	.50	.	.49	.53	.49	.46	.49	.53	.49	.46
		cdlgo	.81	.	.81	.	.85	.88	.85	.87	.83	.88	.83	.87
		ZYGFMT	.82	.	.82	.	.80	.81	.80	.78	.81	.81	.81	.78
		UHTH	.60	.	.60	.	.60	.59	.60	.57	.60	.59	.60	.57
		FB	.93	.	.93	.	.92	.87	.92	.93	.93	.87	.93	.93
		FB2	.88	.	.88	.	.86	.93	.86	.87	.87	.93	.87	.87
		UFIMAI	.44	.	.44	.	.47	.40	.46	.	.46	.40	.45	.

115

Table 13. Index and ratio means, congenitally absent teeth and M3.

MajorG			Female				Male				All			
			Congenitally Absent Teeth		M3 Congenitally Absent		Congenitally Absent Teeth		M3 Congenitally Absent		Congenitally Absent Teeth		M3 Congenitally Absent	
			Absent Mean	Present Mean	Absent Mean	Present Mean	Absent Mean	Present Mean	Absent Mean	Present Mean	Absent Mean	Present Mean	Absent Mean	Present Mean
MajorGeo	English	Cranial Index	79.1	79.6	79.8	75.0	80.8	71.2	80.0	89.7	80.2	76.8	79.9	80.9
		Cranial Module	150.10	145.50	149.82	145.67	153.95	.	153.44	167.67	152.55	145.50	152.05	156.67
		CLHI	71.61	71.70	71.84	67.61	72.79	.	72.82	71.98	72.35	71.70	72.43	69.80
		CBHI	89.74	90.25	90.15	83.80	90.11	.	90.66	85.14	89.98	90.25	90.47	84.80
		Total Facial Index	84.38	82.93	84.25	.	86.79	.	87.34	81.82	85.99	82.93	86.17	81.82
		Upper Facial Index	51.35	50.41	51.29	.	51.89	.	51.96	51.07	51.68	50.41	51.68	51.07
		Maxilloalveolar Index	115.27	121.57	116.20	105.77	113.81	.	114.08	111.86	114.41	121.57	115.03	110.34
		Palatal Index	80.67	79.17	80.60	79.17	79.12	80.00	79.34	77.23	79.66	79.44	79.82	77.62
		Palatal/max ratio	.71	.72	.71	.75	.71	.	.71	.73	.71	.72	.71	.73
		TFHFMT	103.63	100.99	103.41	.	109.22	.	110.39	95.82	107.51	100.99	107.99	95.82
		UFHFMT	61.62	63.39	61.81	.	63.94	67.35	64.47	59.79	63.14	64.71	63.44	59.79
		MAXBCDL	.52	.45	.51	.	.49	.	.49	.51	.50	.45	.50	.51
		cdlgo	.81	.74	.81	.78	.85	.	.85	.85	.83	.74	.83	.83
		ZYGFMT	.83	.82	.83	.	.80	.	.79	.83	.81	.82	.81	.83
		UHTH	.60	.61	.60	.	.59	.	.58	.62	.59	.61	.59	.62
		FB	.90	.98	.90	.	.92	.	.92	.93	.91	.98	.91	.93
		FB2	.91	.83	.90	.89	.87	.	.87	.91	.89	.83	.88	.90
		UFIMAI	.44	.	.44	.	.47	.	.47	.45	.45	.	.45	.45
	Macedonian	Cranial Index	81.3	.	81.3	82.2	80.1	82.3	79.6	84.8	80.7	82.3	80.5	83.8
		Cranial Module	145.17	.	145.20	144.67	153.24	166.00	154.31	150.00	149.08	166.00	149.76	147.33
		CLHI	73.92	.	73.70	77.25	74.21	77.08	74.07	79.41	74.07	77.08	73.89	78.33
		CBHI	90.70	.	90.51	93.48	92.95	93.67	92.98	93.10	91.78	93.67	91.75	93.29
		Total Facial Index	85.09	.	85.52	81.38	83.75	88.89	84.06	.	84.48	88.89	84.79	81.38
		Upper Facial Index	51.91	.	52.18	49.01	51.89	55.56	52.08	.	51.90	55.56	52.13	49.01
		Maxilloalveolar Index	116.68	.	118.11	110.94	116.30	98.33	114.92	.	116.47	98.33	116.14	110.94
		Palatal Index	86.73	.	87.44	80.62	91.86	66.04	91.16	76.47	88.99	66.04	89.19	79.24
		Palatal/max ratio	.72	.	.72	.73	.83	.67	.82	.	.78	.67	.78	.73
		TFHFMT	105.98	.	106.06	105.45	109.72	116.36	110.24	.	107.64	116.36	108.15	105.45
		UFHFMT	63.88	.	63.92	63.57	65.62	72.73	66.13	.	64.55	72.73	64.86	63.57
		MAXBCDL	.48	.	.49	.43	.49	.42	.49	.	.49	.42	.49	.43
		cdlgo	.80	.	.81	.79	.86	.74	.85	.	.83	.74	.83	.79
		ZYGFMT	.82	.	.82	.77	.80	.76	.80	.	.81	.76	.81	.77
		UHTH	.60	.	.60	.60	.62	.63	.62	.	.61	.63	.61	.60
		FB	.96	.	.96	.99	.92	.97	.93	.	.94	.97	.94	.99
		FB2	.85	.	.86	.81	.83	.79	.83	.	.84	.79	.84	.81
		UFIMAI	.45	.	.45	.44	.45	.56	.46	.	.45	.56	.46	.44
	All	Cranial Index	80.4	79.6	80.6	77.9	80.5	76.7	79.8	86.8	80.4	78.2	80.2	82.3
		Cranial Module	147.64	145.50	147.66	145.17	153.71	166.00	153.75	158.83	151.12	152.33	151.12	152.00
		CLHI	72.73	71.70	72.69	72.43	73.31	77.08	73.28	75.69	73.06	73.49	73.03	74.06
		CBHI	90.22	90.25	90.32	88.64	91.06	93.67	91.49	87.13	90.71	91.39	90.99	87.63
		Total Facial Index	84.84	82.93	85.02	81.38	85.44	88.89	85.75	81.82	85.17	85.91	85.42	81.60
		Upper Facial Index	51.69	50.41	51.80	49.01	51.89	55.56	52.02	51.07	51.79	52.98	51.91	50.04
		Maxilloalveolar Index	115.79	121.57	116.81	109.22	114.64	98.33	114.40	111.86	115.13	109.95	115.42	110.54
		Palatal Index	83.47	79.17	83.51	80.14	82.53	73.02	82.69	77.08	82.93	76.09	83.04	78.23
		Palatal/max ratio	.72	.72	.71	.73	.75	.67	.75	.73	.73	.70	.73	.73
		TFHFMT	104.98	100.99	104.79	105.45	109.38	116.36	110.33	95.82	107.57	108.68	108.06	100.63
		UFHFMT	62.87	63.39	62.86	63.57	64.43	70.04	65.00	59.79	63.72	66.71	64.01	61.30
		MAXBCDL	.50	.45	.50	.43	.49	.42	.49	.51	.50	.44	.49	.49
		cdlgo	.81	.74	.81	.78	.85	.74	.85	.85	.83	.74	.83	.82
		ZYGFMT	.82	.82	.82	.77	.80	.76	.80	.83	.81	.79	.81	.81
		UHTH	.60	.61	.60	.60	.60	.63	.60	.62	.60	.62	.60	.61
		FB	.93	.98	.93	.99	.92	.97	.92	.93	.93	.97	.93	.95
		FB2	.88	.83	.89	.86	.86	.79	.86	.91	.87	.81	.87	.89
		UFIMAI	.44	.	.44	.44	.46	.56	.47	.45	.45	.56	.46	.45

Table 14. Index and ratio means, ectopic and impacted teeth and crowding.

			Female				Male				Total			
			Ectopic, heterotopic, impaction		Crowding		Ectopic, heterotopic, impaction		Crowding		Ectopic, heterotopic, impaction		Crowding	
			Absent Mean	Present Mean	Absent Mean	Present Mean	Absent Mean	Present Mean	Absent Mean	Present Mean	Absent Mean	Present Mean	Absent Mean	Present Mean
MajorGeo	English	Cranial Index	78.9	80.4	79.1	80.1	80.9	78.1	80.8	79.7	80.1	79.3	80.0	79.8
		Cranial Module	148.53	154.89	148.60	157.50	154.04	152.83	154.65	151.39	152.02	154.07	152.11	152.92
		Cranial length-height Index	70.60	77.07	70.23	83.47	72.66	74.46	72.83	72.64	71.88	76.03	71.70	75.35
		Cranial breadth-height Index	88.48	96.40	88.02	104.05	89.92	92.79	90.25	89.55	89.42	94.95	89.36	93.18
		Total Facial Index	84.25	84.25	84.03	86.40	86.34	90.82	86.12	88.80	85.59	88.63	85.29	88.40
		Upper Facial Index	51.40	49.61	51.24	51.60	51.83	52.32	52.13	50.96	51.65	51.64	51.75	51.15
		Maxilloalveolar Index	115.63	115.38	115.48	116.78	113.43	117.91	114.44	109.36	114.39	117.07	114.89	112.33
		Palatal Index	80.36	81.81	80.29	82.27	78.77	82.71	78.45	81.66	79.33	82.33	79.17	81.81
		Palatal/max ratio	.72	.69	.72	.69	.71	.72	.71	.71	.71	.71	.71	.71
		TFHFMT	103.60	102.45	103.21	104.37	108.91	112.86	109.05	109.66	107.30	107.65	106.97	108.48
		UFHFMT	62.56	55.42	62.24	59.49	63.85	65.48	64.02	64.11	63.37	62.12	63.33	62.85
		MAXBCDL	.51	.49	.51	.49	.49	.50	.49	.48	.50	.50	.50	.49
		cdlgo	.81	.79	.81	.79	.85	.83	.85	.85	.84	.80	.83	.83
		ZYGFMT	.83	.84	.83	.82	.80	.81	.80	.80	.81	.82	.81	.80
		UHTH	.61	.54	.61	.55	.59	.58	.59	.58	.59	.56	.60	.57
		FB	.90	.87	.90	.92	.92	.93	.92	.93	.91	.91	.91	.93
		FB2	.91	.88	.91	.86	.87	.86	.88	.86	.89	.88	.89	.86
		UFIMAI	.44	.43	.44	.44	.47	.45	.46	.49	.45	.44	.45	.47
	Macedonian	Cranial Index	81.3	81.5	81.3	81.4	80.0	81.1	80.1	80.2	80.7	81.3	80.8	80.7
		Cranial Module	145.72	142.78	144.79	146.00	153.92	154.56	154.37	153.62	149.82	148.67	149.10	150.44
		CLHI	73.79	74.52	73.03	75.89	74.55	73.84	74.58	74.09	74.17	74.13	73.77	74.84
		CBHI	90.53	91.43	89.30	93.77	93.59	90.40	93.20	92.72	92.06	90.91	91.05	93.16
		TFI	84.92	85.99	86.24	82.60	85.54	79.24	83.72	84.54	85.20	82.13	85.14	83.65
		UFI	52.02	51.19	52.30	51.01	52.57	50.23	51.68	52.63	52.25	50.64	52.05	51.87
		MAI	116.68	.	114.20	120.40	110.24	130.51	115.00	114.79	113.46	130.51	114.65	117.29
		Palatal Index	84.47	105.91	87.32	85.07	90.43	89.46	87.15	93.34	87.05	96.04	87.26	90.16
		Palatal/max ratio	.72	.	.75	.68	.86	.69	.80	.84	.79	.68	.77	.77
		TFHFMT	106.55	102.28	104.15	113.31	114.18	97.10	111.90	107.58	109.86	99.17	107.25	109.73
		UFHFMT	64.13	61.52	63.06	67.37	67.40	61.49	63.83	68.43	65.33	61.50	63.29	68.05
		MAXBCDL	.50	.32	.51	.51	.47	.52	.48	.49	.49	.47	.47	.50
		cdlgo	.80	.81	.82	.78	.84	.88	.86	.83	.82	.86	.84	.81
		ZYGFMT	.81	.83	.83	.79	.79	.83	.81	.78	.81	.83	.82	.79
		UHTH	.60	.60	.61	.59	.62	.63	.62	.62	.61	.62	.61	.61
		FB	.96	.95	.97	.94	.93	.92	.92	.94	.95	.93	.95	.94
		FB2	.85	.85	.86	.84	.79	.90	.83	.82	.83	.89	.85	.83
		UFIMAI	.45	.	.45	.44	.49	.39	.46	.47	.47	.39	.46	.45
	Total	Cranial Index	80.3	80.9	80.2	81.1	80.5	79.6	80.5	80.0	80.4	80.2	80.4	80.4
		Cranial Module	147.23	148.83	147.05	149.29	154.00	153.87	154.57	152.59	151.17	151.12	151.07	151.43
		CLHI	72.03	75.80	71.33	78.05	73.29	74.04	73.38	73.42	72.75	74.92	72.42	75.04
		CBHI	89.43	93.91	88.54	96.71	91.08	91.35	91.05	91.26	90.41	92.75	89.92	93.17
		TFI	84.66	85.56	85.28	83.14	86.01	83.10	85.16	86.32	85.39	84.08	85.22	85.15
		UFI	51.75	50.79	51.81	51.14	52.14	51.12	51.97	51.99	51.95	51.00	51.89	51.64
		Maxilloalveolar Index	116.02	115.38	115.13	119.20	112.44	125.47	114.60	112.76	114.08	123.79	114.82	115.52
		Palatal Index	82.20	91.45	83.10	84.02	81.74	85.60	80.15	87.16	81.93	88.04	81.51	86.15
		Palatal/max ratio	.72	.69	.73	.68	.75	.70	.73	.79	.74	.70	.73	.75
		TFHFMT	105.27	102.37	103.72	109.74	110.50	103.40	109.93	108.79	108.35	102.94	107.08	109.07
		UFHFMT	63.39	58.47	62.66	63.99	64.82	63.77	63.98	66.13	64.14	61.84	63.31	65.45
		MAXBCDL	.51	.45	.50	.50	.49	.51	.49	.48	.50	.48	.50	.49
		cdlgo	.81	.80	.81	.79	.85	.86	.85	.84	.83	.83	.84	.82
		ZYGFMT	.82	.83	.83	.80	.80	.82	.80	.79	.81	.82	.82	.79
		UHTH	.61	.57	.61	.58	.60	.62	.60	.60	.60	.60	.60	.59
		FB	.93	.92	.93	.93	.92	.93	.92	.93	.93	.92	.92	.93
		FB2	.88	.88	.89	.85	.86	.89	.87	.84	.87	.88	.88	.84
		UFIMAI	.44	.43	.44	.44	.48	.41	.46	.47	.46	.42	.45	.46

Appendix B

Section 3. Independent T-Tests Results

Part 3. General Craniometrics

Craniometrics, all skulls, Females v Males.

Independent Samples Test

		Levene's Test for Equality of Variances		t-test for Equality of Means					95% Confidence Interval of the Difference	
		F	Sig.	t	df	Sig. (2-tailed)	Mean Difference	Std. Error Difference	Lower	Upper
Max Cranial Length	Equal variances assumed	3.458	.065	4.451	115	.000	6.419	1.442	3.562	9.275
	Equal variances not assumed			4.388	103.281	.000	6.419	1.463	3.518	9.320
Max Cranial Breadth	Equal variances assumed	1.475	.227	3.773	118	.000	4.914	1.302	2.335	7.493
	Equal variances not assumed			3.954	114.383	.000	4.914	1.243	2.452	7.376
Cranial Height	Equal variances assumed	.453	.503	3.564	81	.001	6.227	1.747	2.750	9.703
	Equal variances not assumed			3.364	56.350	.001	6.227	1.851	2.519	9.935
Facial Height n-gn	Equal variances assumed	.337	.563	4.276	74	.000	7.796	1.823	4.163	11.430
	Equal variances not assumed			4.231	62.211	.000	7.796	1.843	4.113	11.480
Facial Width zy-zy	Equal variances assumed	.021	.885	5.921	87	.000	7.299	1.233	4.849	9.749
	Equal variances not assumed			5.902	84.558	.000	7.299	1.237	4.840	9.758
FMT Width	Equal variances assumed	.015	.904	2.017	103	.046	2.377	1.179	.040	4.715
	Equal variances not assumed			2.071	100.980	.041	2.377	1.148	.100	4.654
Upper Facial Height n-pr	Equal variances assumed	.014	.908	4.042	99	.000	3.882	.960	1.976	5.788
	Equal variances not assumed			4.025	92.812	.000	3.882	.964	1.967	5.797
Maxilloalveolar Length pr-alv	Equal variances assumed	.416	.521	3.604	67	.001	3.084	.856	1.376	4.793
	Equal variances not assumed			3.567	58.102	.001	3.084	.865	1.354	4.815
Maxilloalveolar Breadth ect-ect	Equal variances assumed	3.148	.079	3.203	98	.002	3.334	1.041	1.268	5.399
	Equal variances not assumed			3.083	75.761	.003	3.334	1.081	1.180	5.487
Palatal Length ol-sta	Equal variances assumed	.015	.903	2.555	104	.012	2.034	.796	.455	3.612
	Equal variances not assumed			2.551	94.410	.012	2.034	.797	.451	3.616
Palatal Breadth enm-enm	Equal variances assumed	.026	.873	1.208	101	.230	1.158	.958	-.743	3.058
	Equal variances not assumed			1.217	92.898	.227	1.158	.951	-.731	3.047
Bicondylar Breadth cdl-cdl	Equal variances assumed	.020	.888	2.998	82	.004	4.637	1.547	1.560	7.714
	Equal variances not assumed			2.995	73.136	.004	4.637	1.548	1.551	7.722
Bigonial Breadth go-go	Equal variances assumed	.987	.323	5.861	107	.000	8.442	1.440	5.586	11.298
	Equal variances not assumed			6.038	103.435	.000	8.442	1.398	5.669	11.215
Height of Ascending Ramus Right go-cdl	Equal variances assumed	.798	.374	3.435	94	.001	3.444	1.003	1.453	5.434
	Equal variances not assumed			3.534	86.507	.001	3.444	.974	1.507	5.381
Min Breadth of Ascending Ramus Right	Equal variances assumed	.933	.336	3.150	100	.002	1.770	.562	.655	2.886
	Equal variances not assumed			3.244	93.970	.002	1.770	.546	.687	2.854
Height at Mandibular Symphysis gn-idi	Equal variances assumed	.181	.671	4.044	99	.000	3.057	.756	1.557	4.558
	Equal variances not assumed			4.032	82.701	.000	3.057	.758	1.549	4.566

Craniometrics, all skulls, Macedonian versus English.

		Levene's Test for Equality of Variances		t-test for Equality of Means					95% Confidence Interval of the Difference	
		F	Sig.	t	df	Sig. (2-tailed)	Mean Difference	Std. Error Difference	Lower	Upper
Max Cranial Length	Equal variances assumed	.481	.489	2.383	115	.019	3.619	1.519	.611	6.628
	Equal variances not assumed			2.384	114.286	.019	3.619	1.518	.611	6.627
Max Cranial Breadth	Equal variances assumed	2.975	.087	1.419	118	.159	1.931	1.361	-.764	4.625
	Equal variances not assumed			1.460	107.884	.147	1.931	1.322	-.690	4.551
Cranial Height	Equal variances assumed	.067	.796	-.248	81	.805	-.470	1.896	-4.241	3.302
	Equal variances not assumed			-.257	76.131	.798	-.470	1.830	-4.115	3.176
Facial Height n-gn	Equal variances assumed	.513	.476	1.500	74	.138	2.958	1.972	-.972	6.888
	Equal variances not assumed			1.501	73.936	.138	2.958	1.971	-.970	6.885
Facial Width zy-zy	Equal variances assumed	.207	.651	.402	87	.689	.585	1.457	-2.310	3.480
	Equal variances not assumed			.402	86.285	.689	.585	1.458	-2.312	3.483
FMT Width	Equal variances assumed	4.459	.037	2.254	103	.026	2.726	1.210	.327	5.125
	Equal variances not assumed			1.950	51.157	.057	2.726	1.398	-.080	5.532
Upper Facial Height n-pr	Equal variances assumed	.280	.598	-1.188	99	.237	-1.219	1.026	-3.254	.816
	Equal variances not assumed			-1.177	91.970	.242	-1.219	1.036	-3.276	.838
Maxilloalveolar Length pr-alv	Equal variances assumed	.005	.944	-.468	67	.641	-.449	.959	-2.363	1.464
	Equal variances not assumed			-.470	50.445	.641	-.449	.956	-2.369	1.470
Maxilloalveolar Breadth ect-ect	Equal variances assumed	8.683	.004	-.003	98	.998	-.003	1.128	-2.243	2.236
	Equal variances not assumed			-.003	52.367	.998	-.003	1.263	-2.538	2.531
Palatal Length ol-sta	Equal variances assumed	.444	.507	1.874	104	.064	1.579	.842	-.092	3.249
	Equal variances not assumed			1.805	63.945	.076	1.579	.875	-.169	3.326
Palatal Breadth enm-enm	Equal variances assumed	5.054	.027	-2.655	101	.009	-2.562	.965	-4.476	-.648
	Equal variances not assumed			-2.306	49.246	.025	-2.562	1.111	-4.795	-.330
Bicondylar Breadth cdl-cdl	Equal variances assumed	.172	.680	-2.411	82	.018	-3.853	1.598	-7.033	-.673
	Equal variances not assumed			-2.457	69.752	.017	-3.853	1.568	-6.982	-.725
Bigonial Breadth go-go	Equal variances assumed	1.335	.251	-1.153	107	.251	-1.881	1.632	-5.116	1.353
	Equal variances not assumed			-1.171	105.579	.244	-1.881	1.607	-5.068	1.305
Height of Ascending Ramus Right go-cdl	Equal variances assumed	.926	.338	.280	94	.780	.305	1.087	-1.854	2.463
	Equal variances not assumed			.269	60.303	.789	.305	1.133	-1.962	2.571
Min Breadth of Ascending Ramus Right	Equal variances assumed	.028	.867	-.264	100	.792	-.158	.597	-1.343	1.027
	Equal variances not assumed			-.261	74.750	.795	-.158	.605	-1.364	1.048
Height at Mandibular Symphysis gn-idi	Equal variances assumed	3.695	.057	1.511	99	.134	1.231	.815	-.386	2.847
	Equal variances not assumed			1.381	58.255	.173	1.231	.891	-.553	3.014

Craniometrics, normal skulls, Macedonian versus English.

		Levene's Test for Equality of Variances		t-test for Equality of Means					95% Confidence Interval of the Difference	
		F	Sig.	t	df	Sig. (2-tailed)	Mean Difference	Std. Error Difference	Lower	Upper
Max Cranial Length	Equal variances assumed	.056	.814	1.946	48	.058	4.474	2.300	-.150	9.098
	Equal variances not assumed			1.963	46.608	.056	4.474	2.279	-.112	9.060
Max Cranial Breadth	Equal variances assumed	.320	.574	2.417	50	.019	3.270	1.353	.553	5.987
	Equal variances not assumed			2.454	49.437	.018	3.270	1.332	.593	5.947
Cranial Height	Equal variances assumed	1.249	.272	.263	33	.794	.685	2.606	-4.618	5.988
	Equal variances not assumed			.247	18.903	.808	.685	2.778	-5.132	6.501
Facial Height n-gn	Equal variances assumed	1.375	.253	2.030	22	.055	5.343	2.632	-.116	10.802
	Equal variances not assumed			2.220	21.140	.038	5.343	2.407	.339	10.347

Measurement		F	Sig.	t	df	Sig. (2-tailed)	Mean Difference	Std. Error Difference	Lower	Upper
Facial Width zy-zy	Equal variances assumed	2.099	.157	.743	34	.463	1.575	2.120	-2.733	5.883
	Equal variances not assumed			.786	31.472	.438	1.575	2.005	-2.511	5.661
FMT Width	Equal variances assumed	3.354	.074	2.275	42	.028	5.125	2.253	.578	9.672
	Equal variances not assumed			1.856	17.890	.080	5.125	2.762	-.679	10.929
Upper Facial Height enm-enm	Equal variances assumed	1.693	.201	.407	38	.686	.698	1.716	-2.776	4.173
	Equal variances not assumed			.415	36.808	.681	.698	1.682	-2.711	4.107
Maxilloalveolar Length pr-alv	Equal variances assumed	1.925	.175	-1.033	30	.310	-1.673	1.619	-4.980	1.634
	Equal variances not assumed			-1.200	25.442	.241	-1.673	1.394	-4.541	1.196
Maxilloalveolar Breadth ect-ect	Equal variances assumed	2.707	.108	.011	39	.991	.023	2.079	-4.182	4.228
	Equal variances not assumed			.010	17.045	.992	.023	2.290	-4.807	4.853
Palatal Length ol-sta	Equal variances assumed	1.919	.173	2.168	41	.036	3.384	1.561	.232	6.535
	Equal variances not assumed			1.819	13.497	.091	3.384	1.860	-.620	7.387
Palatal Breadth enm-enm	Equal variances assumed	.986	.326	-1.110	41	.274	-1.634	1.473	-4.609	1.340
	Equal variances not assumed			-1.040	17.767	.312	-1.634	1.572	-4.939	1.671
Bicondylar Breadth cdl-cdl	Equal variances assumed	.197	.661	-.830	25	.414	-2.389	2.877	-8.315	3.537
	Equal variances not assumed			-.847	16.961	.409	-2.389	2.822	-8.343	3.565
Bigonial Breadth go-go	Equal variances assumed	.688	.412	.681	36	.500	1.617	2.375	-3.199	6.434
	Equal variances not assumed			.706	33.488	.485	1.617	2.291	-3.040	6.275
Height of Ascending Ramus Right go-cdl	Equal variances assumed	.177	.677	.720	33	.476	1.235	1.714	-2.253	4.723
	Equal variances not assumed			.767	22.834	.451	1.235	1.609	-2.095	4.565
Min Breadth of Ascending Ramus Right	Equal variances assumed	.495	.486	.573	35	.571	.523	.914	-1.332	2.379
	Equal variances not assumed			.612	25.898	.546	.523	.855	-1.235	2.282
Height at Mandibular Symphysis gn-idi	Equal variances assumed	.542	.467	2.382	36	.023	3.077	1.292	.457	5.698
	Equal variances not assumed			2.464	30.197	.020	3.077	1.249	.527	5.628

English v. Macedonian craniometrics, by sex.

Sex				Levene's Test for Equality of Variances		t-test for Equality of Means				95% Confidence Interval of the Difference	
				F	Sig.	t	df	Sig. (2-tailed)	Mean Difference	Std. Error Difference	Lower	Upper
Female	Max Cranial Length		Equal variances assumed	2.140	.150	2.813	51	.007	6.097	2.167	1.746	10.448
			Equal variances not assumed			2.763	43.361	.008	6.097	2.206	1.649	10.546
	Max Cranial Breadth		Equal variances assumed	3.891	.054	.895	51	.375	1.326	1.481	-1.647	4.298
			Equal variances not assumed			.870	37.421	.390	1.326	1.524	-1.761	4.413
	Cranial Height		Equal variances assumed	.266	.610	.617	33	.541	2.000	3.240	-4.591	8.591
			Equal variances not assumed			.646	29.077	.523	2.000	3.094	-4.327	8.327
	Facial Height n-gn		Equal variances assumed	1.367	.252	-.167	29	.869	-.504	3.026	-6.694	5.685
			Equal variances not assumed			-.177	27.590	.861	-.504	2.857	-6.361	5.352
	Facial Width zy-zy		Equal variances assumed	.975	.329	.443	40	.660	.833	1.882	-2.970	4.637
			Equal variances not assumed			.419	28.045	.679	.833	1.990	-3.242	4.909
	FMT Width		Equal variances assumed	1.372	.248	2.173	46	.035	2.993	1.377	.221	5.765
			Equal variances not assumed			2.118	37.800	.041	2.993	1.413	.131	5.855

	Measurement											
	Upper Facial Height n-pr	Equal variances assumed	1.223	.275	-.637	43	.528	-.947	1.488	-3.948	2.053
		Equal variances not assumed			-.666	42.967	.509	-.947	1.422	-3.815	1.920
	Maxilloalveolar Length pr-alv	Equal variances assumed	1.331	.259	-1.095	27	.283	-1.520	1.388	-4.368	1.328
		Equal variances not assumed			-1.047	18.343	.309	-1.520	1.452	-4.567	1.527
	Maxilloalveolar Breadth ect-ect	Equal variances assumed	3.597	.065	.068	41	.946	.125	1.839	-3.589	3.839
		Equal variances not assumed			.065	29.326	.949	.125	1.932	-3.824	4.074
	Palatal Length ol-sta	Equal variances assumed	.017	.897	.873	43	.387	1.077	1.233	-1.410	3.564
		Equal variances not assumed			.887	40.983	.380	1.077	1.214	-1.374	3.528
	Palatal Breadth enm-enm	Equal variances assumed	.118	.733	-1.522	41	.136	-2.151	1.413	-5.005	.703
		Equal variances not assumed			-1.476	33.004	.150	-2.151	1.458	-5.118	.815
	Bicondylar Breadth cdl-cdl	Equal variances assumed	3.988	.054	-2.133	33	.040	-4.829	2.264	-9.436	-.222
		Equal variances not assumed			-2.233	29.081	.033	-4.829	2.162	-9.251	-.407
	Bigonial Breadth go-go	Equal variances assumed	.029	.866	-1.090	43	.282	-2.156	1.979	-6.146	1.834
		Equal variances not assumed			-1.090	42.963	.282	-2.156	1.978	-6.145	1.833
	Height of Ascending Ramus Right go-cdl	Equal variances assumed	2.003	.166	.922	36	.362	1.328	1.439	-1.592	4.247
		Equal variances not assumed			.894	28.790	.379	1.328	1.486	-1.712	4.368
	Min Breadth of Ascending Ramus Right	Equal variances assumed	.064	.801	-.864	39	.393	-.687	.795	-2.294	.921
		Equal variances not assumed			-.853	35.575	.399	-.687	.805	-2.319	.946
	Height at Mandibular Symphysis gn-idi	Equal variances assumed	5.103	.030	1.739	38	.090	2.020	1.162	-.331	4.372
		Equal variances not assumed			1.650	25.761	.111	2.020	1.224	-.497	4.538
Male	Max Cranial Length	Equal variances assumed	.141	.709	.286	62	.776	.524	1.831	-3.137	4.185
		Equal variances not assumed			.287	59.182	.775	.524	1.823	-3.123	4.171
	Max Cranial Breadth	Equal variances assumed	.712	.402	.727	65	.470	1.479	2.035	-2.585	5.543
		Equal variances not assumed			.780	64.194	.438	1.479	1.896	-2.308	5.266
	Cranial Height	Equal variances assumed	1.822	.184	-1.905	46	.063	-3.615	1.898	-7.435	.205
		Equal variances not assumed			-2.050	40.427	.047	-3.615	1.764	-7.178	-.052
	Facial Height n-gn	Equal variances assumed	1.113	.297	1.178	43	.245	2.722	2.311	-1.939	7.383
		Equal variances not assumed			1.208	39.569	.234	2.722	2.254	-1.834	7.279
	Facial Width zy-zy	Equal variances assumed	.006	.939	-.814	45	.420	-1.353	1.663	-4.704	1.997
		Equal variances not assumed			-.820	44.016	.417	-1.353	1.651	-4.681	1.974
	FMT Width	Equal variances assumed	1.308	.258	.904	55	.370	1.781	1.969	-2.165	5.727
		Equal variances not assumed			.673	18.501	.509	1.781	2.645	-3.765	7.327
	Upper Facial Height n-pr	Equal variances assumed	1.669	.202	-2.436	54	.018	-3.038	1.247	-5.539	-.537
		Equal variances not assumed			-2.557	48.615	.014	-3.038	1.188	-5.426	-.650
	Maxilloalveolar Length pr-alv	Equal variances assumed	.105	.748	.163	38	.871	.187	1.145	-2.132	2.505
		Equal variances not assumed			.162	26.313	.872	.187	1.152	-2.179	2.553

		Levene's Test for Equality of Variances		t-test for Equality of Means						
		F	Sig.	t	df	Sig. (2-tailed)	Mean Difference	Std. Error Difference	95% Confidence Interval of the Difference	
									Lower	Upper
Maxilloalveolar Breadth ect-ect	Equal variances assumed	4.155	.046	-.844	55	.402	-1.101	1.305	-3.717	1.514
	Equal variances not assumed			-.737	23.176	.469	-1.101	1.495	-4.193	1.990
Palatal Length ol-sta	Equal variances assumed	.697	.407	1.292	59	.201	1.480	1.145	-.812	3.772
	Equal variances not assumed			1.119	22.724	.275	1.480	1.322	-1.257	4.217
Palatal Breadth enm-enm	Equal variances assumed	7.037	.010	-2.567	58	.013	-3.430	1.336	-6.104	-.755
	Equal variances not assumed			-1.968	19.391	.064	-3.430	1.743	-7.072	.213
Bicondylar Breadth cdl-cdl	Equal variances assumed	.882	.352	-2.115	47	.040	-4.339	2.051	-8.465	-.213
	Equal variances not assumed			-1.945	24.323	.063	-4.339	2.230	-8.939	.261
Bigonial Breadth go-go	Equal variances assumed	3.849	.054	-1.755	62	.084	-3.490	1.989	-7.465	.485
	Equal variances not assumed			-1.909	61.826	.061	-3.490	1.828	-7.145	.164
Height of Ascending Ramus Right go-cdl	Equal variances assumed	.096	.757	-1.028	56	.308	-1.496	1.455	-4.412	1.419
	Equal variances not assumed			-1.056	31.804	.299	-1.496	1.417	-4.383	1.390
Min Breadth of Ascending Ramus Right	Equal variances assumed	.165	.686	-.314	59	.755	-.257	.819	-1.896	1.382
	Equal variances not assumed			-.305	32.577	.763	-.257	.843	-1.973	1.459
Height at Mandibular Symphysis gn-idi	Equal variances assumed	1.933	.170	.011	59	.991	.011	1.016	-2.022	2.044
	Equal variances not assumed			.010	31.634	.992	.011	1.092	-2.215	2.237

Macedonian v. English Indices and Ratios, all skulls.

		Levene's Test for Equality of Variances		t-test for Equality of Means						
		F	Sig.	t	df	Sig. (2-tailed)	Mean Difference	Std. Error Difference	95% Confidence Interval of the Difference	
									Lower	Upper
Cranial Index	Equal variances assumed	1.685	.197	-.848	112	.398	-.7605	.8964	-2.5367	1.0157
	Equal variances not assumed			-.857	106.823	.393	-.7605	.8873	-2.5196	.9986
Cranial Module	Equal variances assumed	.018	.893	1.859	76	.067	2.64221	1.42167	-.18930	5.47372
	Equal variances not assumed			1.881	69.609	.064	2.64221	1.40440	-.15905	5.44347
Cranial length-height Index	Equal variances assumed	1.065	.305	-1.992	78	.050	-1.84185	.92452	-3.68242	-.00128
	Equal variances not assumed			-2.129	77.912	.036	-1.84185	.86524	-3.56443	-.11927
Cranial breadth-height Index	Equal variances assumed	2.473	.120	-1.406	78	.164	-1.84897	1.31472	-4.46637	.76842
	Equal variances not assumed			-1.528	77.963	.131	-1.84897	1.21033	-4.25857	.56063
Total Facial Index	Equal variances assumed	.657	.421	.849	65	.399	1.28723	1.51598	-1.74040	4.31485
	Equal variances not assumed			.866	64.270	.390	1.28723	1.48705	-1.68325	4.25771
Upper Facial Index	Equal variances assumed	.333	.566	-.511	80	.611	-.33741	.66050	-1.65184	.97701
	Equal variances not assumed			-.513	79.358	.610	-.33741	.65823	-1.64750	.97267
Maxilloalveolar Index	Equal variances assumed	.274	.602	-.375	63	.709	-1.10023	2.93653	-6.96841	4.76796
	Equal variances not assumed			-.362	41.047	.719	-1.10023	3.04035	-7.24011	5.03966
Palatal Index	Equal variances assumed	7.094	.009	-3.378	99	.001	-8.68402	2.57055	-13.78455	-3.58349
	Equal variances not assumed			-2.829	44.254	.007	-8.68402	3.06942	-14.86902	-2.49901
Palatal/max ratio	Equal variances assumed	8.282	.006	-1.816	61	.074	-.05886	.03241	-.12366	.00594
	Equal variances not assumed			-1.458	25.005	.157	-.05886	.04036	-.14199	.02427
TFHFMT	Equal variances assumed	.881	.351	-.209	63	.835	-.61906	2.96063	-6.53541	5.29729
	Equal variances not assumed			-.193	37.981	.848	-.61906	3.21072	-7.11892	5.88080
UFHFMT	Equal variances assumed	.642	.425	-1.527	85	.130	-1.55549	1.01850	-3.58054	.46956
	Equal variances not assumed			-1.490	66.670	.141	-1.55549	1.04422	-3.63995	.52897
MAXBCDL	Equal variances assumed	3.432	.069	1.145	63	.257	.01489	.01301	-.01110	.04088
	Equal variances not assumed			.961	24.473	.346	.01489	.01549	-.01706	.04683
cdlgo	Equal variances assumed	.869	.354	.375	82	.708	.00491	.01307	-.02109	.03091
	Equal variances not assumed			.358	56.309	.721	.00491	.01369	-.02251	.03233
ZYGFMT	Equal variances assumed	.311	.579	.104	75	.917	.00098	.00940	-.01775	.01971

		F	Sig.	t	df	Sig.	Mean Difference	Std. Error Difference	Lower	Upper
	Equal variances not assumed			.105	71.931	.916	.00098	.00928	-.01753	.01949
UHTH	Equal variances assumed	.045	.833	-2.540	72	.013	-.02095	.00825	-.03740	-.00451
	Equal variances not assumed			-2.548	71.799	.013	-.02095	.00822	-.03735	-.00456
FB	Equal variances assumed	.777	.382	-3.234	58	.002	-.03201	.00990	-.05183	-.01220
	Equal variances not assumed			-3.274	57.889	.002	-.03201	.00978	-.05159	-.01244
FB2	Equal variances assumed	1.377	.245	2.394	66	.020	.04339	.01813	.00720	.07958
	Equal variances not assumed			1.952	26.832	.061	.04339	.02222	-.00222	.08900
UFIMAI	Equal variances assumed	3.321	.075	-.136	49	.893	-.00184	.01360	-.02917	.02548
	Equal variances not assumed			-.122	27.973	.904	-.00184	.01508	-.03273	.02905

Macedonian v. English indices and ratios, by sex

Sex			Levene's Test for Equality of Variances		t-test for Equality of Means					95% Confidence Interval of the Difference	
			F	Sig.	t	df	Sig. (2-tailed)	Mean Difference	Std. Error Difference	Lower	Upper
Female	Cranial Index	Equal variances assumed	1.309	.258	-2.195	50	.033	-2.1662	.9867	-4.1481	-.1843
		Equal variances not assumed			-2.134	39.826	.039	-2.1662	1.0149	-4.2177	-.1147
	Cranial Module	Equal variances assumed	1.775	.192	2.412	32	.022	4.42593	1.83463	.68891	8.16294
		Equal variances not assumed			2.492	27.029	.019	4.42593	1.77620	.78166	8.07019
	Cranial length-height Index	Equal variances assumed	.882	.354	-1.336	33	.191	-2.30404	1.72408	-5.81171	1.20362
		Equal variances not assumed			-1.398	29.293	.173	-2.30404	1.64800	-5.67312	1.06503
	Cranial breadth-height Index	Equal variances assumed	.457	.504	-.412	32	.683	-.89494	2.17002	-5.31513	3.52526
		Equal variances not assumed			-.421	30.589	.677	-.89494	2.12699	-5.23534	3.44546
	Total Facial Index	Equal variances assumed	1.254	.272	-.302	28	.765	-.83941	2.77718	-6.52820	4.84937
		Equal variances not assumed			-.336	27.259	.740	-.83941	2.49949	-5.96566	4.28683
	Upper Facial Index	Equal variances assumed	.949	.336	-.646	37	.522	-.62137	.96240	-2.57139	1.32864
		Equal variances not assumed			-.694	36.949	.492	-.62137	.89574	-2.43639	1.19365
	Maxilloalveolar Index	Equal variances assumed	.132	.719	-.236	26	.815	-1.05840	4.48470	-10.27682	8.16003
		Equal variances not assumed			-.230	17.453	.820	-1.05840	4.59353	-10.73079	8.61399
	Palatal Index	Equal variances assumed	.238	.628	-1.778	41	.083	-6.18353	3.47707	-13.20561	.83855
		Equal variances not assumed			-1.710	31.312	.097	-6.18353	3.61684	-13.55714	1.19008
	Palatal/max ratio	Equal variances assumed	.018	.895	-.089	25	.930	-.00312	.03516	-.07553	.06929
		Equal variances not assumed			-.093	21.553	.927	-.00312	.03368	-.07305	.06681
	TFHFMT	Equal variances assumed	.213	.648	-.795	25	.434	-2.57130	3.23604	-9.23605	4.09344
		Equal variances not assumed			-.800	24.261	.432	-2.57130	3.21437	-9.20167	4.05906
	UFHFMT	Equal variances assumed	1.104	.300	-1.364	38	.181	-2.07524	1.52168	-5.15571	1.00524
		Equal variances not assumed			-1.378	37.560	.176	-2.07524	1.50544	-5.12402	.97355
	MAXBCDL	Equal variances assumed	1.402	.247	1.401	26	.173	.02831	.02020	-.01322	.06984
		Equal variances not assumed			1.256	14.495	.229	.02831	.02254	-.01988	.07651
	cdlgo	Equal variances assumed	.180	.674	.219	33	.828	.00373	.01703	-.03092	.03839
		Equal variances not assumed			.218	31.498	.829	.00373	.01710	-.03111	.03858
	ZYGFMT	Equal variances assumed	.020	.889	.764	34	.450	.01119	.01465	-.01859	.04097
		Equal variances not assumed			.764	33.191	.451	.01119	.01465	-.01862	.04099
	UHTH	Equal variances assumed	.167	.686	-.144	29	.887	-.00216	.01506	-.03297	.02864
		Equal variances not assumed			-.145	24.314	.886	-.00216	.01491	-.03292	.02859
	FB	Equal variances assumed	6.032	.021	-3.963	28	.000	-.05641	.01423	-.08556	-.02725
		Equal variances not assumed			-3.806	18.820	.001	-.05641	.01482	-.08744	-.02537

Male	FB2	Equal variances assumed	.513	.480	2.517	28	.018	.04783	.01900	.00890	.08676
		Equal variances not assumed			2.514	23.629	.019	.04783	.01903	.00853	.08714
	UFIMAI	Equal variances assumed	3.374	.080	-.420	21	.678	-.00608	.01446	-.03615	.02399
		Equal variances not assumed			-.372	11.151	.717	-.00608	.01636	-.04202	.02986
	Cranial Index	Equal variances assumed	.353	.554	.285	60	.776	.4096	1.4361	-2.4630	3.2823
		Equal variances not assumed			.293	59.860	.770	.4096	1.3967	-2.3844	3.2036
	Cranial Module	Equal variances assumed	1.473	.232	-.054	42	.957	-.08929	1.63855	-3.39600	3.21743
		Equal variances not assumed			-.059	39.099	.953	-.08929	1.50876	-3.14079	2.96222
	Cranial length-height Index	Equal variances assumed	.224	.639	-1.648	43	.107	-1.59004	.96472	-3.53557	.35550
		Equal variances not assumed			-1.712	37.951	.095	-1.59004	.92892	-3.47062	.29054
	Cranial breadth-height Index	Equal variances assumed	4.146	.048	-1.733	44	.090	-2.88059	1.66243	-6.23101	.46982
		Equal variances not assumed			-2.122	43.458	.040	-2.88059	1.35750	-5.61742	-.14377
	Total Facial Index	Equal variances assumed	.359	.553	1.609	35	.117	2.73337	1.69897	-.71571	6.18246
		Equal variances not assumed			1.606	33.803	.118	2.73337	1.70193	-.72611	6.19286
	Upper Facial Index	Equal variances assumed	.059	.810	-.201	41	.841	-.19028	.94450	-2.09774	1.71718
		Equal variances not assumed			-.202	39.079	.841	-.19028	.94244	-2.09642	1.71586
	Maxilloalveolar Index	Equal variances assumed	.414	.524	-.280	35	.781	-1.11248	3.97390	-9.17992	6.95496
		Equal variances not assumed			-.266	21.491	.792	-1.11248	4.17642	-9.78574	7.56078
	Palatal Index	Equal variances assumed	12.174	.001	-2.892	56	.005	-11.10441	3.84001	-18.79687	-3.41195
		Equal variances not assumed			-2.071	17.046	.054	-11.10441	5.36088	-22.41257	.20375
	Palatal/max ratio	Equal variances assumed	16.636	.000	-2.115	34	.042	-.10501	.04964	-.20589	-.00413
		Equal variances not assumed			-1.556	11.829	.146	-.10501	.06750	-.25230	.04229
	TFHFMT	Equal variances assumed	2.208	.146	-.218	36	.829	-1.01347	4.64948	-10.44306	8.41611
		Equal variances not assumed			-.168	13.594	.869	-1.01347	6.02620	-13.97474	11.94779
	UFHFMT	Equal variances assumed	.012	.915	-1.494	45	.142	-2.08770	1.39764	-4.90270	.72730
		Equal variances not assumed			-1.480	24.091	.152	-2.08770	1.41026	-4.99775	.82235
	MAXBCDL	Equal variances assumed	2.545	.120	.343	35	.733	.00606	.01765	-.02977	.04188
		Equal variances not assumed			.275	8.834	.790	.00606	.02207	-.04400	.05612
	cdlgo	Equal variances assumed	1.855	.180	-.233	47	.817	-.00415	.01778	-.03991	.03162
		Equal variances not assumed			-.209	23.051	.836	-.00415	.01981	-.04512	.03683
	ZYGFMT	Equal variances assumed	.082	.777	-.239	39	.812	-.00275	.01149	-.02600	.02049
		Equal variances not assumed			-.236	28.162	.815	-.00275	.01165	-.02661	.02110
	UHTH	Equal variances assumed	1.927	.173	-3.776	41	.001	-.03582	.00949	-.05498	-.01666
		Equal variances not assumed			-4.310	40.990	.000	-.03582	.00831	-.05261	-.01904
	FB	Equal variances assumed	1.024	.320	-.424	28	.675	-.00539	.01272	-.03144	.02066
		Equal variances not assumed			-.411	21.294	.685	-.00539	.01310	-.03261	.02184
	FB2	Equal variances assumed	5.115	.030	1.590	36	.121	.04755	.02990	-.01310	.10819
		Equal variances not assumed			1.074	9.896	.308	.04755	.04425	-.05119	.14629
	UFIMAI	Equal variances assumed	3.325	.080	.080	26	.937	.00170	.02134	-.04217	.04557
		Equal variances not assumed			.071	14.220	.944	.00170	.02394	-.04958	.05298

Macedonian v. English indices and ratios, normal skulls.

Sex			Levene's Test for Equality of Variances		t-test for Equality of Means					95% Confidence Interval of the Difference	
			F	Sig.	t	df	Sig. (2-tailed)	Mean Difference	Std. Error Difference	Lower	Upper
Female	Max Cranial Length	Equal variances assumed	.429	.520	2.066	20	.052	5.783	2.799	-.055	11.621
		Equal variances not assumed			2.082	19.747	.051	5.783	2.778	-.016	11.583
	Max Cranial Breadth	Equal variances assumed	.045	.834	1.136	19	.270	1.722	1.516	-1.451	4.895
		Equal variances not assumed			1.167	18.717	.258	1.722	1.476	-1.370	4.814
	Cranial Height	Equal variances assumed	1.514	.242	.229	12	.823	.833	3.646	-7.110	8.777
		Equal variances not assumed			.215	8.241	.835	.833	3.870	-8.046	9.713
	Facial Height n-gn	Equal variances assumed	22.615	.009	-.481	4	.656	-2.250	4.679	-15.240	10.740
		Equal variances not assumed			-.316	1.064	.802	-2.250	7.111	-80.648	76.148
	Facial Width zy-zy	Equal variances assumed	3.318	.090	.037	14	.971	.125	3.396	-7.159	7.409
		Equal variances not assumed			.037	7.917	.972	.125	3.396	-7.721	7.971
	FMT Width	Equal variances assumed	3.161	.092	1.205	18	.244	2.500	2.074	-1.858	6.858
		Equal variances not assumed			1.205	14.992	.247	2.500	2.074	-1.922	6.922
	Upper Facial Height enm-enm	Equal variances assumed	.285	.601	-.436	15	.669	-1.057	2.422	-6.221	4.106
		Equal variances not assumed			-.474	14.891	.643	-1.057	2.231	-5.816	3.701
	Maxilloalveolar Length pr-alv	Equal variances assumed	.003	.954	-1.391	9	.198	-3.929	2.824	-10.317	2.460
		Equal variances not assumed			-1.412	6.652	.203	-3.929	2.783	-10.579	2.722
	Maxilloalveolar Breadth ect-ect	Equal variances assumed	.071	.793	-.958	14	.354	-3.233	3.376	-10.473	4.007
		Equal variances not assumed			-.924	9.538	.378	-3.233	3.497	-11.078	4.611
	Palatal Length ol-sta	Equal variances assumed	.014	.909	.676	15	.510	1.515	2.243	-3.266	6.296
		Equal variances not assumed			.670	10.139	.518	1.515	2.263	-3.517	6.547
	Palatal Breadth enm-enm	Equal variances assumed	.000	.990	-.718	15	.484	-1.818	2.533	-7.217	3.581
		Equal variances not assumed			-.738	11.266	.475	-1.818	2.462	-7.222	3.586
	Bicondylar Breadth cdl-cdl	Equal variances assumed	4.552	.065	-.773	8	.462	-3.600	4.658	-14.342	7.142
		Equal variances not assumed			-.773	4.491	.478	-3.600	4.658	-15.994	8.794
	Bigonial Breadth go-go	Equal variances assumed	.078	.784	.151	12	.883	.571	3.793	-7.693	8.836
		Equal variances not assumed			.151	11.273	.883	.571	3.793	-7.753	8.895
	Height of Ascending Ramus Right go-cdl	Equal variances assumed	.813	.389	.582	10	.573	1.429	2.454	-4.040	6.898
		Equal variances not assumed			.604	9.725	.560	1.429	2.366	-3.863	6.721
	Min Breadth of Ascending Ramus Right	Equal variances assumed	.061	.809	-.532	11	.605	-.810	1.521	-4.157	2.538
		Equal variances not assumed			-.524	9.753	.612	-.810	1.546	-4.265	2.646
	Height at Mandibular Symphysis gn-idi	Equal variances assumed	1.918	.191	1.396	12	.188	2.286	1.637	-1.281	5.853
		Equal variances not assumed			1.396	11.043	.190	2.286	1.637	-1.316	5.887
Male	Max Cranial Length	Equal variances assumed	1.105	.303	.519	26	.608	1.789	3.444	-5.291	8.868
		Equal variances not assumed			.553	22.297	.586	1.789	3.236	-4.917	8.494
	Max Cranial Breadth	Equal variances assumed	.033	.857	1.608	29	.119	3.200	1.990	-.870	7.270
		Equal variances not assumed			1.639	21.906	.115	3.200	1.952	-.850	7.250
	Cranial Height	Equal variances assumed	2.016	.172	-.820	19	.423	-2.000	2.440	-7.106	3.106
		Equal variances not assumed			-1.062	17.160	.303	-2.000	1.883	-5.970	1.970
	Facial Height n-gn	Equal variances assumed	.711	.412	1.929	16	.072	5.333	2.765	-.527	11.194
		Equal variances not assumed			2.130	13.133	.053	5.333	2.504	-.070	10.737

125

Variable	Variance	F	Sig.	t	df	Sig. (2-tailed)	Mean Difference	Std. Error Difference	Lower	Upper
Facial Width zy-zy	Equal variances assumed	.480	.497	.801	18	.434	1.625	2.030	-2.639	5.889
	Equal variances not assumed			.810	15.768	.430	1.625	2.005	-2.631	5.881
FMT Width	Equal variances assumed	7.149	.014	2.072	22	.050	8.556	4.130	-.009	17.120
	Equal variances not assumed			1.278	5.289	.255	8.556	6.695	-8.376	25.487
Upper Facial Height enm-enm	Equal variances assumed	2.339	.141	-.061	21	.952	-.143	2.325	-4.978	4.693
	Equal variances not assumed			-.081	20.923	.936	-.143	1.762	-3.809	3.523
Maxilloalveolar Length pr-alv	Equal variances assumed	2.236	.151	-.456	19	.653	-.800	1.754	-4.470	2.870
	Equal variances not assumed			-.584	16.715	.567	-.800	1.370	-3.695	2.095
Maxilloalveolar Breadth ect-ect	Equal variances assumed	10.258	.004	.642	23	.527	1.579	2.460	-3.510	6.668
	Equal variances not assumed			.479	6.037	.649	1.579	3.295	-6.472	9.629
Palatal Length ol-sta	Equal variances assumed	3.905	.060	2.067	24	.050	4.629	2.239	.007	9.250
	Equal variances not assumed			1.349	4.460	.242	4.629	3.430	-4.520	13.777
Palatal Breadth enm-enm	Equal variances assumed	1.785	.194	-.992	24	.331	-1.833	1.848	-5.648	1.981
	Equal variances not assumed			-.803	6.449	.451	-1.833	2.283	-7.327	3.660
Bicondylar Breadth cdl-cdl	Equal variances assumed	1.276	.276	-.776	15	.450	-3.115	4.016	-11.676	5.445
	Equal variances not assumed			-.574	3.624	.600	-3.115	5.426	-18.817	12.586
Bigonial Breadth go-go	Equal variances assumed	.628	.437	.225	22	.824	.625	2.775	-5.131	6.381
	Equal variances not assumed			.244	17.373	.810	.625	2.566	-4.781	6.031
Height of Ascending Ramus Right go-cdl	Equal variances assumed	1.012	.326	.104	21	.918	.235	2.254	-4.452	4.922
	Equal variances not assumed			.118	11.255	.908	.235	1.998	-4.151	4.621
Min Breadth of Ascending Ramus Right	Equal variances assumed	1.575	.223	.776	22	.446	.889	1.145	-1.486	3.263
	Equal variances not assumed			1.027	16.078	.320	.889	.866	-.946	2.724
Height at Mandibular Symphysis gn-idi	Equal variances assumed	.010	.920	1.595	22	.125	3.025	1.897	-.909	6.960
	Equal variances not assumed			1.553	10.640	.150	3.025	1.948	-1.281	7.331

Part 4. Craniometrics with anomalies Independent Samples T-tests.

a. All skulls, anomalies and craniometrics

T-Test Supplemental teeth

Independent Samples Test

		Levene's Test for Equality of Variances		t-test for Equality of Means					
								95% Confidence Interval of the Difference	
		F	Sig.	t	df	Sig. (2-tailed)	Mean Difference	Std. Error Difference	
								Lower	Upper
Max Cranial Length	Equal variances assumed	.092	.763	-.504	115	.615	-3.022	5.990	-14.887	8.843
	Equal variances not assumed			-.544	1.041	.680	-3.022	5.556	-67.368	61.324
Max Cranial Breadth	Equal variances assumed	1.723	.192	1.553	118	.123	8.220	5.294	-2.263	18.704
	Equal variances not assumed			.820	1.009	.562	8.220	10.023	-116.434	132.875
Facial Height n-gn	Equal variances assumed			.676	74	.501	5.920	8.755	-11.525	23.365
	Equal variances not assumed						5.920			
Facial Width zy-zy	Equal variances assumed			-.727	87	.469	-5.011	6.894	-18.715	8.692
	Equal variances not assumed						-5.011			
FMT Width	Equal variances assumed	.362	.549	.106	103	.915	.466	4.379	-8.219	9.152
	Equal variances not assumed			.077	1.020	.951	.466	6.030	-72.658	73.590
Upper Facial Height n-pr	Equal variances assumed	1.292	.258	.623	99	.535	2.298	3.691	-5.026	9.622
	Equal variances not assumed			1.447	1.256	.348	2.298	1.588	-10.338	14.934
Maxilloalveolar Length pr-alv	Equal variances assumed			-.328	67	.744	-1.265	3.859	-8.967	6.438
	Equal variances not assumed						-1.265			
Maxilloalveolar Breadth ect-ect	Equal variances assumed	2.855	.094	-.802	98	.425	-3.092	3.856	-10.744	4.561
	Equal variances not assumed			-5.641	97.000	.000	-3.092	.548	-4.180	-2.004
Palatal Length ol-sta	Equal variances assumed	2.771	.099	-.413	104	.680	-1.231	2.979	-7.137	4.676
	Equal variances not assumed			-2.994	103.000	.003	-1.231	.411	-2.046	-.415
Palatal Breadth enm-enm	Equal variances assumed	1.731	.191	.000	101	1.000	.000	3.449	-6.842	6.842
	Equal variances not assumed			.000	100.000	1.000	.000	.483	-.958	.958
Bicondylar Breadth cdl-cdl	Equal variances assumed			.456	82	.650	3.373	7.397	-11.342	18.089
	Equal variances not assumed						3.373			
Bigonial Breadth go-go	Equal variances assumed	6.073	.015	1.869	107	.064	11.173	5.977	-.675	23.021
	Equal variances not assumed			.769	1.006	.582	11.173	14.522	-170.782	193.127
Height of Ascending Ramus Right go-cdl	Equal variances assumed	.039	.843	1.085	94	.281	3.926	3.619	-3.261	11.112
	Equal variances not assumed			.867	1.027	.542	3.926	4.530	-50.183	58.034
Min Breadth of Ascending Ramus Right	Equal variances assumed	.025	.876	-.461	100	.646	-.960	2.082	-5.090	3.170
	Equal variances not assumed			-.475	1.043	.715	-.960	2.021	-24.271	22.351
Height at Mandibular Symphysis gn-idi	Equal variances assumed	2.441	.121	.480	99	.632	1.374	2.862	-4.304	7.052
	Equal variances not assumed			3.394	98.000	.001	1.374	.405	.571	2.177

T-Test Rotations

Independent Samples Test

		Levene's Test for Equality of Variances		t-test for Equality of Means					
								95% Confidence Interval of the Difference	
		F	Sig.	t	df	Sig. (2-tailed)	Mean Difference	Std. Error Difference	Lower	Upper
Max Cranial Length	Equal variances assumed	.145	.704	2.260	115	.026	3.819	1.690	.471	7.167
	Equal variances not assumed			2.230	57.070	.030	3.819	1.712	.391	7.248
Max Cranial Breadth	Equal variances assumed	2.183	.142	.453	118	.651	.682	1.505	-2.298	3.663
	Equal variances not assumed			.364	43.327	.717	.682	1.873	-3.095	4.460

Measurement		F	Sig.	t	df	Sig. (2-tailed)	Mean Difference	Std. Error Difference	Lower	Upper
Cranial Height	Equal variances assumed	.469	.496	2.195	81	.031	4.366	1.989	.409	8.323
	Equal variances not assumed			2.471	56.317	.017	4.366	1.767	.827	7.905
Facial Height n-gn	Equal variances assumed	.115	.736	2.492	74	.015	4.930	1.979	.988	8.873
	Equal variances not assumed			2.518	61.479	.014	4.930	1.958	1.016	8.844
Facial Width zy-zy	Equal variances assumed	.104	.748	2.313	87	.023	3.435	1.485	.483	6.386
	Equal variances not assumed			2.260	57.480	.028	3.435	1.520	.392	6.478
FMT Width	Equal variances assumed	.103	.749	1.155	103	.251	1.537	1.330	-1.102	4.175
	Equal variances not assumed			1.273	62.628	.208	1.537	1.207	-.876	3.950
Upper Facial Height n-pr	Equal variances assumed	1.887	.173	1.064	99	.290	1.163	1.092	-1.005	3.330
	Equal variances not assumed			1.145	76.873	.256	1.163	1.015	-.859	3.184
Maxilloalveolar Length pr-alv	Equal variances assumed	.490	.486	1.197	67	.235	1.245	1.040	-.831	3.321
	Equal variances not assumed			1.294	34.798	.204	1.245	.962	-.709	3.199
Maxilloalveolar Breadth ect-ect	Equal variances assumed	1.899	.171	-.035	98	.972	-.042	1.194	-2.411	2.326
	Equal variances not assumed			-.040	70.510	.968	-.042	1.050	-2.136	2.051
Palatal Length ol-sta	Equal variances assumed	.419	.519	1.910	104	.059	1.708	.894	-.065	3.481
	Equal variances not assumed			2.052	58.613	.045	1.708	.833	.042	3.374
Palatal Breadth enm-enm	Equal variances assumed	.090	.765	.505	101	.615	.540	1.068	-1.580	2.659
	Equal variances not assumed			.561	60.752	.577	.540	.962	-1.383	2.463
Bicondylar Breadth cdl-cdl	Equal variances assumed	.000	.983	3.676	82	.000	5.804	1.579	2.663	8.945
	Equal variances not assumed			3.669	53.866	.001	5.804	1.582	2.632	8.975
Bigonial Breadth go-go	Equal variances assumed	.734	.394	1.648	107	.102	2.888	1.752	-.586	6.361
	Equal variances not assumed			1.564	54.283	.124	2.888	1.847	-.815	6.590
Height of Ascending Ramus Right go-cdl	Equal variances assumed	1.045	.309	2.913	94	.004	3.161	1.085	1.006	5.315
	Equal variances not assumed			2.722	46.017	.009	3.161	1.161	.823	5.498
Min Breadth of Ascending Ramus Right	Equal variances assumed	.073	.787	2.958	100	.004	1.817	.614	.598	3.035
	Equal variances not assumed			2.821	46.883	.007	1.817	.644	.521	3.113
Height at Mandibular Symphysis gn-idi	Equal variances assumed	.009	.924	2.376	99	.019	2.061	.867	.340	3.781
	Equal variances not assumed			2.317	46.628	.025	2.061	.889	.271	3.850

T-Test Reversals

Independent Samples Test

Measurement		Levene's Test for Equality of Variances		t-test for Equality of Means					95% Confidence Interval of the Difference	
		F	Sig.	t	df	Sig. (2-tailed)	Mean Difference	Std. Error Difference	Lower	Upper
Max Cranial Length	Equal variances assumed	.015	.904	2.169	115	.032	12.748	5.878	1.106	24.390
	Equal variances not assumed			2.107	1.033	.276	12.748	6.049	-58.537	84.033
Max Cranial Breadth	Equal variances assumed	1.461	.229	1.067	118	.288	5.678	5.322	-4.862	16.218
	Equal variances not assumed			6.663	8.182	.000	5.678	.852	3.721	7.635
Cranial Height	Equal variances assumed	1.807	.183	.286	81	.776	1.728	6.049	-10.306	13.763
	Equal variances not assumed			1.256	3.545	.285	1.728	1.376	-2.292	5.749
Facial Height n-gn	Equal variances assumed	1.606	.209	-.355	74	.724	-2.216	6.246	-14.662	10.230
	Equal variances not assumed			-.987	1.586	.450	-2.216	2.245	-14.746	10.314
Facial Width zy-zy	Equal variances assumed	.238	.627	.322	87	.749	1.580	4.915	-8.189	11.350
	Equal variances not assumed			.442	1.091	.730	1.580	3.577	-35.816	38.977
FMT Width	Equal variances assumed	.119	.731	.573	103	.568	2.505	4.373	-6.167	11.177
	Equal variances not assumed			.818	1.083	.555	2.505	3.060	-30.001	35.011
Upper Facial Height n-pr	Equal variances assumed	3.329	.071	.208	99	.836	.768	3.698	-6.569	8.105
	Equal variances not assumed			1.468	98.000	.145	.768	.523	-.270	1.806
Maxilloalveolar Length pr-alv	Equal variances assumed	.427	.516	.659	67	.512	1.806	2.742	-3.668	7.280
	Equal variances not assumed			.449	1.027	.730	1.806	4.027	-46.293	49.905

		F	Sig.	t	df	Sig. (2-tailed)	Mean Difference	Std. Error Difference	95% Confidence Interval of the Difference	
									Lower	Upper
Maxilloalveolar Breadth ect-ect	Equal variances assumed	2.880	.093	-.536	98	.593	-2.071	3.863	-9.738	5.595
	Equal variances not assumed			-3.772	97.000	.000	-2.071	.549	-3.161	-.982
Palatal Length ol-sta	Equal variances assumed	.007	.935	.271	104	.787	.808	2.980	-5.102	6.717
	Equal variances not assumed			.267	1.038	.833	.808	3.028	-34.524	36.139
Palatal Breadth enm-enm	Equal variances assumed	1.235	.269	-.148	101	.883	-.510	3.448	-7.351	6.331
	Equal variances not assumed			-.734	3.703	.507	-.510	.695	-2.502	1.483
Bicondylar Breadth cdl-cdl	Equal variances assumed	.367	.546	-.130	82	.897	-.683	5.268	-11.164	9.798
	Equal variances not assumed			-.167	1.085	.893	-.683	4.082	-43.893	42.527
Bigonial Breadth go-go	Equal variances assumed	2.708	.103	1.348	107	.181	8.117	6.023	-3.822	20.056
	Equal variances not assumed			4.749	1.684	.057	8.117	1.709	-.729	16.963
Height of Ascending Ramus Right go-cdl	Equal variances assumed	3.951	.050	-.184	94	.854	-.670	3.641	-7.900	6.560
	Equal variances not assumed			-1.268	93.000	.208	-.670	.528	-1.720	.379
Min Breadth of Ascending Ramus Right	Equal variances assumed	.856	.357	.029	100	.977	.060	2.084	-4.075	4.195
	Equal variances not assumed			.058	1.179	.962	.060	1.042	-9.260	9.380
Height at Mandibular Symphysis gn-idi	Equal variances assumed	.	.	-.164	99	.870	-.660	4.031	-8.658	7.338
	Equal variances not assumed			.	.	.	-.660	.	.	.

T-Test Misshape Teeth

Independent Samples Test

		Levene's Test for Equality of Variances		t-test for Equality of Means						
		F	Sig.	t	df	Sig. (2-tailed)	Mean Difference	Std. Error Difference	95% Confidence Interval of the Difference	
									Lower	Upper
Max Cranial Length	Equal variances assumed	.178	.674	-1.576	115	.118	-7.667	4.865	-17.304	1.971
	Equal variances not assumed			-1.863	2.152	.195	-7.667	4.116	-24.230	8.897
Max Cranial Breadth	Equal variances assumed	.699	.405	-1.961	118	.052	-8.462	4.315	-17.007	.084
	Equal variances not assumed			-4.276	2.585	.031	-8.462	1.979	-15.372	-1.551
Cranial Height	Equal variances assumed	.301	.585	-1.115	81	.268	-4.794	4.300	-13.350	3.762
	Equal variances not assumed			-1.459	3.573	.227	-4.794	3.287	-14.366	4.777
Facial Height n-gn	Equal variances assumed	.187	.667	-1.227	74	.224	-5.444	4.437	-14.285	3.396
	Equal variances not assumed			-1.388	3.453	.248	-5.444	3.922	-17.048	6.159
Facial Width zy-zy	Equal variances assumed	.417	.520	-.616	87	.539	-3.023	4.907	-12.777	6.731
	Equal variances not assumed			-.978	1.125	.492	-3.023	3.090	-33.348	27.302
FMT Width	Equal variances assumed	1.139	.288	.418	103	.677	1.500	3.590	-5.621	8.621
	Equal variances not assumed			1.279	3.771	.274	1.500	1.173	-1.835	4.835
Upper Facial Height n-pr	Equal variances assumed	1.334	.251	.198	99	.843	.523	2.642	-4.718	5.765
	Equal variances not assumed			.320	3.746	.766	.523	1.636	-4.144	5.191
Maxilloalveolar Length pr-alv	Equal variances assumed	.	.	.461	67	.646	1.779	3.856	-5.917	9.476
	Equal variances not assumed			.	.	.	1.779	.	.	.
Maxilloalveolar Breadth ect-ect	Equal variances assumed	1.693	.196	-.272	98	.786	-1.051	3.867	-8.726	6.624
	Equal variances not assumed			-.921	1.694	.469	-1.051	1.141	-6.918	4.816
Palatal Length ol-sta	Equal variances assumed	.245	.621	-.101	104	.919	-.216	2.128	-4.436	4.005
	Equal variances not assumed			-.141	3.499	.896	-.216	1.530	-4.714	4.283
Palatal Breadth enm-enm	Equal variances assumed	1.864	.175	-.317	101	.752	-.780	2.462	-5.664	4.104
	Equal variances not assumed			-.977	7.704	.358	-.780	.799	-2.635	1.074
Bicondylar Breadth cdl-cdl	Equal variances assumed	.025	.875	.721	82	.473	3.111	4.315	-5.473	11.695
	Equal variances not assumed			.590	2.098	.612	3.111	5.269	-18.576	24.799
Bigonial Breadth go-go	Equal variances assumed	.290	.591	-.662	107	.510	-3.289	4.972	-13.146	6.567
	Equal variances not assumed			-.513	2.067	.658	-3.289	6.412	-30.040	23.461
Height of Ascending Ramus Right go-cdl	Equal variances assumed	.333	.565	-1.174	94	.244	-3.033	2.584	-8.164	2.098
	Equal variances not assumed			-1.355	3.366	.259	-3.033	2.238	-9.737	3.672

		F	Sig.	t	df	Sig. (2-tailed)	Mean Difference	Std. Error Difference	Lower	Upper
Min Breadth of Ascending Ramus Right	Equal variances assumed	.249	.619	-.134	100	.894	-.199	1.488	-3.152	2.754
	Equal variances not assumed			-.173	3.445	.872	-.199	1.148	-3.599	3.201
Height at Mandibular Symphysis gn-idi	Equal variances assumed	1.696	.196	-.588	99	.558	-1.201	2.043	-5.255	2.853
	Equal variances not assumed			-1.253	4.502	.272	-1.201	.959	-3.750	1.348

T-Test congenitally absent teeth

Independent Samples Test

		Levene's Test for Equality of Variances		t-test for Equality of Means					95% Confidence Interval of the Difference	
		F	Sig.	t	df	Sig. (2-tailed)	Mean Difference	Std. Error Difference	Lower	Upper
Max Cranial Length	Equal variances assumed	.436	.511	.068	115	.946	.290	4.277	-8.183	8.763
	Equal variances not assumed			.051	3.116	.963	.290	5.716	-17.526	18.105
Max Cranial Breadth	Equal variances assumed	2.197	.141	1.113	118	.268	4.224	3.794	-3.289	11.738
	Equal variances not assumed			.629	3.061	.573	4.224	6.717	-16.913	25.362
Cranial Height	Equal variances assumed	1.783	.185	-.344	81	.732	-1.708	4.968	-11.594	8.177
	Equal variances not assumed			-.215	2.055	.849	-1.708	7.935	-34.982	31.566
Facial Height n-gn	Equal variances assumed	2.870	.094	-.520	74	.605	-3.243	6.240	-15.677	9.191
	Equal variances not assumed			-.249	1.012	.844	-3.243	13.037	-164.483	157.997
Facial Width zy-zy	Equal variances assumed	3.010	.086	-.721	87	.473	-3.534	4.903	-13.280	6.211
	Equal variances not assumed			-.336	1.009	.793	-3.534	10.525	-134.354	127.285
FMT Width	Equal variances assumed	.022	.882	.402	103	.689	1.255	3.125	-4.943	7.453
	Equal variances not assumed			.476	3.353	.663	1.255	2.634	-6.650	9.160
Upper Facial Height n-pr	Equal variances assumed	.887	.349	-.889	99	.376	-2.340	2.632	-7.562	2.881
	Equal variances not assumed			-.599	3.106	.590	-2.340	3.907	-14.536	9.856
Maxilloalveolar Length pr-alv	Equal variances assumed	.952	.333	-1.423	67	.159	-3.858	2.710	-9.268	1.552
	Equal variances not assumed			-.853	1.021	.548	-3.858	4.523	-58.664	50.948
Maxilloalveolar Breadth ect-ect	Equal variances assumed	.657	.420	-.106	98	.916	-.292	2.764	-5.776	5.193
	Equal variances not assumed			-.148	3.545	.890	-.292	1.968	-6.044	5.460
Palatal Length ol-sta	Equal variances assumed	1.145	.287	-.468	104	.641	-.995	2.126	-5.211	3.221
	Equal variances not assumed			-.794	3.793	.474	-.995	1.253	-4.550	2.560
Palatal Breadth enm-enm	Equal variances assumed	.000	.999	.955	101	.342	2.341	2.452	-2.524	7.205
	Equal variances not assumed			1.176	3.391	.316	2.341	1.991	-3.602	8.284
Bicondylar Breadth cdl-cdl	Equal variances assumed	1.194	.278	-1.715	82	.090	-8.878	5.177	-19.177	1.421
	Equal variances not assumed			-.983	1.015	.504	-8.878	9.034	-119.637	101.880
Bigonial Breadth go-go	Equal variances assumed	1.078	.302	2.357	107	.020	11.450	4.858	1.820	21.080
	Equal variances not assumed			1.409	2.038	.292	11.450	8.128	-22.899	45.798
Height of Ascending Ramus Right go-cdl	Equal variances assumed	1.291	.259	-.227	94	.821	-.677	2.989	-6.612	5.257
	Equal variances not assumed			-.137	2.044	.904	-.677	4.960	-21.581	20.226
Min Breadth of Ascending Ramus Right	Equal variances assumed	3.124	.080	-1.800	100	.075	-3.030	1.683	-6.370	.309
	Equal variances not assumed			-.988	2.034	.426	-3.030	3.068	-16.021	9.960
Height at Mandibular Symphysis gn-idi	Equal variances assumed	.975	.326	-.874	99	.384	-2.048	2.342	-6.695	2.599
	Equal variances not assumed			-.610	2.058	.602	-2.048	3.357	-16.111	12.015

T-Test absent M3

Independent Samples Test

		Levene's Test for Equality of Variances		t-test for Equality of Means					95% Confidence Interval of the Difference	
		F	Sig.	t	df	Sig. (2-tailed)	Mean Difference	Std. Error Difference	Lower	Upper
Max Cranial Length	Equal variances assumed	.028	.867	.484	115	.629	1.345	2.777	-4.157	6.846

		F	Sig.	t	df	Sig. (2-tailed)	Mean Difference	Std. Error Difference	Lower	Upper
	Equal variances not assumed			.520	11.094	.613	1.345	2.587	-4.342	7.032
Max Cranial Breadth	Equal variances assumed	10.942	.001	-.691	118	.491	-1.574	2.278	-6.084	2.936
	Equal variances not assumed			-.346	11.371	.735	-1.574	4.544	-11.536	8.388
Cranial Height	Equal variances assumed	1.392	.242	.408	81	.685	1.459	3.580	-5.664	8.582
	Equal variances not assumed			.589	7.012	.574	1.459	2.478	-4.398	7.315
Facial Height n-gn	Equal variances assumed	2.072	.154	2.407	74	.019	10.389	4.316	1.790	18.988
	Equal variances not assumed			5.296	5.505	.002	10.389	1.962	5.482	15.296
Facial Width zy-zy	Equal variances assumed	.058	.810	1.094	87	.277	3.438	3.144	-2.811	9.687
	Equal variances not assumed			1.348	4.795	.238	3.438	2.550	-3.203	10.080
FMT Width	Equal variances assumed	.001	.972	.405	103	.687	.865	2.137	-3.373	5.102
	Equal variances not assumed			.423	9.749	.681	.865	2.043	-3.703	5.432
Upper Facial Height n-pr	Equal variances assumed	.222	.639	1.355	99	.179	2.926	2.160	-1.359	7.212
	Equal variances not assumed			1.415	5.719	.209	2.926	2.068	-2.196	8.049
Maxilloalveolar Length pr-alv	Equal variances assumed	2.722	.104	-.165	67	.870	-.270	1.638	-3.539	2.999
	Equal variances not assumed			-.282	9.287	.784	-.270	.956	-2.422	1.882
Maxilloalveolar Breadth ect-ect	Equal variances assumed	.030	.863	.597	98	.552	1.190	1.993	-2.764	5.145
	Equal variances not assumed			.662	8.631	.525	1.190	1.798	-2.903	5.283
Palatal Length ol-sta	Equal variances assumed	.615	.435	-.490	104	.625	-.712	1.453	-3.595	2.170
	Equal variances not assumed			-.625	10.863	.545	-.712	1.140	-3.226	1.801
Palatal Breadth enm-enm	Equal variances assumed	.354	.553	1.229	101	.222	2.168	1.765	-1.333	5.669
	Equal variances not assumed			1.673	9.654	.126	2.168	1.296	-.733	5.070
Bicondylar Breadth cdl-cdl	Equal variances assumed	1.720	.193	.751	82	.455	2.333	3.108	-3.850	8.517
	Equal variances not assumed			1.175	7.451	.276	2.333	1.987	-2.307	6.974
Bigonial Breadth go-go	Equal variances assumed	1.012	.317	.490	107	.625	1.275	2.601	-3.882	6.432
	Equal variances not assumed			.564	15.189	.581	1.275	2.260	-3.537	6.087
Height of Ascending Ramus Right go-cdl	Equal variances assumed	.319	.574	1.113	94	.269	1.973	1.773	-1.547	5.493
	Equal variances not assumed			1.284	10.501	.227	1.973	1.537	-1.428	5.375
Min Breadth of Ascending Ramus Right	Equal variances assumed	.595	.442	.290	100	.773	.270	.931	-1.578	2.117
	Equal variances not assumed			.337	13.833	.741	.270	.799	-1.446	1.986
Height at Mandibular Symphysis gn-idi	Equal variances assumed	.369	.545	.383	99	.702	.491	1.280	-2.049	3.031
	Equal variances not assumed			.422	13.320	.680	.491	1.164	-2.017	2.999

T-Test ectopic and impacted teeth

Independent Samples Test

		Levene's Test for Equality of Variances		t-test for Equality of Means					95% Confidence Interval of the Difference	
		F	Sig.	t	df	Sig. (2-tailed)	Mean Difference	Std. Error Difference	Lower	Upper
Max Cranial Length	Equal variances assumed	.877	.351	.303	115	.762	.686	2.261	-3.793	5.166
	Equal variances not assumed			.321	20.937	.752	.686	2.139	-3.763	5.135
Max Cranial Breadth	Equal variances assumed	.102	.750	.896	118	.372	1.848	2.063	-2.238	5.933
	Equal variances not assumed			.887	18.124	.387	1.848	2.083	-2.526	6.222
Cranial Height	Equal variances assumed	4.372	.040	-1.449	81	.151	-3.776	2.605	-8.959	1.408
	Equal variances not assumed			-.923	11.993	.374	-3.776	4.090	-12.689	5.137
Facial Height n-gn	Equal variances assumed	.019	.890	1.567	74	.121	4.386	2.798	-1.190	9.962
	Equal variances not assumed			1.604	13.863	.131	4.386	2.735	-1.485	10.257
Facial Width zy-zy	Equal variances assumed	.266	.607	.586	87	.559	1.296	2.210	-3.097	5.689
	Equal variances not assumed			.463	11.556	.652	1.296	2.798	-4.827	7.419
FMT Width	Equal variances assumed	.015	.903	.432	103	.666	.785	1.816	-2.816	4.387
	Equal variances not assumed			.468	16.473	.646	.785	1.678	-2.765	4.335
Upper Facial Height n-pr	Equal variances assumed	.180	.672	1.555	99	.123	2.365	1.520	-.652	5.381

131

		F	Sig.	t	df	Sig. (2-tailed)	Mean Difference	Std. Error Difference	Lower	Upper
	Equal variances not assumed			1.487	15.314	.157	2.365	1.590	-1.019	5.748
Maxilloalveolar Length pr-alv	Equal variances assumed	1.023	.316	1.300	67	.198	2.103	1.618	-1.126	5.332
	Equal variances not assumed			1.869	7.551	.101	2.103	1.125	-.518	4.725
Maxilloalveolar Breadth ect-ect	Equal variances assumed	1.109	.295	.720	98	.473	1.197	1.662	-2.102	4.496
	Equal variances not assumed			.537	12.416	.601	1.197	2.229	-3.641	6.035
Palatal Length ol-sta	Equal variances assumed	.025	.874	1.454	104	.149	1.780	1.224	-.647	4.207
	Equal variances not assumed			1.388	15.122	.185	1.780	1.282	-.951	4.511
Palatal Breadth enm-enm	Equal variances assumed	.116	.734	-.573	101	.568	-.849	1.481	-3.787	2.089
	Equal variances not assumed			-.455	12.639	.657	-.849	1.865	-4.890	3.192
Bicondylar Breadth cdl-cdl	Equal variances assumed	.924	.339	-.068	82	.946	-.152	2.221	-4.570	4.267
	Equal variances not assumed			-.076	18.624	.940	-.152	1.986	-4.314	4.011
Bigonial Breadth go-go	Equal variances assumed	1.847	.177	.985	107	.327	2.321	2.355	-2.349	6.990
	Equal variances not assumed			.770	16.327	.452	2.321	3.014	-4.059	8.700
Height of Ascending Ramus Right go-cdl	Equal variances assumed	.613	.436	1.364	94	.176	1.991	1.459	-.906	4.889
	Equal variances not assumed			1.132	15.731	.274	1.991	1.759	-1.742	5.724
Min Breadth of Ascending Ramus Right	Equal variances assumed	1.084	.300	.377	100	.707	.317	.839	-1.348	1.981
	Equal variances not assumed			.463	21.080	.648	.317	.683	-1.104	1.737
Height at Mandibular Symphysis gn-idi	Equal variances assumed	1.593	.210	1.440	99	.153	1.646	1.143	-.622	3.914
	Equal variances not assumed			1.790	21.512	.088	1.646	.920	-.264	3.556

T-Test Crowding

Independent Samples Test

		Levene's Test for Equality of Variances		t-test for Equality of Means					95% Confidence Interval of the Difference	
		F	Sig.	t	df	Sig. (2-tailed)	Mean Difference	Std. Error Difference	Lower	Upper
Max Cranial Length	Equal variances assumed	3.957	.049	.872	115	.385	1.604	1.839	-2.039	5.246
	Equal variances not assumed			1.047	60.212	.299	1.604	1.532	-1.460	4.668
Max Cranial Breadth	Equal variances assumed	.079	.779	.416	118	.678	.681	1.638	-2.563	3.925
	Equal variances not assumed			.442	46.464	.661	.681	1.542	-2.423	3.785
Cranial Height	Equal variances assumed	.006	.941	-1.676	81	.098	-3.575	2.133	-7.819	.670
	Equal variances not assumed			-1.403	25.293	.173	-3.575	2.548	-8.820	1.671
Facial Height n-gn	Equal variances assumed	1.283	.261	-.653	74	.516	-1.438	2.200	-5.822	2.946
	Equal variances not assumed			-.711	47.419	.480	-1.438	2.021	-5.503	2.627
Facial Width zy-zy	Equal variances assumed	.001	.969	-1.189	87	.238	-1.993	1.676	-5.325	1.338
	Equal variances not assumed			-1.252	39.247	.218	-1.993	1.592	-5.213	1.226
FMT Width	Equal variances assumed	2.120	.148	.264	103	.792	.377	1.425	-2.450	3.203
	Equal variances not assumed			.345	64.428	.731	.377	1.092	-1.805	2.559
Upper Facial Height n-pr	Equal variances assumed	.179	.673	-1.120	99	.265	-1.281	1.144	-3.551	.988
	Equal variances not assumed			-1.024	41.596	.312	-1.281	1.251	-3.807	1.245
Maxilloalveolar Length pr-alv	Equal variances assumed	1.091	.300	-.899	67	.372	-1.026	1.141	-3.303	1.251
	Equal variances not assumed			-1.003	23.511	.326	-1.026	1.023	-3.140	1.088
Maxilloalveolar Breadth ect-ect	Equal variances assumed	4.843	.030	-1.876	98	.064	-2.275	1.213	-4.683	.132
	Equal variances not assumed			-2.247	64.805	.028	-2.275	1.013	-4.298	-.253
Palatal Length ol-sta	Equal variances assumed	.141	.708	.792	104	.430	.744	.940	-1.119	2.608
	Equal variances not assumed			.774	40.963	.443	.744	.961	-1.197	2.685
Palatal Breadth enm-enm	Equal variances assumed	.217	.642	-1.520	101	.132	-1.646	1.083	-3.795	.502
	Equal variances not assumed			-1.329	35.285	.192	-1.646	1.239	-4.161	.868
Bicondylar Breadth cdl-cdl	Equal variances assumed	1.390	.242	-1.530	82	.130	-2.683	1.753	-6.171	.805
	Equal variances not assumed			-1.669	51.592	.101	-2.683	1.608	-5.910	.544
Bigonial Breadth go-go	Equal variances assumed	.550	.460	.632	107	.529	1.151	1.822	-2.460	4.763

		Equal variances not assumed			.596	46.914	.554	1.151	1.933	-2.738	5.041
Height of Ascending Ramus Right go-cdl	Equal variances assumed	.683	.411	-.405	94	.686	-.486	1.200	-2.869	1.897
	Equal variances not assumed			-.417	41.499	.679	-.486	1.166	-2.841	1.869
Min Breadth of Ascending Ramus Right	Equal variances assumed	.894	.347	-1.993	100	.049	-1.280	.642	-2.554	-.006
	Equal variances not assumed			-1.827	39.690	.075	-1.280	.701	-2.697	.137
Height at Mandibular Symphysis gn-idi	Equal variances assumed	.066	.797	-1.668	99	.099	-1.502	.900	-3.288	.285
	Equal variances not assumed			-1.801	50.537	.078	-1.502	.834	-3.176	.173

b. By sex, craniometrics with anomalies

T-Test Supplemental Teeth

Independent Samples Test[a]

Sex			Levene's Test for Equality of Variances		t-test for Equality of Means					95% Confidence Interval of the Difference	
			F	Sig.	t	df	Sig. (2-tailed)	Mean Difference	Std. Error Difference	Lower	Upper
Male	Max Cranial Length	Equal variances assumed	.000	.990	-.012	62	.990	-.065	5.225	-10.510	10.381
		Equal variances not assumed			-.012	1.057	.993	-.065	5.577	-62.496	62.367
	Max Cranial Breadth	Equal variances assumed	1.297	.259	1.830	65	.072	10.569	5.775	-.964	22.102
		Equal variances not assumed			1.052	1.019	.481	10.569	10.048	-111.516	132.654
	Facial Height n-gn	Equal variances assumed	.	.	1.202	43	.236	9.227	7.677	-6.254	24.709
		Equal variances not assumed			.	.	.	9.227	.	.	.
	Facial Width zy-zy	Equal variances assumed	.	.	-.268	45	.790	-1.543	5.768	-13.161	10.074
		Equal variances not assumed			.	.	.	-1.543	.	.	.
	FMT Width	Equal variances assumed	.311	.579	.325	55	.747	1.600	4.928	-8.275	11.475
		Equal variances not assumed			.264	1.047	.834	1.600	6.070	-67.747	70.947
	Upper Facial Height n-pr	Equal variances assumed	.961	.331	1.221	54	.227	4.130	3.382	-2.651	10.910
		Equal variances not assumed			2.530	1.402	.178	4.130	1.632	-6.718	14.977
	Maxilloalveolar Length pr-alv	Equal variances assumed	.	.	.015	38	.988	.051	3.500	-7.034	7.137
		Equal variances not assumed			.	.	.	.051	.	.	.
	Maxilloalveolar Breadth ect-ect	Equal variances assumed	3.445	.069	-.508	55	.614	-1.655	3.258	-8.183	4.874
		Equal variances not assumed			-2.687	54.000	.010	-1.655	.616	-2.889	-.420
	Palatal Length ol-sta	Equal variances assumed	2.667	.108	-.122	59	.904	-.356	2.924	-6.206	5.494
		Equal variances not assumed			-.667	58.000	.508	-.356	.534	-1.425	.713
	Palatal Breadth enm-enm	Equal variances assumed	1.692	.198	.141	58	.888	.500	3.539	-6.584	7.584
		Equal variances not assumed			.767	57.000	.446	.500	.652	-.805	1.805
	Bicondylar Breadth cdl-cdl	Equal variances assumed	.	.	.760	47	.451	5.375	7.076	-8.860	19.610
		Equal variances not assumed			.	.	.	5.375	.	.	.
	Bigonial Breadth go-go	Equal variances assumed	9.213	.004	2.768	62	.007	14.919	5.390	4.145	25.693
		Equal variances not assumed			1.027	1.008	.490	14.919	14.528	-166.361	196.200
	Height of Ascending Ramus Right go-cdl	Equal variances assumed	.057	.811	1.501	56	.139	5.393	3.593	-1.804	12.590
		Equal variances not assumed			1.186	1.044	.440	5.393	4.549	-46.961	57.747
	Min Breadth of Ascending Ramus Right	Equal variances assumed	.069	.794	-.111	59	.912	-.237	2.132	-4.503	4.028
		Equal variances not assumed			-.116	1.076	.925	-.237	2.037	-22.176	21.701
	Height at Mandibular Symphysis gn-idi	Equal variances assumed	3.114	.083	.995	59	.324	2.644	2.657	-2.672	7.960
		Equal variances not assumed			5.450	58.000	.000	2.644	.485	1.673	3.615

a. No statistics are computed for one or more split files

T-Test Rotations

Independent Samples Test

Sex			Levene's Test for Equality of Variances		t-test for Equality of Means					95% Confidence Interval of the Difference	
			F	Sig.	t	df	Sig. (2-tailed)	Mean Difference	Std. Error Difference	Lower	Upper
Female	Max Cranial Length	Equal variances assumed	1.305	.259	1.728	51	.090	4.185	2.421	-.676	9.046
		Equal variances not assumed			1.557	24.741	.132	4.185	2.688	-1.355	9.724
	Max Cranial Breadth	Equal variances assumed	4.155	.047	-.584	51	.562	-.916	1.568	-4.063	2.231
		Equal variances not assumed			-.503	23.756	.620	-.916	1.821	-4.677	2.846
	Cranial Height	Equal variances assumed	1.025	.319	.919	33	.365	3.174	3.452	-3.850	10.198
		Equal variances not assumed			1.193	33.000	.242	3.174	2.662	-2.241	8.589
	Facial Height n-gn	Equal variances assumed	3.080	.090	.345	29	.732	1.021	2.957	-5.028	7.070
		Equal variances not assumed			.358	28.017	.723	1.021	2.848	-4.813	6.855
	Facial Width zy-zy	Equal variances assumed	.393	.534	.961	40	.343	1.792	1.865	-1.978	5.562
		Equal variances not assumed			.945	34.403	.351	1.792	1.896	-2.059	5.642
	FMT Width	Equal variances assumed	.258	.614	1.184	46	.243	1.849	1.562	-1.295	4.993
		Equal variances not assumed			1.097	20.859	.285	1.849	1.686	-1.658	5.355
	Upper Facial Height n-pr	Equal variances assumed	.040	.841	-.630	43	.532	-.944	1.500	-3.970	2.081
		Equal variances not assumed			-.632	37.035	.531	-.944	1.495	-3.973	2.084
	Maxilloalveolar Length pr-alv	Equal variances assumed	1.708	.202	1.547	27	.134	2.206	1.426	-.720	5.131
		Equal variances not assumed			1.810	22.935	.083	2.206	1.218	-.315	4.727
	Maxilloalveolar Breadth ect-ect	Equal variances assumed	1.653	.206	-.751	41	.457	-1.429	1.903	-5.273	2.415
		Equal variances not assumed			-.838	38.227	.407	-1.429	1.704	-4.877	2.020
	Palatal Length ol-sta	Equal variances assumed	2.821	.100	2.124	43	.040	2.633	1.240	.133	5.134
		Equal variances not assumed			2.512	41.762	.016	2.633	1.048	.518	4.749
	Palatal Breadth enm-enm	Equal variances assumed	2.000	.165	.176	41	.861	.271	1.539	-2.837	3.379
		Equal variances not assumed			.218	40.827	.829	.271	1.243	-2.240	2.782
	Bicondylar Breadth cdl-cdl	Equal variances assumed	.112	.740	2.798	33	.009	6.117	2.186	1.670	10.564
		Equal variances not assumed			2.766	28.938	.010	6.117	2.211	1.594	10.640
	Bigonial Breadth go-go	Equal variances assumed	.028	.867	.281	43	.780	.574	2.045	-3.550	4.698
		Equal variances not assumed			.280	36.180	.781	.574	2.051	-3.586	4.734
	Height of Ascending Ramus Right go-cdl	Equal variances assumed	.799	.377	2.037	36	.049	2.858	1.403	.013	5.703
		Equal variances not assumed			1.967	26.517	.060	2.858	1.453	-.126	5.842
	Min Breadth of Ascending Ramus Right	Equal variances assumed	1.481	.231	1.566	39	.126	1.262	.806	-.368	2.891
		Equal variances not assumed			1.448	23.159	.161	1.262	.871	-.540	3.063
	Height at Mandibular Symphysis gn-idi	Equal variances assumed	1.007	.322	1.529	38	.135	1.868	1.222	-.605	4.342
		Equal variances not assumed			1.374	19.982	.185	1.868	1.360	-.969	4.705
Male	Max Cranial Length	Equal variances assumed	5.415	.023	1.164	62	.249	2.417	2.077	-1.735	6.569
		Equal variances not assumed			1.581	51.256	.120	2.417	1.529	-.652	5.486
	Max Cranial Breadth	Equal variances assumed	3.325	.073	.522	65	.603	1.207	2.311	-3.408	5.822
		Equal variances not assumed			.368	18.217	.717	1.207	3.276	-5.670	8.084
	Cranial Height	Equal variances assumed	.679	.414	2.374	46	.022	4.754	2.002	.724	8.784
		Equal variances not assumed			2.138	17.988	.046	4.754	2.223	.083	9.425
	Facial Height n-gn	Equal variances assumed	2.136	.151	1.826	43	.075	4.576	2.506	-.478	9.630
		Equal variances not assumed			2.283	32.569	.029	4.576	2.005	.495	8.656

			F	Sig.	t	df	Sig. (2-tailed)	Mean Difference	Std. Error Difference	Lower	Upper
	Facial Width zy-zy	Equal variances assumed	.196	.660	1.545	45	.129	2.803	1.815	-.852	6.458
		Equal variances not assumed			1.414	18.561	.174	2.803	1.983	-1.353	6.960
	FMT Width	Equal variances assumed	.096	.758	.535	55	.595	1.100	2.056	-3.020	5.220
		Equal variances not assumed			.673	41.441	.505	1.100	1.635	-2.202	4.402
	Upper Facial Height n-pr	Equal variances assumed	1.114	.296	1.503	54	.139	2.115	1.407	-.706	4.937
		Equal variances not assumed			1.713	33.033	.096	2.115	1.235	-.398	4.628
	Maxilloalveolar Length pr-alv	Equal variances assumed	2.741	.106	-.170	38	.866	-.222	1.308	-2.870	2.426
		Equal variances not assumed			-.229	23.908	.821	-.222	.971	-2.227	1.783
	Maxilloalveolar Breadth ect-ect	Equal variances assumed	.820	.369	.316	55	.753	.440	1.395	-2.355	3.235
		Equal variances not assumed			.351	27.021	.728	.440	1.253	-2.130	3.010
	Palatal Length ol-sta	Equal variances assumed	.121	.729	.313	59	.755	.388	1.237	-2.088	2.863
		Equal variances not assumed			.327	22.877	.746	.388	1.184	-2.063	2.838
	Palatal Breadth enm-enm	Equal variances assumed	.935	.338	.358	58	.722	.537	1.501	-2.467	3.541
		Equal variances not assumed			.350	20.830	.730	.537	1.535	-2.656	3.731
	Bicondylar Breadth cdl-cdl	Equal variances assumed	.124	.726	1.930	47	.060	4.235	2.195	-.180	8.650
		Equal variances not assumed			2.037	23.683	.053	4.235	2.079	-.058	8.528
	Bigonial Breadth go-go	Equal variances assumed	1.873	.176	.870	62	.388	2.029	2.332	-2.634	6.691
		Equal variances not assumed			.712	18.169	.485	2.029	2.849	-3.953	8.010
	Height of Ascending Ramus Right go-cdl	Equal variances assumed	1.652	.204	1.596	56	.116	2.438	1.528	-.623	5.500
		Equal variances not assumed			1.408	18.410	.176	2.438	1.731	-1.193	6.070
	Min Breadth of Ascending Ramus Right	Equal variances assumed	.128	.722	2.107	59	.039	1.834	.871	.092	3.577
		Equal variances not assumed			1.986	19.674	.061	1.834	.924	-.095	3.763
	Height at Mandibular Symphysis gn-idi	Equal variances assumed	.613	.437	1.310	59	.195	1.465	1.118	-.773	3.703
		Equal variances not assumed			1.528	28.138	.138	1.465	.959	-.498	3.428

T-Test Reversals

			Levene's Test for Equality of Variances		t-test for Equality of Means						
										95% Confidence Interval of the Difference	
Sex			F	Sig.	t	df	Sig. (2-tailed)	Mean Difference	Std. Error Difference	Lower	Upper
Female	Max Cranial Length	Equal variances assumed	.098	.755	1.573	51	.122	9.373	5.960	-2.592	21.337
		Equal variances not assumed			1.534	1.076	.355	9.373	6.111	-56.473	75.218
	Max Cranial Breadth	Equal variances assumed	2.273	.138	.759	51	.451	2.951	3.887	-4.853	10.755
		Equal variances not assumed			3.236	9.981	.009	2.951	.912	.919	4.983
	Cranial Height	Equal variances assumed	.890	.352	-.291	33	.773	-2.030	6.984	-16.239	12.178
		Equal variances not assumed			-1.032	11.920	.323	-2.030	1.968	-6.321	2.260
	Facial Height n-gn	Equal variances assumed	1.874	.182	-1.238	29	.226	-7.241	5.851	-19.207	4.725
		Equal variances not assumed			-2.890	2.435	.081	-7.241	2.505	-16.372	1.889
	Facial Width zy-zy	Equal variances assumed	.047	.829	-.555	40	.582	-2.425	4.367	-11.252	6.402
		Equal variances not assumed			-.668	1.155	.612	-2.425	3.628	-36.200	31.350
	FMT Width	Equal variances assumed	.216	.644	.338	46	.737	1.217	3.602	-6.033	8.468
		Equal variances not assumed			.394	1.124	.755	1.217	3.089	-29.123	31.558
	Upper Facial Height n-pr	Equal variances assumed	2.851	.099	-.410	43	.684	-1.465	3.576	-8.676	5.746
		Equal variances not assumed			-1.921	42.000	.062	-1.465	.763	-3.004	.074
	Maxilloalveolar Length pr-alv	Equal variances assumed	.573	.456	-.014	27	.989	-.037	2.716	-5.611	5.536

			F	Sig.	t	df	Sig. (2-tailed)	Mean Difference	Std. Error Difference	Lower	Upper
		Equal variances not assumed			-.009	1.061	.994	-.037	4.060	-45.095	45.021
	Maxilloalveolar Breadth ect-ect	Equal variances assumed	3.350	.074	-.961	41	.342	-4.122	4.289	-12.784	4.540
		Equal variances not assumed			-4.401	40.000	.000	-4.122	.937	-6.015	-2.229
	Palatal Length ol-sta	Equal variances assumed	.001	.970	-.133	43	.895	-.395	2.981	-6.407	5.616
		Equal variances not assumed			-.129	1.090	.917	-.395	3.065	-32.536	31.746
	Palatal Breadth enm-enm	Equal variances assumed	1.230	.274	-.360	41	.721	-1.232	3.420	-8.139	5.675
		Equal variances not assumed			-1.371	9.276	.203	-1.232	.899	-3.255	.792
	Bicondylar Breadth cdl-cdl	Equal variances assumed	.359	.553	-.695	33	.492	-3.576	5.146	-14.046	6.894
		Equal variances not assumed			-.854	1.200	.530	-3.576	4.187	-39.782	32.631
	Bigonial Breadth go-go	Equal variances assumed	1.638	.208	.651	43	.519	3.151	4.842	-6.613	12.915
		Equal variances not assumed			1.731	2.158	.216	3.151	1.820	-4.157	10.459
	Height of Ascending Ramus Right go-cdl	Equal variances assumed	3.569	.067	-.901	36	.374	-2.889	3.207	-9.393	3.615
		Equal variances not assumed			-3.872	35.000	.000	-2.889	.746	-4.404	-1.374
	Min Breadth of Ascending Ramus Right	Equal variances assumed	.957	.334	-.568	39	.573	-1.051	1.850	-4.793	2.690
		Equal variances not assumed			-.972	1.368	.471	-1.051	1.082	-8.518	6.415
	Height at Mandibular Symphysis gn-idi	Equal variances assumed	.	.	-.671	38	.507	-2.564	3.823	-10.304	5.176
		Equal variances not assumed	.	.	.	.	.	-2.564	.	.	.

a. No statistics are computed for one or more split files

T-Test Misshapen teeth

			Levene's Test for Equality of Variances		t-test for Equality of Means						
										95% Confidence Interval of the Difference	
Sex			F	Sig.	t	df	Sig. (2-tailed)	Mean Difference	Std. Error Difference	Lower	Upper
Male	Max Cranial Length	Equal variances assumed	.000	.993	-1.124	62	.265	-4.787	4.258	-13.299	3.725
		Equal variances not assumed			-1.155	2.214	.358	-4.787	4.145	-21.070	11.497
	Max Cranial Breadth	Equal variances assumed	.563	.456	-1.324	65	.190	-6.365	4.808	-15.968	3.238
		Equal variances not assumed			-2.998	3.415	.049	-6.365	2.123	-12.680	-.049
	Cranial Height	Equal variances assumed	.029	.866	-.622	46	.537	-2.114	3.397	-8.951	4.723
		Equal variances not assumed			-.641	3.612	.560	-2.114	3.296	-11.665	7.438
	Facial Height n-gn	Equal variances assumed	.018	.894	-.539	43	.593	-2.171	4.029	-10.296	5.954
		Equal variances not assumed			-.546	3.633	.617	-2.171	3.972	-13.653	9.312
	Facial Width zy-zy	Equal variances assumed	.248	.621	.124	45	.902	.511	4.126	-7.800	8.822
		Equal variances not assumed			.164	1.169	.894	.511	3.120	-27.845	28.867
	FMT Width	Equal variances assumed	.581	.449	.663	55	.510	2.685	4.048	-5.428	10.798
		Equal variances not assumed			1.952	6.957	.092	2.685	1.376	-.572	5.943
	Upper Facial Height n-pr	Equal variances assumed	.911	.344	.982	54	.331	2.404	2.449	-2.505	7.313
		Equal variances not assumed			1.427	4.202	.224	2.404	1.685	-2.186	6.994
	Maxilloalveolar Length pr-alv	Equal variances assumed	.	.	.903	38	.372	3.128	3.463	-3.883	10.139
		Equal variances not assumed			.	.	.	3.128	.	.	.
	Maxilloalveolar Breadth ect-ect	Equal variances assumed	1.839	.181	.128	55	.899	.418	3.265	-6.125	6.961
		Equal variances not assumed			.356	1.900	.757	.418	1.175	-4.900	5.737
	Palatal Length ol-sta	Equal variances assumed	.153	.698	.334	59	.740	.702	2.102	-3.503	4.907
		Equal variances not assumed			.447	3.875	.679	.702	1.570	-3.712	5.116
	Palatal Breadth enm-enm	Equal variances assumed	1.906	.173	-.112	58	.911	-.286	2.547	-5.384	4.813
		Equal variances not assumed			-.310	12.916	.762	-.286	.922	-2.279	1.708

Measurement	Variances	F	Sig.	t	df	Sig. (2-tailed)	Mean Difference	Std. Error Difference	Lower	Upper
Bicondylar Breadth cdl-cdl	Equal variances assumed	.059	.809	1.273	47	.209	5.254	4.128	-3.051	13.559
	Equal variances not assumed			.991	2.152	.420	5.254	5.303	-16.088	26.595
Bigonial Breadth go-go	Equal variances assumed	.708	.403	.064	62	.949	.301	4.703	-9.100	9.701
	Equal variances not assumed			.047	2.101	.967	.301	6.438	-26.167	26.769
Height of Ascending Ramus Right go-cdl	Equal variances assumed	.333	.566	-.630	56	.531	-1.657	2.629	-6.925	3.610
	Equal variances not assumed			-.726	3.643	.512	-1.657	2.283	-8.249	4.934
Min Breadth of Ascending Ramus Right	Equal variances assumed	.464	.498	.364	59	.717	.557	1.532	-2.509	3.623
	Equal variances not assumed			.473	3.815	.662	.557	1.178	-2.776	3.890
Height at Mandibular Symphysis gn-idi	Equal variances assumed	2.235	.140	.032	59	.975	.061	1.927	-3.795	3.918
	Equal variances not assumed			.061	5.341	.953	.061	1.002	-2.465	2.588

a. No statistics are computed for one or more split files

T-Test congenitally absent teeth

Sex	Measurement	Variances	F	Sig.	t	df	Sig. (2-tailed)	Mean Difference	Std. Error Difference	Lower	Upper
Female	Max Cranial Length	Equal variances assumed	.402	.529	.344	51	.732	2.098	6.095	-10.139	14.335
		Equal variances not assumed			.231	1.034	.854	2.098	9.076	-104.628	108.824
	Max Cranial Breadth	Equal variances assumed	.792	.378	.895	51	.375	3.471	3.879	-4.316	11.258
		Equal variances not assumed			1.622	1.308	.306	3.471	2.139	-12.406	19.347
	Cranial Height	Equal variances assumed	.725	.401	.393	33	.697	2.742	6.976	-11.451	16.936
		Equal variances not assumed			1.213	4.917	.280	2.742	2.261	-3.100	8.585
	Facial Height n-gn	Equal variances assumed	.	.	.652	29	.520	5.400	8.287	-11.548	22.348
		Equal variances not assumed			.	.	.	5.400	.	.	.
	Facial Width zy-zy	Equal variances assumed	.	.	.536	40	.595	3.268	6.102	-9.065	15.601
		Equal variances not assumed			.	.	.	3.268	.	.	.
	FMT Width	Equal variances assumed	1.475	.231	.193	46	.848	.696	3.605	-6.561	7.952
		Equal variances not assumed			.416	1.548	.728	.696	1.674	-8.948	10.340
	Upper Facial Height n-pr	Equal variances assumed	.107	.745	-.117	43	.908	-.419	3.582	-7.643	6.805
		Equal variances not assumed			-.135	1.131	.912	-.419	3.094	-30.423	29.586
	Maxilloalveolar Length pr-alv	Equal variances assumed	.	.	-.284	27	.778	-1.071	3.767	-8.800	6.657
		Equal variances not assumed			.	.	.	-1.071	.	.	.
	Maxilloalveolar Breadth ect-ect	Equal variances assumed	.073	.788	-.225	41	.823	-.976	4.335	-9.729	7.778
		Equal variances not assumed			-.237	1.112	.848	-.976	4.108	-42.217	40.266
	Palatal Length ol-sta	Equal variances assumed	2.881	.097	-.133	43	.895	-.395	2.981	-6.407	5.616
		Equal variances not assumed			-.622	42.000	.537	-.395	.636	-1.679	.888
	Palatal Breadth enm-enm	Equal variances assumed	.127	.723	.407	41	.686	1.390	3.419	-5.514	8.294
		Equal variances not assumed			.342	1.068	.787	1.390	4.067	-43.092	45.873
	Bicondylar Breadth cdl-cdl	Equal variances assumed	.	.	-.339	33	.737	-2.441	7.210	-17.110	12.227
		Equal variances not assumed			.	.	.	-2.441	.	.	.
	Bigonial Breadth go-go	Equal variances assumed	.	.	.835	43	.408	5.636	6.747	-7.971	19.244
		Equal variances not assumed			.	.	.	5.636	.	.	.
	Height of Ascending Ramus Right go-cdl	Equal variances assumed	.	.	-.857	36	.397	-3.838	4.478	-12.921	5.245
		Equal variances not assumed			.	.	.	-3.838	.	.	.

137

Sex			F	Sig.	t	df	Sig. (2-tailed)	Mean Difference	Std. Error Difference	95% Confidence Interval of the Difference Lower	Upper
	Min Breadth of Ascending Ramus Right	Equal variances assumed	.	.	-.797	39	.430	-2.050	2.573	-7.254	3.154
		Equal variances not assumed			.	.	.	-2.050	.	.	.
	Height at Mandibular Symphysis gn-idi	Equal variances assumed	.	.	-.133	38	.895	-.513	3.845	-8.297	7.271
		Equal variances not assumed			.	.	.	-.513	.	.	.
Male	Max Cranial Length	Equal variances assumed	.395	.532	-.408	62	.685	-2.129	5.218	-12.560	8.302
		Equal variances not assumed			-.282	1.030	.824	-2.129	7.555	-91.786	87.528
	Max Cranial Breadth	Equal variances assumed	6.773	.011	.744	65	.460	4.385	5.897	-7.392	16.161
		Equal variances not assumed			.274	1.007	.830	4.385	16.029	-195.835	204.604
	Cranial Height	Equal variances assumed	.	.	-2.412	46	.020	-15.000	6.219	-27.518	-2.482
		Equal variances not assumed			.	.	.	-15.000	.	.	.
	Facial Height n-gn	Equal variances assumed	.	.	-1.761	43	.085	-13.273	7.538	-28.474	1.928
		Equal variances not assumed			.	.	.	-13.273	.	.	.
	Facial Width zy-zy	Equal variances assumed	.	.	-1.936	45	.059	-10.739	5.546	-21.910	.432
		Equal variances not assumed			.	.	.	-10.739	.	.	.
	FMT Width	Equal variances assumed	.311	.579	.325	55	.747	1.600	4.928	-8.275	11.475
		Equal variances not assumed			.264	1.047	.834	1.600	6.070	-67.747	70.947
	Upper Facial Height n-pr	Equal variances assumed	3.063	.086	-1.391	54	.170	-4.685	3.368	-11.439	2.068
		Equal variances not assumed			-.667	1.016	.624	-4.685	7.027	-90.812	81.442
	Maxilloalveolar Length pr-alv	Equal variances assumed	.	.	-2.158	38	.037	-7.128	3.304	-13.816	-.440
		Equal variances not assumed			.	.	.	-7.128	.	.	.
	Maxilloalveolar Breadth ect-ect	Equal variances assumed	1.178	.283	-.031	55	.976	-.100	3.265	-6.644	6.444
		Equal variances not assumed			-.062	1.365	.959	-.100	1.622	-11.328	11.128
	Palatal Length ol-sta	Equal variances assumed	.652	.423	-.654	59	.515	-1.907	2.913	-7.736	3.923
		Equal variances not assumed			-1.198	1.266	.409	-1.907	1.591	-14.401	10.587
	Palatal Breadth enm-enm	Equal variances assumed	.087	.770	.878	58	.384	3.086	3.516	-3.953	10.125
		Equal variances not assumed			1.195	1.137	.424	3.086	2.582	-21.691	27.864
	Bicondylar Breadth cdl-cdl	Equal variances assumed	.	.	-2.389	47	.021	-16.063	6.723	-29.587	-2.538
		Equal variances not assumed			.	.	.	-16.063	.	.	.
	Bigonial Breadth go-go	Equal variances assumed	8.135	.006	2.876	62	.006	15.435	5.366	4.708	26.163
		Equal variances not assumed			1.100	1.008	.468	15.435	14.029	-159.392	190.263
	Height of Ascending Ramus Right go-cdl	Equal variances assumed	5.059	.028	.341	56	.734	1.250	3.661	-6.083	8.583
		Equal variances not assumed			.147	1.012	.907	1.250	8.525	-104.139	106.639
	Min Breadth of Ascending Ramus Right	Equal variances assumed	5.635	.021	-1.600	59	.115	-3.339	2.087	-7.516	.838
		Equal variances not assumed			-.666	1.010	.625	-3.339	5.013	-65.495	58.817
	Height at Mandibular Symphysis gn-idi	Equal variances assumed	1.879	.176	-.950	59	.346	-2.525	2.659	-7.845	2.794
		Equal variances not assumed			-.503	1.018	.702	-2.525	5.022	-63.764	58.713

T-Test Absent M3

			Levene's Test for Equality of Variances		t-test for Equality of Means						
Sex			F	Sig.	t	df	Sig. (2-tailed)	Mean Difference	Std. Error Difference	95% Confidence Interval of the Difference Lower	Upper
Female	Max Cranial Length	Equal variances assumed	.200	.657	-.608	51	.546	-2.408	3.964	-10.366	5.550
		Equal variances not assumed			-.569	4.740	.595	-2.408	4.231	-13.467	8.650
	Max Cranial Breadth	Equal variances assumed	.078	.781	1.294	51	.201	3.246	2.508	-1.788	8.280

		Equal variances not assumed			1.364	4.997	.231	3.246	2.379	-2.870	9.362
	Cranial Height	Equal variances assumed	.031	.861	.470	33	.642	3.273	6.969	-10.906	17.452
		Equal variances not assumed			.621	1.237	.630	3.273	5.274	-39.842	46.388
	Facial Height n-gn	Equal variances assumed	2.902	.099	1.228	29	.229	7.190	5.853	-4.781	19.160
		Equal variances not assumed			4.513	25.823	.000	7.190	1.593	3.914	10.466
	Facial Width zy-zy	Equal variances assumed	.759	.389	.648	40	.521	2.825	4.361	-5.990	11.640
		Equal variances not assumed			1.585	1.984	.255	2.825	1.782	-4.902	10.552
	FMT Width	Equal variances assumed	.784	.381	.650	46	.519	1.526	2.348	-3.201	6.253
		Equal variances not assumed			.481	4.450	.653	1.526	3.172	-6.942	9.993
	Upper Facial Height n-pr	Equal variances assumed	.896	.349	1.218	43	.230	4.291	3.522	-2.813	11.394
		Equal variances not assumed			2.559	1.560	.159	4.291	1.677	-5.275	13.857
	Maxilloalveolar Length pr-alv	Equal variances assumed	2.238	.146	-.347	27	.731	-.782	2.255	-5.409	3.845
		Equal variances not assumed			-.676	5.689	.526	-.782	1.157	-3.651	2.087
	Maxilloalveolar Breadth ect-ect	Equal variances assumed	1.999	.165	.522	41	.604	1.867	3.573	-5.350	9.083
		Equal variances not assumed			1.071	4.105	.343	1.867	1.743	-2.925	6.659
	Palatal Length ol-sta	Equal variances assumed	.039	.844	-.834	43	.409	-1.787	2.142	-6.106	2.533
		Equal variances not assumed			-.753	3.475	.499	-1.787	2.373	-8.786	5.212
	Palatal Breadth enm-enm	Equal variances assumed	1.093	.302	.633	41	.530	1.783	2.818	-3.908	7.474
		Equal variances not assumed			1.531	5.921	.177	1.783	1.165	-1.076	4.643
	Bicondylar Breadth cdl-cdl	Equal variances assumed	1.422	.242	-.956	33	.346	-4.052	4.240	-12.678	4.574
		Equal variances not assumed			-1.603	3.550	.193	-4.052	2.528	-11.435	3.331
	Bigonial Breadth go-go	Equal variances assumed	.993	.325	.463	43	.645	1.475	3.182	-4.943	7.893
		Equal variances not assumed			.708	7.530	.500	1.475	2.083	-3.382	6.332
	Height of Ascending Ramus Right go-cdl	Equal variances assumed	1.053	.312	-.709	36	.483	-1.662	2.343	-6.414	3.091
		Equal variances not assumed			-.566	3.417	.606	-1.662	2.934	-10.385	7.062
	Min Breadth of Ascending Ramus Right	Equal variances assumed	2.133	.152	-.186	39	.853	-.228	1.222	-2.700	2.244
		Equal variances not assumed			-.266	7.291	.798	-.228	.857	-2.238	1.782
	Height at Mandibular Symphysis gn-idi	Equal variances assumed	.448	.507	-.189	38	.851	-.343	1.815	-4.017	3.331
		Equal variances not assumed			-.244	6.513	.815	-.343	1.405	-3.716	3.031
Male	Max Cranial Length	Equal variances assumed	.165	.686	1.311	62	.195	4.380	3.342	-2.300	11.060
		Equal variances not assumed			1.290	4.678	.257	4.380	3.396	-4.533	13.292
	Max Cranial Breadth	Equal variances assumed	21.491	.000	-1.488	65	.142	-4.821	3.240	-11.292	1.649
		Equal variances not assumed			-.670	6.142	.527	-4.821	7.193	-22.324	12.681
	Cranial Height	Equal variances assumed	2.492	.121	.421	46	.676	1.432	3.404	-5.421	8.284
		Equal variances not assumed			.873	7.611	.409	1.432	1.640	-2.384	5.247
	Facial Height n-gn	Equal variances assumed	.407	.527	2.288	43	.027	12.058	5.271	1.428	22.688
		Equal variances not assumed			3.282	1.214	.152	12.058	3.674	-19.028	43.144
	Facial Width zy-zy	Equal variances assumed	.038	.847	1.439	45	.157	4.795	3.332	-1.916	11.507
		Equal variances not assumed			1.296	2.221	.313	4.795	3.701	-9.704	19.295
	FMT Width	Equal variances assumed	.242	.625	-.138	55	.891	-.491	3.552	-7.609	6.628
		Equal variances not assumed			-.233	4.768	.825	-.491	2.103	-5.976	4.995
	Upper Facial Height n-pr	Equal variances assumed	.005	.942	1.207	54	.233	2.942	2.438	-1.945	7.830
		Equal variances not assumed			1.114	3.395	.338	2.942	2.642	-4.939	10.824
	Maxilloalveolar Length pr-alv	Equal variances assumed	1.257	.269	-.148	38	.883	-.306	2.074	-4.505	3.893

						-.290	4.067	.786	-.306	1.056	-3.219	2.606
	Maxilloalveolar Breadth ect-ect	Equal variances assumed	.439	.511	.519	55	.606	1.100	2.119	-3.146	5.346
		Equal variances not assumed			.437	4.524	.682	1.100	2.518	-5.582	7.782
	Palatal Length ol-sta	Equal variances assumed	1.363	.248	.032	59	.975	.061	1.898	-3.737	3.859
		Equal variances not assumed			.056	7.349	.957	.061	1.082	-2.474	2.595
	Palatal Breadth enm-enm	Equal variances assumed	.007	.934	1.095	58	.278	2.491	2.276	-2.064	7.046
		Equal variances not assumed			1.219	4.987	.277	2.491	2.044	-2.768	7.749
	Bicondylar Breadth cdl-cdl	Equal variances assumed	3.722	.060	1.914	47	.062	7.739	4.044	-.397	15.875
		Equal variances not assumed			5.021	6.180	.002	7.739	1.541	3.994	11.484
	Bigonial Breadth go-go	Equal variances assumed	.264	.609	.336	62	.738	1.070	3.182	-5.291	7.431
		Equal variances not assumed			.381	8.163	.713	1.070	2.811	-5.388	7.529
	Height of Ascending Ramus Right go-cdl	Equal variances assumed	1.317	.256	1.950	56	.056	4.494	2.305	-.124	9.112
		Equal variances not assumed			2.821	6.049	.030	4.494	1.593	.603	8.385
	Min Breadth of Ascending Ramus Right	Equal variances assumed	.089	.767	.381	59	.705	.485	1.273	-2.063	3.033
		Equal variances not assumed			.375	6.101	.720	.485	1.292	-2.665	3.634
	Height at Mandibular Symphysis gn-idi	Equal variances assumed	.109	.742	.502	59	.617	.803	1.598	-2.396	4.002
		Equal variances not assumed			.453	5.880	.667	.803	1.772	-3.554	5.160

T-Test ectopic, impacted teeth

			Levene's Test for Equality of Variances		t-test for Equality of Means						
										95% Confidence Interval of the Difference	
Sex			F	Sig.	t	df	Sig. (2-tailed)	Mean Difference	Std. Error Difference	Lower	Upper
Female	Max Cranial Length	Equal variances assumed	.419	.520	.535	51	.595	1.832	3.425	-5.044	8.708
		Equal variances not assumed			.577	8.399	.579	1.832	3.178	-5.436	9.101
	Max Cranial Breadth	Equal variances assumed	.016	.901	.178	51	.860	.391	2.199	-4.024	4.807
		Equal variances not assumed			.167	7.628	.872	.391	2.342	-5.054	5.837
	Cranial Height	Equal variances assumed	9.213	.005	-1.470	33	.151	-6.132	4.172	-14.621	2.356
		Equal variances not assumed			-.757	5.177	.482	-6.132	8.101	-26.744	14.480
	Facial Height n-gn	Equal variances assumed	.416	.524	.789	29	.436	3.131	3.967	-4.984	11.245
		Equal variances not assumed			.903	6.509	.399	3.131	3.467	-5.193	11.455
	Facial Width zy-zy	Equal variances assumed	.819	.371	1.591	40	.119	4.908	3.085	-1.326	11.142
		Equal variances not assumed			1.160	3.300	.323	4.908	4.230	-7.889	17.705
	FMT Width	Equal variances assumed	.056	.813	.881	46	.383	1.905	2.161	-2.445	6.254
		Equal variances not assumed			.861	6.419	.420	1.905	2.213	-3.425	7.235
	Upper Facial Height n-pr	Equal variances assumed	.008	.930	2.339	43	.024	5.175	2.213	.712	9.638
		Equal variances not assumed			2.240	4.941	.076	5.175	2.310	-.786	11.136
	Maxilloalveolar Length pr-alv	Equal variances assumed	.	.	-.562	27	.579	-2.107	3.750	-9.802	5.588
		Equal variances not assumed			.	.	.	-2.107	.	.	.
	Maxilloalveolar Breadth ect-ect	Equal variances assumed	2.882	.097	1.848	41	.072	5.058	2.738	-.471	10.587
		Equal variances not assumed			1.167	4.319	.303	5.058	4.332	-6.628	16.743
	Palatal Length ol-sta	Equal variances assumed	2.123	.152	.505	43	.616	.910	1.802	-2.724	4.545
		Equal variances not assumed			.358	5.617	.733	.910	2.542	-5.414	7.234
	Palatal Breadth enm-enm	Equal variances assumed	7.774	.008	-.849	41	.401	-1.895	2.231	-6.400	2.611
		Equal variances not assumed			-.420	4.144	.695	-1.895	4.512	-14.252	10.463

	Measurement		F	Sig.	t	df	Sig. (2-tailed)	Mean Diff	Std Error Diff	Lower	Upper
	Bicondylar Breadth cdl-cdl	Equal variances assumed	2.077	.159	.049	33	.962	.155	3.192	-6.340	6.650
		Equal variances not assumed			.065	10.861	.949	.155	2.388	-5.109	5.419
	Bigonial Breadth go-go	Equal variances assumed	1.192	.281	.775	43	.443	2.128	2.747	-3.413	7.668
		Equal variances not assumed			1.036	11.979	.321	2.128	2.053	-2.347	6.602
	Height of Ascending Ramus Right go-cdl	Equal variances assumed	.127	.723	1.719	36	.094	3.281	1.909	-.591	7.153
		Equal variances not assumed			1.587	6.584	.159	3.281	2.067	-1.670	8.232
	Min Breadth of Ascending Ramus Right	Equal variances assumed	4.574	.039	.173	39	.864	.195	1.132	-2.094	2.484
		Equal variances not assumed			.295	16.372	.771	.195	.661	-1.204	1.594
	Height at Mandibular Symphysis gn-idi	Equal variances assumed	.194	.662	.944	38	.351	1.569	1.662	-1.796	4.934
		Equal variances not assumed			1.030	7.448	.335	1.569	1.523	-1.990	5.128
Male	Max Cranial Length	Equal variances assumed	1.498	.226	-.003	62	.998	-.008	2.615	-5.236	5.220
		Equal variances not assumed			-.003	11.957	.997	-.008	2.322	-5.068	5.052
	Max Cranial Breadth	Equal variances assumed	.142	.708	.921	65	.361	2.843	3.088	-3.323	9.010
		Equal variances not assumed			.848	8.605	.419	2.843	3.353	-4.796	10.482
	Cranial Height	Equal variances assumed	.213	.647	-.953	46	.346	-2.690	2.823	-8.372	2.992
		Equal variances not assumed			-1.116	7.357	.300	-2.690	2.411	-8.336	2.955
	Facial Height n-gn	Equal variances assumed	.003	.960	1.402	43	.168	4.641	3.309	-2.033	11.315
		Equal variances not assumed			1.213	6.089	.270	4.641	3.828	-4.692	13.974
	Facial Width zy-zy	Equal variances assumed	.065	.799	.246	45	.807	.575	2.338	-4.135	5.285
		Equal variances not assumed			.213	7.472	.837	.575	2.700	-5.728	6.878
	FMT Width	Equal variances assumed	.000	.986	-.070	55	.944	-.194	2.765	-5.735	5.347
		Equal variances not assumed			-.083	8.864	.935	-.194	2.332	-5.483	5.094
	Upper Facial Height n-pr	Equal variances assumed	1.507	.225	.552	54	.584	1.000	1.813	-2.635	4.635
		Equal variances not assumed			.740	13.123	.472	1.000	1.351	-1.916	3.916
	Maxilloalveolar Length pr-alv	Equal variances assumed	.743	.394	2.767	38	.009	4.171	1.507	1.120	7.223
		Equal variances not assumed			3.344	6.063	.015	4.171	1.248	1.127	7.216
	Maxilloalveolar Breadth ect-ect	Equal variances assumed	6.105	.017	-.821	55	.415	-1.494	1.819	-5.141	2.152
		Equal variances not assumed			-1.702	28.028	.100	-1.494	.878	-3.292	.304
	Palatal Length ol-sta	Equal variances assumed	.890	.349	1.467	59	.148	2.354	1.605	-.856	5.565
		Equal variances not assumed			2.023	10.058	.070	2.354	1.164	-.237	4.946
	Palatal Breadth enm-enm	Equal variances assumed	2.002	.162	-.050	58	.960	-.100	1.979	-4.062	3.862
		Equal variances not assumed			-.093	17.379	.927	-.100	1.077	-2.368	2.168
	Bicondylar Breadth cdl-cdl	Equal variances assumed	.002	.969	-.298	47	.767	-.857	2.874	-6.639	4.924
		Equal variances not assumed			-.306	8.294	.767	-.857	2.803	-7.281	5.567
	Bigonial Breadth go-go	Equal variances assumed	5.291	.025	.506	62	.615	1.518	3.000	-4.478	7.514
		Equal variances not assumed			.304	7.491	.769	1.518	4.986	-10.118	13.154
	Height of Ascending Ramus Right go-cdl	Equal variances assumed	1.574	.215	.424	56	.673	.820	1.936	-3.058	4.698
		Equal variances not assumed			.342	8.291	.741	.820	2.399	-4.679	6.319
	Min Breadth of Ascending Ramus Right	Equal variances assumed	.112	.739	.277	59	.783	.311	1.124	-1.938	2.560
		Equal variances not assumed			.302	9.869	.769	.311	1.031	-1.990	2.612
	Height at Mandibular Symphysis gn-idi	Equal variances assumed	3.238	.077	1.075	59	.287	1.505	1.400	-1.296	4.305
		Equal variances not assumed			1.674	15.845	.114	1.505	.899	-.402	3.411

141

T-Test Crowding

Sex			Levene's Test for Equality of Variances		t-test for Equality of Means					95% Confidence Interval of the Difference	
			F	Sig.	t	df	Sig. (2-tailed)	Mean Difference	Std. Error Difference	Lower	Upper
Female	Max Cranial Length	Equal variances assumed	.689	.410	.790	51	.433	2.432	3.078	-3.748	8.612
		Equal variances not assumed			.842	12.301	.416	2.432	2.889	-3.846	8.710
	Max Cranial Breadth	Equal variances assumed	3.109	.084	-.755	51	.453	-1.430	1.893	-5.231	2.371
		Equal variances not assumed			-.615	11.261	.551	-1.430	2.326	-6.534	3.674
	Cranial Height	Equal variances assumed	5.599	.024	-2.813	33	.008	-10.250	3.644	-17.665	-2.835
		Equal variances not assumed			-1.648	6.376	.147	-10.250	6.219	-25.252	4.752
	Facial Height n-gn	Equal variances assumed	1.213	.280	-.613	29	.544	-2.054	3.349	-8.903	4.795
		Equal variances not assumed			-.692	15.585	.499	-2.054	2.971	-8.366	4.257
	Facial Width zy-zy	Equal variances assumed	.574	.453	-.833	40	.410	-1.879	2.256	-6.438	2.681
		Equal variances not assumed			-1.072	20.156	.296	-1.879	1.753	-5.533	1.775
	FMT Width	Equal variances assumed	3.380	.072	1.008	46	.319	2.035	2.020	-2.031	6.100
		Equal variances not assumed			1.606	16.119	.128	2.035	1.267	-.650	4.719
	Upper Facial Height n-pr	Equal variances assumed	.658	.422	.363	43	.719	.643	1.773	-2.933	4.219
		Equal variances not assumed			.303	11.852	.767	.643	2.118	-3.979	5.265
	Maxilloalveolar Length pr-alv	Equal variances assumed	.031	.862	-1.167	27	.253	-1.935	1.658	-5.337	1.467
		Equal variances not assumed			-1.239	8.490	.248	-1.935	1.561	-5.500	1.630
	Maxilloalveolar Breadth ect-ect	Equal variances assumed	3.197	.081	-1.298	41	.202	-2.986	2.300	-7.631	1.660
		Equal variances not assumed			-1.883	20.126	.074	-2.986	1.586	-6.292	.321
	Palatal Length ol-sta	Equal variances assumed	6.802	.012	.568	43	.573	.909	1.601	-2.320	4.138
		Equal variances not assumed			.412	8.133	.691	.909	2.207	-4.166	5.983
	Palatal Breadth enm-enm	Equal variances assumed	1.229	.274	.216	41	.830	.400	1.853	-3.342	4.142
		Equal variances not assumed			.296	17.507	.771	.400	1.351	-2.444	3.244
	Bicondylar Breadth cdl-cdl	Equal variances assumed	1.543	.223	-.510	33	.614	-1.397	2.742	-6.977	4.182
		Equal variances not assumed			-.624	21.634	.539	-1.397	2.241	-6.050	3.255
	Bigonial Breadth go-go	Equal variances assumed	1.019	.318	1.482	43	.146	3.486	2.352	-1.258	8.230
		Equal variances not assumed			1.697	18.240	.107	3.486	2.055	-.827	7.798
	Height of Ascending Ramus Right go-cdl	Equal variances assumed	1.599	.214	.267	36	.791	.498	1.866	-3.287	4.282
		Equal variances not assumed			.336	12.406	.743	.498	1.483	-2.721	3.717
	Min Breadth of Ascending Ramus Right	Equal variances assumed	.094	.761	-1.093	39	.281	-1.087	.995	-3.099	.925
		Equal variances not assumed			-1.173	11.670	.264	-1.087	.927	-3.113	.938
	Height at Mandibular Symphysis gn-idi	Equal variances assumed	.454	.504	-.942	38	.352	-1.472	1.562	-4.634	1.690
		Equal variances not assumed			-1.261	13.332	.229	-1.472	1.167	-3.987	1.044
Male	Max Cranial Length	Equal variances assumed	6.116	.016	1.393	62	.169	2.773	1.991	-1.207	6.753
		Equal variances not assumed			1.802	56.602	.077	2.773	1.539	-.309	5.855
	Max Cranial Breadth	Equal variances assumed	.045	.832	1.216	65	.229	2.784	2.290	-1.790	7.357
		Equal variances not assumed			1.343	33.587	.188	2.784	2.073	-1.431	6.998
	Cranial Height	Equal variances assumed	.109	.743	.602	46	.550	1.273	2.113	-2.981	5.526
		Equal variances not assumed			.599	21.290	.556	1.273	2.125	-3.143	5.688
	Facial Height n-gn	Equal variances assumed	.253	.617	-.112	43	.911	-.279	2.485	-5.290	4.732

		Equal variances not assumed			-.118	28.368	.907	-.279	2.367	-5.124	4.566
	Facial Width zy-zy	Equal variances assumed	.136	.715	-.552	45	.584	-1.025	1.856	-4.763	2.713
		Equal variances not assumed			-.518	19.333	.610	-1.025	1.979	-5.162	3.113
	FMT Width	Equal variances assumed	.937	.337	.179	55	.858	.356	1.983	-3.619	4.330
		Equal variances not assumed			.230	53.127	.819	.356	1.549	-2.751	3.463
	Upper Facial Height n-pr	Equal variances assumed	.000	.993	-1.301	54	.199	-1.746	1.341	-4.435	.944
		Equal variances not assumed			-1.285	32.413	.208	-1.746	1.359	-4.512	1.021
	Maxilloalveolar Length pr-alv	Equal variances assumed	.102	.751	-.298	38	.768	-.406	1.365	-3.169	2.356
		Equal variances not assumed			-.315	11.582	.759	-.406	1.291	-3.231	2.419
	Maxilloalveolar Breadth ect-ect	Equal variances assumed	.615	.436	-.869	55	.389	-1.115	1.284	-3.688	1.457
		Equal variances not assumed			-.913	37.594	.367	-1.115	1.221	-3.588	1.357
	Palatal Length ol-sta	Equal variances assumed	.962	.331	1.031	59	.307	1.167	1.132	-1.098	3.431
		Equal variances not assumed			1.143	40.771	.260	1.167	1.021	-.896	3.229
	Palatal Breadth enm-enm	Equal variances assumed	2.552	.116	-1.843	58	.070	-2.484	1.348	-5.182	.213
		Equal variances not assumed			-1.514	22.351	.144	-2.484	1.641	-5.884	.916
	Bicondylar Breadth cdl-cdl	Equal variances assumed	2.002	.164	-1.439	47	.157	-3.076	2.138	-7.377	1.224
		Equal variances not assumed			-1.547	32.006	.132	-3.076	1.989	-7.128	.975
	Bigonial Breadth go-go	Equal variances assumed	.274	.602	.614	62	.541	1.314	2.138	-2.960	5.588
		Equal variances not assumed			.569	30.956	.574	1.314	2.310	-3.397	6.024
	Height of Ascending Ramus Right go-cdl	Equal variances assumed	.227	.635	-.169	56	.866	-.248	1.469	-3.190	2.694
		Equal variances not assumed			-.170	30.475	.866	-.248	1.457	-3.222	2.726
	Min Breadth of Ascending Ramus Right	Equal variances assumed	3.163	.080	-1.262	59	.212	-1.021	.809	-2.640	.597
		Equal variances not assumed			-1.128	27.290	.269	-1.021	.906	-2.878	.836
	Height at Mandibular Symphysis gn-idi	Equal variances assumed	.207	.651	-.776	59	.441	-.796	1.025	-2.847	1.255
		Equal variances not assumed			-.783	35.559	.439	-.796	1.016	-2.858	1.266

c. By sex and population, craniometrics with anomalies

T-Test Supplemental

Independent Samples Test

				Levene's Test for Equality of Variances		t-test for Equality of Means					95% Confidence Interval of the Difference	
Sex	MajorGeo			F	Sig.	t	df	Sig. (2-tailed)	Mean Difference	Std. Error Difference	Lower	Upper
Male	English	Max Cranial Length	Equal variances assumed	.003	.959	.032	34	.974	.176	5.453	-10.906	11.259
			Equal variances not assumed			.031	1.112	.980	.176	5.648	-56.586	56.939
		Max Cranial Breadth	Equal variances assumed	.787	.381	1.708	37	.096	11.459	6.708	-2.133	25.051
			Equal variances not assumed			1.133	1.045	.454	11.459	10.110	-104.665	127.584
		Facial Height n-gn	Equal variances assumed	.	.	1.314	25	.201	10.500	7.989	-5.954	26.954
			Equal variances not assumed			.	.	.	10.500	.	.	.
		Facial Width zy-zy	Equal variances assumed	.	.	-.363	24	.720	-2.200	6.062	-14.711	10.311
			Equal variances not assumed			.	.	.	-2.200	.	.	.
		FMT Width	Equal variances assumed	1.848	.182	.670	38	.507	2.184	3.261	-4.417	8.785
			Equal variances not assumed			.362	1.028	.778	2.184	6.041	-69.859	74.227
		Upper Facial Height n-pr	Equal variances assumed	1.336	.256	.857	33	.398	3.015	3.519	-4.145	10.175

143

		Equal variances not assumed			1.748	1.743	.241	3.015	1.725	-5.559	11.589
	Maxilloalveolar Length pr-alv	Equal variances assumed	.	.	.034	24	.973	.120	3.573	-7.255	7.495
		Equal variances not assumed	.	.	.	.	.	.120	.	.	.
	Maxilloalveolar Breadth ect-ect	Equal variances assumed	3.017	.091	-.698	38	.490	-2.026	2.904	-7.906	3.853
		Equal variances not assumed			-3.079	37.000	.004	-2.026	.658	-3.360	-.693
	Palatal Length ol-sta	Equal variances assumed	3.595	.065	.027	42	.978	.071	2.626	-5.227	5.370
		Equal variances not assumed			.126	41.000	.900	.071	.567	-1.073	1.216
	Palatal Breadth enm-enm	Equal variances assumed	3.338	.075	-.200	41	.842	-.512	2.560	-5.681	4.657
		Equal variances not assumed			-.916	40.000	.365	-.512	.559	-1.642	.617
	Bicondylar Breadth cdl-cdl	Equal variances assumed	.	.	.629	31	.534	3.969	6.310	-8.901	16.838
		Equal variances not assumed	.	.	.	.	.	3.969	.	.	.
	Bigonial Breadth go-go	Equal variances assumed	7.937	.008	2.291	37	.028	13.797	6.022	1.595	26.000
		Equal variances not assumed			.948	1.015	.515	13.797	14.555	-164.709	192.303
	Height of Ascending Ramus Right go-cdl	Equal variances assumed	.040	.843	1.361	39	.181	5.013	3.683	-2.436	12.462
		Equal variances not assumed			1.096	1.065	.462	5.013	4.572	-45.297	55.322
	Min Breadth of Ascending Ramus Right	Equal variances assumed	.046	.832	-.153	40	.879	-.325	2.121	-4.612	3.962
		Equal variances not assumed			-.158	1.110	.898	-.325	2.053	-21.025	20.375
	Height at Mandibular Symphysis gn-idi	Equal variances assumed	2.559	.118	1.079	39	.287	2.692	2.496	-2.357	7.741
		Equal variances not assumed			4.820	38.000	.000	2.692	.559	1.562	3.823

a. No statistics are computed for one or more split files

T-Test Rotations

Independent Samples Test

				Levene's Test for Equality of Variances		t-test for Equality of Means						
											95% Confidence Interval of the Difference	
Sex	MajorGeo			F	Sig.	t	df	Sig. (2-tailed)	Mean Difference	Std. Error Difference	Lower	Upper
Female	English	Max Cranial Length	Equal variances assumed	12.768	.002	1.601	23	.123	6.286	3.927	-1.837	14.409
			Equal variances not assumed			1.153	6.907	.287	6.286	5.450	-6.636	19.207
		Max Cranial Breadth	Equal variances assumed	3.650	.069	-.484	23	.633	-1.412	2.916	-7.445	4.621
			Equal variances not assumed			-.386	8.771	.708	-1.412	3.655	-9.712	6.889
		Cranial Height	Equal variances assumed	.410	.530	.763	17	.456	4.385	5.747	-7.741	16.510
			Equal variances not assumed			1.009	16.947	.327	4.385	4.344	-4.782	13.551
		Facial Height n-gn	Equal variances assumed	2.459	.148	.441	10	.668	1.857	4.210	-7.522	11.237
			Equal variances not assumed			.480	9.855	.642	1.857	3.870	-6.783	10.497
		Facial Width zy-zy	Equal variances assumed	.084	.776	.337	16	.740	1.200	3.557	-6.340	8.740
			Equal variances not assumed			.347	15.997	.733	1.200	3.455	-6.125	8.525
		FMT Width	Equal variances assumed	3.324	.081	1.554	24	.133	2.583	1.663	-.848	6.015
			Equal variances not assumed			1.252	8.995	.242	2.583	2.063	-2.085	7.251
		Upper Facial Height n-pr	Equal variances assumed	.102	.753	-.741	17	.469	-1.420	1.918	-5.467	2.626
			Equal variances not assumed			-.779	16.990	.447	-1.420	1.823	-5.267	2.426
		Maxilloalveolar Length pr-alv	Equal variances assumed	2.404	.141	.814	16	.427	1.338	1.642	-2.144	4.819
			Equal variances not assumed			.953	14.821	.356	1.338	1.403	-1.656	4.331
		Maxilloalveolar Breadth ect-ect	Equal variances assumed	4.140	.054	-1.011	22	.323	-2.063	2.039	-6.292	2.167
			Equal variances not assumed			-1.251	21.989	.224	-2.063	1.649	-5.481	1.356
		Palatal Length ol-sta	Equal variances assumed	2.428	.132	1.725	24	.097	3.000	1.739	-.589	6.589
			Equal variances assumed									

Group	Measurement		F	Sig.	t	df	Sig. (2-tailed)	Mean Difference	Std. Error Difference	Lower	Upper
		Equal variances not assumed			2.346	23.698	.028	3.000	1.279	.359	5.641
	Palatal Breadth enm-enm	Equal variances assumed	.972	.335	-.370	22	.715	-.681	1.840	-4.497	3.135
		Equal variances not assumed			-.445	17.556	.662	-.681	1.530	-3.901	2.540
	Bicondylar Breadth cdl-cdl	Equal variances assumed	.004	.949	2.526	17	.022	8.284	3.279	1.365	15.203
		Equal variances not assumed			2.596	16.498	.019	8.284	3.192	1.535	15.034
	Bigonial Breadth go-go	Equal variances assumed	.697	.414	1.549	20	.137	4.375	2.824	-1.515	10.265
		Equal variances not assumed			1.711	19.014	.103	4.375	2.557	-.976	9.726
	Height of Ascending Ramus Right go-cdl	Equal variances assumed	.091	.766	1.058	19	.303	1.788	1.690	-1.749	5.326
		Equal variances not assumed			1.093	16.488	.290	1.788	1.637	-1.673	5.250
	Min Breadth of Ascending Ramus Right	Equal variances assumed	.230	.637	2.145	20	.044	2.054	.957	.057	4.050
		Equal variances not assumed			2.218	16.210	.041	2.054	.926	.093	4.014
	Height at Mandibular Symphysis gn-idi	Equal variances assumed	.375	.547	1.622	20	.121	1.821	1.123	-.521	4.164
		Equal variances not assumed			1.721	17.404	.103	1.821	1.058	-.407	4.050
Macedonian	Max Cranial Length	Equal variances assumed	.279	.602	.616	26	.543	1.622	2.635	-3.794	7.039
		Equal variances not assumed			.628	19.842	.537	1.622	2.583	-3.768	7.012
	Max Cranial Breadth	Equal variances assumed	.979	.331	-.388	26	.701	-.600	1.546	-3.777	2.577
		Equal variances not assumed			-.370	16.286	.716	-.600	1.622	-4.033	2.833
	Cranial Height	Equal variances assumed	2.479	.138	.489	14	.633	1.745	3.571	-5.913	9.403
		Equal variances not assumed			.583	12.153	.571	1.745	2.994	-4.769	8.260
	Facial Height n-gn	Equal variances assumed	1.114	.306	.111	17	.913	.467	4.208	-8.411	9.344
		Equal variances not assumed			.113	15.981	.911	.467	4.125	-8.278	9.211
	Facial Width zy-zy	Equal variances assumed	2.458	.131	1.135	22	.269	2.286	2.015	-1.892	6.464
		Equal variances not assumed			1.018	12.051	.329	2.286	2.246	-2.605	7.177
	FMT Width	Equal variances assumed	.022	.883	.450	20	.658	1.208	2.685	-4.392	6.809
		Equal variances not assumed			.433	8.407	.676	1.208	2.792	-5.175	7.592
	Upper Facial Height n-pr	Equal variances assumed	.202	.657	-.290	24	.775	-.650	2.244	-5.280	3.980
		Equal variances not assumed			-.281	17.383	.782	-.650	2.313	-5.522	4.222
	Maxilloalveolar Length pr-alv	Equal variances assumed	.511	.493	1.144	9	.282	3.556	3.108	-3.474	10.585
		Equal variances not assumed			.849	1.199	.532	3.556	4.187	-32.706	39.817
	Maxilloalveolar Breadth ect-ect	Equal variances assumed	.168	.687	-.190	17	.852	-.679	3.570	-8.211	6.854
		Equal variances not assumed			-.204	15.517	.841	-.679	3.319	-7.733	6.376
	Palatal Length ol-sta	Equal variances assumed	.418	.527	1.121	17	.278	2.036	1.815	-1.794	5.866
		Equal variances not assumed			1.168	14.309	.262	2.036	1.742	-1.694	5.765
	Palatal Breadth enm-enm	Equal variances assumed	1.440	.247	.685	17	.502	1.738	2.536	-3.612	7.089
		Equal variances not assumed			.825	16.329	.421	1.738	2.106	-2.720	6.196
	Bicondylar Breadth cdl-cdl	Equal variances assumed	.360	.558	1.760	14	.100	3.746	2.129	-.819	8.311
		Equal variances not assumed			1.716	11.601	.113	3.746	2.183	-1.029	8.521
	Bigonial Breadth go-go	Equal variances assumed	.122	.730	-.899	21	.379	-2.538	2.825	-8.413	3.336
		Equal variances not assumed			-.891	18.879	.384	-2.538	2.848	-8.502	3.425
	Height of Ascending Ramus Right go-cdl	Equal variances assumed	1.594	.226	1.708	15	.108	4.057	2.375	-1.006	9.120
		Equal variances not assumed			1.614	10.387	.137	4.057	2.514	-1.516	9.631
	Min Breadth of Ascending Ramus Right	Equal variances assumed	1.386	.255	.266	17	.794	.357	1.344	-2.479	3.194
		Equal variances not assumed			.233	8.657	.821	.357	1.530	-3.126	3.840
	Height at Mandibular	Equal variances assumed	1.917	.185	.897	16	.383	2.083	2.321	-2.838	7.005

145

				F	Sig.	t	df	Sig. (2-tailed)	Mean Diff	Std. Error Diff	Lower	Upper
		Symphysis gn-idi	Equal variances not assumed			.729	6.395	.492	2.083	2.859	-4.810	8.977
Male	English	Max Cranial Length	Equal variances assumed	7.482	.010	1.858	34	.072	4.938	2.657	-.462	10.339
			Equal variances not assumed			2.789	32.600	.009	4.938	1.771	1.334	8.543
		Max Cranial Breadth	Equal variances assumed	6.171	.018	.096	37	.924	.328	3.415	-6.591	7.247
			Equal variances not assumed			.066	10.871	.949	.328	4.994	-10.680	11.336
		Cranial Height	Equal variances assumed	1.049	.314	2.049	29	.050	5.067	2.473	.010	10.124
			Equal variances not assumed			1.826	13.677	.090	5.067	2.775	-.898	11.031
		Facial Height n-gn	Equal variances assumed	1.252	.274	1.641	25	.113	5.550	3.382	-1.416	12.516
			Equal variances not assumed			1.998	16.172	.063	5.550	2.778	-.333	11.433
		Facial Width zy-zy	Equal variances assumed	.490	.491	.950	24	.352	2.361	2.486	-2.771	7.493
			Equal variances not assumed			.818	9.993	.433	2.361	2.888	-4.074	8.796
		FMT Width	Equal variances assumed	1.075	.306	1.265	38	.213	1.984	1.568	-1.191	5.159
			Equal variances not assumed			1.140	15.078	.272	1.984	1.740	-1.723	5.692
		Upper Facial Height n-pr	Equal variances assumed	1.858	.182	1.456	33	.155	2.580	1.772	-1.026	6.186
			Equal variances not assumed			1.754	25.909	.091	2.580	1.471	-.444	5.604
		Maxilloalveolar Length pr-alv	Equal variances assumed	2.090	.161	-.174	24	.863	-.283	1.630	-3.647	3.081
			Equal variances not assumed			-.219	12.942	.830	-.283	1.294	-3.081	2.514
		Maxilloalveolar Breadth ect-ect	Equal variances assumed	.004	.949	-.545	38	.589	-.774	1.421	-3.651	2.103
			Equal variances not assumed			-.556	18.867	.585	-.774	1.392	-3.689	2.140
		Palatal Length ol-sta	Equal variances assumed	.750	.391	.971	42	.337	1.253	1.291	-1.352	3.858
			Equal variances not assumed			1.070	17.291	.299	1.253	1.170	-1.213	3.719
		Palatal Breadth enm-enm	Equal variances assumed	2.186	.147	.260	41	.796	.321	1.235	-2.173	2.815
			Equal variances not assumed			.231	14.545	.820	.321	1.387	-2.643	3.286
		Bicondylar Breadth cdl-cdl	Equal variances assumed	.276	.603	1.394	31	.173	3.306	2.371	-1.530	8.141
			Equal variances not assumed			1.307	12.845	.214	3.306	2.528	-2.163	8.775
		Bigonial Breadth go-go	Equal variances assumed	1.816	.186	1.132	37	.265	3.617	3.196	-2.858	10.093
			Equal variances not assumed			.923	11.772	.375	3.617	3.920	-4.942	12.176
		Height of Ascending Ramus Right go-cdl	Equal variances assumed	.567	.456	1.532	39	.133	2.727	1.780	-.872	6.327
			Equal variances not assumed			1.415	15.543	.177	2.727	1.928	-1.370	6.824
		Min Breadth of Ascending Ramus Right	Equal variances assumed	.020	.889	1.820	40	.076	1.798	.988	-.198	3.794
			Equal variances not assumed			1.645	14.940	.121	1.798	1.093	-.533	4.128
		Height at Mandibular Symphysis gn-idi	Equal variances assumed	.294	.591	2.152	39	.038	2.506	1.164	.151	4.861
			Equal variances not assumed			2.450	23.572	.022	2.506	1.023	.393	4.619
	Macedonian	Max Cranial Length	Equal variances assumed	.380	.543	-.392	26	.699	-1.303	3.328	-8.144	5.537
			Equal variances not assumed			-.488	11.659	.635	-1.303	2.672	-7.144	4.538
		Max Cranial Breadth	Equal variances assumed	1.630	.213	1.103	26	.280	3.045	2.762	-2.632	8.723
			Equal variances not assumed			1.595	17.142	.129	3.045	1.909	-.980	7.071
		Cranial Height	Equal variances assumed	3.317	.089	.584	15	.568	2.000	3.422	-5.294	9.294
			Equal variances not assumed			1.216	14.987	.243	2.000	1.645	-1.507	5.507
		Facial Height n-gn	Equal variances assumed	.658	.429	.812	16	.429	3.031	3.733	-4.883	10.944
			Equal variances not assumed			1.018	12.510	.328	3.031	2.976	-3.424	9.486
		Facial Width zy-zy	Equal variances assumed	.089	.769	1.156	19	.262	3.200	2.769	-2.595	8.995
			Equal variances not assumed			1.224	7.378	.259	3.200	2.615	-2.921	9.321
		FMT Width	Equal variances assumed	.879	.363	-.149	15	.884	-.923	6.202	-14.143	12.296

			Equal variances not assumed			-.262	14.018	.797	-.923	3.520	-8.472	6.626
	Upper Facial Height n-pr	Equal variances assumed	.423	.523	.367	19	.718	.763	2.079	-3.588	5.113
		Equal variances not assumed			.448	9.924	.664	.763	1.702	-3.035	4.560
	Maxilloalveolar Length pr-alv	Equal variances assumed	.659	.433	-.038	12	.970	-.091	2.370	-5.255	5.073
		Equal variances not assumed			-.059	8.240	.955	-.091	1.546	-3.638	3.456
	Maxilloalveolar Breadth ect-ect	Equal variances assumed	1.009	.331	1.090	15	.293	3.857	3.537	-3.683	11.397
		Equal variances not assumed			1.523	4.872	.190	3.857	2.533	-2.706	10.420
	Palatal Length ol-sta	Equal variances assumed	.150	.704	-.637	15	.534	-1.846	2.899	-8.026	4.334
		Equal variances not assumed			-.579	4.410	.591	-1.846	3.188	-10.383	6.690
	Palatal Breadth enm-enm	Equal variances assumed	.021	.888	-.016	15	.988	-.071	4.495	-9.653	9.510
		Equal variances not assumed			-.014	2.680	.990	-.071	4.974	-17.026	16.883
	Bicondylar Breadth cdl-cdl	Equal variances assumed	.637	.438	1.344	14	.200	5.917	4.401	-3.522	15.355
		Equal variances not assumed			1.639	7.801	.141	5.917	3.611	-2.447	14.280
	Bigonial Breadth go-go	Equal variances assumed	.062	.805	-.554	23	.585	-1.650	2.980	-7.814	4.514
		Equal variances not assumed			-.630	7.401	.547	-1.650	2.617	-7.771	4.471
	Height of Ascending Ramus Right go-cdl	Equal variances assumed	1.111	.309	.294	15	.773	.929	3.155	-5.797	7.654
		Equal variances not assumed			.206	2.304	.854	.929	4.517	-16.245	18.102
	Min Breadth of Ascending Ramus Right	Equal variances assumed	.085	.774	.976	17	.343	1.917	1.964	-2.227	6.060
		Equal variances not assumed			.993	2.850	.397	1.917	1.930	-4.411	8.244
	Height at Mandibular Symphysis gn-idi	Equal variances assumed	1.026	.324	-.631	18	.536	-1.706	2.704	-7.386	3.974
		Equal variances not assumed			-.910	4.399	.410	-1.706	1.875	-6.731	3.319

T-Test Reversals

Independent Samples Test[a]

				Levene's Test for Equality of Variances		t-test for Equality of Means						
											95% Confidence Interval of the Difference	
Sex	MajorGeo			F	Sig.	t	df	Sig. (2-tailed)	Mean Difference	Std. Error Difference	Lower	Upper
Female	Macedonian	Max Cranial Length	Equal variances assumed	.089	.768	1.388	26	.177	6.615	4.765	-3.178	16.409
			Equal variances not assumed			1.079	1.089	.464	6.615	6.130	-57.683	70.914
		Max Cranial Breadth	Equal variances assumed	3.284	.082	.838	26	.410	2.385	2.846	-3.466	8.235
			Equal variances not assumed			2.585	9.412	.028	2.385	.922	.312	4.458
		Cranial Height	Equal variances assumed	3.068	.102	-.691	14	.501	-3.429	4.963	-14.073	7.216
			Equal variances not assumed			-1.653	10.070	.129	-3.429	2.075	-8.047	1.190
		Facial Height n-gn	Equal variances assumed	2.449	.136	-1.112	17	.282	-7.353	6.612	-21.303	6.597
			Equal variances not assumed			-2.470	4.492	.062	-7.353	2.977	-15.272	.566
		Facial Width zy-zy	Equal variances assumed	.001	.970	-.798	22	.433	-2.909	3.645	-10.468	4.650
			Equal variances not assumed			-.796	1.188	.554	-2.909	3.655	-35.102	29.284
		FMT Width	Equal variances assumed	.278	.604	-.120	20	.906	-.500	4.179	-9.217	8.217
			Equal variances not assumed			-.153	1.391	.897	-.500	3.259	-22.415	21.415
		Upper Facial Height n-pr	Equal variances assumed	2.885	.102	-.264	24	.794	-1.083	4.097	-9.540	7.373
			Equal variances not assumed			-.933	23.000	.360	-1.083	1.161	-3.485	1.318
		Maxilloalveolar Length pr-alv	Equal variances assumed	.254	.626	.336	9	.744	1.111	3.305	-6.366	8.588
			Equal variances not assumed			.263	1.234	.829	1.111	4.218	-33.522	35.745
		Maxilloalveolar Breadth ect-ect	Equal variances assumed	3.605	.075	-.811	17	.429	-4.471	5.512	-16.100	7.159
			Equal variances not assumed			-2.425	16.000	.027	-4.471	1.843	-8.378	-.563

147

	Palatal Length ol-sta	Equal variances assumed	.002	.969	-.380	17	.709	-1.118	2.945	-7.330	5.095
		Equal variances not assumed			-.355	1.210	.774	-1.118	3.147	-27.913	25.678
	Palatal Breadth enm-enm	Equal variances assumed	1.241	.281	.007	17	.994	.029	4.041	-8.496	8.555
		Equal variances not assumed			.020	15.906	.984	.029	1.440	-3.025	3.084
	Bicondylar Breadth cdl-cdl	Equal variances assumed	.025	.876	-.243	14	.811	-.857	3.521	-8.409	6.694
		Equal variances not assumed			-.205	1.195	.867	-.857	4.182	-37.343	35.628
	Bigonial Breadth go-go	Equal variances assumed	1.395	.251	.896	21	.381	4.452	4.971	-5.885	14.789
		Equal variances not assumed			2.100	3.802	.107	4.452	2.120	-1.557	10.462
	Height of Ascending Ramus Right go-cdl	Equal variances assumed	3.781	.071	-1.026	15	.321	-3.933	3.833	-12.103	4.237
		Equal variances not assumed			-2.890	14.000	.012	-3.933	1.361	-6.852	-1.014
	Min Breadth of Ascending Ramus Right	Equal variances assumed	.838	.373	-.334	17	.742	-.706	2.111	-5.159	3.747
		Equal variances not assumed			-.578	2.190	.617	-.706	1.221	-5.546	4.135
	Height at Mandibular Symphysis gn-idi	Equal variances assumed	.	.	-.796	16	.438	-3.824	4.802	-14.004	6.357
		Equal variances not assumed			.	.	.	-3.824	.	.	.

a. No statistics are computed for one or more split files

T-Test misshapen teeth

Independent Samples Test

				Levene's Test for Equality of Variances		t-test for Equality of Means					95% Confidence Interval of the Difference	
Sex	MajorGeo			F	Sig.	t	df	Sig. (2-tailed)	Mean Difference	Std. Error Difference	Lower	Upper
Male	English	Max Cranial Length	Equal variances assumed	.003	.959	-1.063	34	.295	-4.727	4.446	-13.763	4.309
			Equal variances not assumed			-1.115	2.425	.363	-4.727	4.242	-20.230	10.776
		Max Cranial Breadth	Equal variances assumed	.523	.474	-1.041	37	.305	-5.917	5.685	-17.435	5.602
			Equal variances not assumed			-2.404	5.986	.053	-5.917	2.461	-11.942	.108
		Cranial Height	Equal variances assumed	.113	.739	-1.019	29	.317	-3.694	3.625	-11.108	3.719
			Equal variances not assumed			-1.084	4.120	.338	-3.694	3.408	-13.050	5.661
		Facial Height n-gn	Equal variances assumed	.183	.673	-.238	25	.814	-1.043	4.386	-10.077	7.990
			Equal variances not assumed			-.251	4.312	.813	-1.043	4.151	-12.247	10.160
		Facial Width zy-zy	Equal variances assumed	.219	.644	-.028	24	.978	-.125	4.387	-9.179	8.929
			Equal variances not assumed			-.039	1.363	.974	-.125	3.242	-22.641	22.391
		FMT Width	Equal variances assumed	1.383	.247	1.250	38	.219	3.324	2.660	-2.061	8.709
			Equal variances not assumed			2.665	4.758	.047	3.324	1.247	.069	6.580
		Upper Facial Height n-pr	Equal variances assumed	1.493	.230	.477	33	.637	1.234	2.587	-4.030	6.497
			Equal variances not assumed			.689	5.312	.520	1.234	1.791	-3.289	5.757
		Maxilloalveolar Length pr-alv	Equal variances assumed	.	.	.923	24	.365	3.240	3.512	-4.007	10.487
			Equal variances not assumed			.	.	.	3.240	.	.	.
		Maxilloalveolar Breadth ect-ect	Equal variances assumed	1.477	.232	.027	38	.979	.079	2.923	-5.838	5.996
			Equal variances not assumed			.066	2.055	.953	.079	1.199	-4.949	5.107
		Palatal Length ol-sta	Equal variances assumed	.090	.766	.620	42	.538	1.175	1.894	-2.647	4.997
			Equal variances not assumed			.743	3.990	.499	1.175	1.581	-3.220	5.570
		Palatal Breadth enm-enm	Equal variances assumed	3.186	.082	-.740	41	.463	-1.365	1.844	-5.090	2.359
			Equal variances not assumed			-1.594	9.755	.143	-1.365	.857	-3.281	.550
		Bicondylar Breadth cdl-cdl	Equal variances assumed	.447	.509	1.039	31	.307	3.867	3.722	-3.725	11.458
			Equal variances not assumed			.727	2.174	.537	3.867	5.317	-17.339	25.072

		F	Sig.	t	df	Sig. (2-tailed)	Mean Difference	Std. Error Difference	Lower	Upper
Bigonial Breadth go-go	Equal variances assumed	.258	.614	-.219	37	.828	-1.167	5.323	-11.953	9.620
	Equal variances not assumed			-.179	2.214	.873	-1.167	6.524	-26.789	24.456
Height of Ascending Ramus Right go-cdl	Equal variances assumed	.392	.535	-.809	39	.423	-2.196	2.714	-7.685	3.293
	Equal variances not assumed			-.939	3.998	.401	-2.196	2.338	-8.688	4.296
Min Breadth of Ascending Ramus Right	Equal variances assumed	.388	.537	.317	40	.753	.487	1.537	-2.620	3.594
	Equal variances not assumed			.403	4.232	.707	.487	1.209	-2.799	3.773
Height at Mandibular Symphysis gn-idi	Equal variances assumed	1.647	.207	.037	39	.971	.068	1.839	-3.652	3.787
	Equal variances not assumed			.064	6.346	.951	.068	1.049	-2.466	2.601

a. No statistics are computed for one or more split files

T-Test congenitally absent teeth

Independent Samples Test

				Levene's Test for Equality of Variances		t-test for Equality of Means					95% Confidence Interval of the Difference	
Sex	MajorGeo			F	Sig.	t	df	Sig. (2-tailed)	Mean Difference	Std. Error Difference	Lower	Upper
Female	English	Max Cranial Length	Equal variances assumed	.288	.597	.844	23	.407	5.696	6.748	-8.263	19.654
			Equal variances not assumed			.620	1.088	.640	5.696	9.192	-90.999	102.390
		Max Cranial Breadth	Equal variances assumed	.906	.351	.886	23	.385	4.391	4.956	-5.861	14.644
			Equal variances not assumed			1.787	2.252	.202	4.391	2.457	-5.124	13.906
		Cranial Height	Equal variances assumed	.577	.458	.444	17	.662	3.912	8.802	-14.658	22.481
			Equal variances not assumed			1.185	12.197	.259	3.912	3.301	-3.268	11.091
		Facial Height n-gn	Equal variances assumed	.	.	.726	10	.485	5.364	7.390	-11.101	21.829
			Equal variances not assumed			.	.	.	5.364	.	.	.
		Facial Width zy-zy	Equal variances assumed	.	.	.505	16	.620	3.882	7.682	-12.403	20.168
			Equal variances not assumed			.	.	.	3.882	.	.	.
		FMT Width	Equal variances assumed	1.325	.261	.739	24	.467	2.208	2.988	-3.958	8.374
			Equal variances not assumed			1.284	1.721	.345	2.208	1.720	-6.468	10.885
		Upper Facial Height n-pr	Equal variances assumed	.000	.999	-.339	17	.739	-1.059	3.124	-7.650	5.533
			Equal variances not assumed			-.334	1.240	.786	-1.059	3.166	-26.850	24.732
		Maxilloalveolar Length pr-alv	Equal variances assumed	.	.	-.482	16	.637	-1.706	3.542	-9.214	5.802
			Equal variances not assumed			.	.	.	-1.706	.	.	.
		Maxilloalveolar Breadth ect-ect	Equal variances assumed	.014	.908	-.269	22	.791	-.955	3.552	-8.322	6.412
			Equal variances not assumed			-.231	1.133	.852	-.955	4.127	-40.868	38.959
		Palatal Length ol-sta	Equal variances assumed	2.164	.154	.026	24	.979	.083	3.193	-6.507	6.674
			Equal variances not assumed			.092	23.000	.927	.083	.905	-1.788	1.955
		Palatal Breadth enm-enm	Equal variances assumed	.294	.593	.135	22	.894	.409	3.034	-5.883	6.702
			Equal variances not assumed			.100	1.094	.935	.409	4.091	-42.133	42.951
		Bicondylar Breadth cdl-cdl	Equal variances assumed	.	.	-.574	17	.574	-4.833	8.423	-22.603	12.937
			Equal variances not assumed			.	.	.	-4.833	.	.	.
		Bigonial Breadth go-go	Equal variances assumed	.	.	.677	20	.506	4.619	6.824	-9.615	18.853
			Equal variances not assumed			.	.	.	4.619	.	.	.
		Height of Ascending Ramus Right go-cdl	Equal variances assumed	.	.	-.848	19	.407	-3.300	3.893	-11.448	4.848
			Equal variances not assumed			.	.	.	-3.300	.	.	.
		Min Breadth of Ascending Ramus Right	Equal variances assumed	.	.	-1.016	20	.322	-2.429	2.391	-7.416	2.559
			Equal variances not assumed			.	.	.	-2.429	.	.	.

						F	df	Sig.	Mean Diff	Std. Error	Lower	Upper
Male	English	Height at Mandibular Symphysis gn-idi	Equal variances assumed			.155	20	.878	.429	2.757	-5.323	6.180
			Equal variances not assumed						.429			
		Max Cranial Length	Equal variances assumed			.773	34	.445	5.829	7.535	-9.485	21.142
			Equal variances not assumed						5.829			
		Max Cranial Breadth	Equal variances assumed			2.364	37	.023	21.421	9.063	3.057	39.785
			Equal variances not assumed						21.421			
		FMT Width	Equal variances assumed			1.892	38	.066	8.282	4.377	-.579	17.143
			Equal variances not assumed						8.282			
		Upper Facial Height n-pr	Equal variances assumed			.279	33	.782	1.382	4.952	-8.692	11.457
			Equal variances not assumed						1.382			
		Maxilloalveolar Breadth ect-ect	Equal variances assumed			-.485	38	.630	-1.974	4.067	-10.209	6.260
			Equal variances not assumed						-1.974			
		Palatal Length ol-sta	Equal variances assumed			.019	42	.985	.070	3.670	-7.336	7.476
			Equal variances not assumed						.070			
		Palatal Breadth enm-enm	Equal variances assumed			-.140	41	.890	-.500	3.577	-7.725	6.725
			Equal variances not assumed						-.500			
		Bigonial Breadth go-go	Equal variances assumed			3.687	37	.001	28.316	7.680	12.755	43.876
			Equal variances not assumed						28.316			
		Height of Ascending Ramus Right go-cdl	Equal variances assumed			1.885	39	.067	9.500	5.039	-.692	19.692
			Equal variances not assumed						9.500			
		Min Breadth of Ascending Ramus Right	Equal variances assumed			.587	40	.561	1.732	2.951	-4.233	7.696
			Equal variances not assumed						1.732			
		Height at Mandibular Symphysis gn-idi	Equal variances assumed			.747	39	.459	2.625	3.512	-4.479	9.729
			Equal variances not assumed						2.625			
	Macedonian	Max Cranial Length	Equal variances assumed			-1.439	26	.162	-10.222	7.102	-24.821	4.377
			Equal variances not assumed						-10.222			
		Max Cranial Breadth	Equal variances assumed			-2.295	26	.030	-13.074	5.697	-24.785	-1.363
			Equal variances not assumed						-13.074			
		Cranial Height	Equal variances assumed			-2.938	15	.010	-13.125	4.467	-22.647	-3.603
			Equal variances not assumed						-13.125			
		Facial Height n-gn	Equal variances assumed			-2.431	16	.027	-15.471	6.365	-28.964	-1.977
			Equal variances not assumed						-15.471			
		Facial Width zy-zy	Equal variances assumed			-1.962	19	.065	-10.250	5.224	-21.183	.683
			Equal variances not assumed						-10.250			
		FMT Width	Equal variances assumed			-.547	15	.592	-6.063	11.079	-29.677	17.552
			Equal variances not assumed						-6.063			
		Upper Facial Height n-pr	Equal variances assumed			-2.911	19	.009	-10.100	3.469	-17.361	-2.839
			Equal variances not assumed						-10.100			
		Maxilloalveolar Length pr-alv	Equal variances assumed			-2.480	12	.029	-7.615	3.071	-14.306	-.925
			Equal variances not assumed						-7.615			
		Maxilloalveolar Breadth ect-ect	Equal variances assumed			.390	15	.702	2.313	5.924	-10.314	14.939
			Equal variances not assumed						2.313			
		Palatal Length ol-sta	Equal variances assumed			-.909	15	.378	-4.688	5.157	-15.679	6.304
			Equal variances not assumed						-4.688			

					t	df	Sig. (2-tailed)	Mean Difference	Std. Error Difference	Lower	Upper
	Palatal Breadth enm-enm	Equal variances assumed	.	.	1.214	15	.244	8.438	6.950	-6.376	23.251
		Equal variances not assumed	.	.	.	.	.	8.438	.	.	.
	Bicondylar Breadth cdl-cdl	Equal variances assumed	.	.	-1.816	14	.091	-13.667	7.526	-29.808	2.474
		Equal variances not assumed	.	.	.	.	.	-13.667	.	.	.
	Bigonial Breadth go-go	Equal variances assumed	.	.	.527	23	.603	3.208	6.086	-9.383	15.799
		Equal variances not assumed	.	.	.	.	.	3.208	.	.	.
	Height of Ascending Ramus Right go-cdl	Equal variances assumed	.	.	-1.371	15	.191	-6.625	4.833	-16.926	3.676
		Equal variances not assumed	.	.	.	.	.	-6.625	.	.	.
	Min Breadth of Ascending Ramus Right	Equal variances assumed	.	.	-3.305	17	.004	-8.500	2.572	-13.925	-3.075
		Equal variances not assumed	.	.	.	.	.	-8.500	.	.	.
	Height at Mandibular Symphysis gn-idi	Equal variances assumed	.	.	-1.923	18	.071	-7.842	4.079	-16.412	.728
		Equal variances not assumed	.	.	.	.	.	-7.842	.	.	.

a. No statistics are computed for one or more split files

T-Test absent M3

Independent Samples Test

Sex	MajorGeo			Levene's Test for Equality of Variances		t-test for Equality of Means					95% Confidence Interval of the Difference	
				F	Sig.	t	df	Sig. (2-tailed)	Mean Difference	Std. Error Difference	Lower	Upper
Female	English	Max Cranial Length	Equal variances assumed	.157	.695	-.688	23	.498	-3.894	5.662	-15.607	7.819
			Equal variances not assumed			-.749	2.727	.513	-3.894	5.198	-21.415	13.627
		Max Cranial Breadth	Equal variances assumed	.182	.674	1.523	23	.141	6.106	4.010	-2.190	14.402
			Equal variances not assumed			1.756	2.851	.182	6.106	3.478	-5.296	17.509
		Cranial Height	Equal variances assumed	.	.	.795	17	.437	9.500	11.946	-15.705	34.705
			Equal variances not assumed			.	.	.	9.500	.	.	.
		FMT Width	Equal variances assumed	.913	.349	-.662	24	.515	-1.652	2.497	-6.806	3.502
			Equal variances not assumed			-.853	3.106	.454	-1.652	1.936	-7.697	4.392
		Maxilloalveolar Length pr-alv	Equal variances assumed	.	.	-.790	16	.441	-2.765	3.500	-10.183	4.654
			Equal variances not assumed			.	.	.	-2.765	.	.	.
		Maxilloalveolar Breadth ect-ect	Equal variances assumed	.	.	.453	22	.655	2.217	4.899	-7.942	12.376
			Equal variances not assumed			.	.	.	2.217	.	.	.
		Palatal Length ol-sta	Equal variances assumed	.298	.590	-1.383	24	.179	-4.250	3.073	-10.593	2.093
			Equal variances not assumed			-1.040	1.089	.476	-4.250	4.087	-47.117	38.617
		Palatal Breadth enm-enm	Equal variances assumed	.	.	.093	22	.927	.391	4.198	-8.314	9.097
			Equal variances not assumed			.	.	.	.391	.	.	.
		Bicondylar Breadth cdl-cdl	Equal variances assumed	.664	.427	-.941	17	.360	-5.676	6.032	-18.403	7.051
			Equal variances not assumed			-1.409	1.744	.311	-5.676	4.029	-25.695	14.342
		Bigonial Breadth go-go	Equal variances assumed	.483	.495	.113	20	.911	.474	4.188	-8.262	9.209
			Equal variances not assumed			.159	3.862	.882	.474	2.980	-7.918	8.865
		Height of Ascending Ramus Right go-cdl	Equal variances assumed	1.046	.319	.137	19	.892	.395	2.876	-5.624	6.413
			Equal variances not assumed			.086	1.072	.945	.395	4.579	-49.357	50.146
		Min Breadth of Ascending Ramus Right	Equal variances assumed	.444	.513	-.778	20	.446	-1.140	1.466	-4.199	1.918
			Equal variances not assumed			-.863	2.904	.453	-1.140	1.321	-5.423	3.143
		Height at Mandibular Symphysis gn-idi	Equal variances assumed	1.723	.204	-.410	20	.686	-.684	1.668	-4.163	2.794
			Equal variances not assumed			-.791	8.608	.450	-.684	.865	-2.655	1.287

				F	Sig.	t	df	Sig. (2-tailed)	Mean Difference	Std. Error Difference	Lower	Upper
	Macedonian	Max Cranial Length	Equal variances assumed	.085	.773	.359	26	.722	1.769	4.926	-8.356	11.895
			Equal variances not assumed			.377	1.179	.763	1.769	4.689	-40.174	43.713
		Max Cranial Breadth	Equal variances assumed	.018	.895	-.107	26	.916	-.308	2.884	-6.235	5.620
			Equal variances not assumed			-.099	1.135	.935	-.308	3.097	-30.138	29.523
		Cranial Height	Equal variances assumed	.	.	-.468	14	.647	-3.200	6.842	-17.874	11.474
			Equal variances not assumed			.	.	.	-3.200	.	.	.
		FMT Width	Equal variances assumed	.033	.857	1.702	20	.104	6.650	3.907	-1.500	14.800
			Equal variances not assumed			1.431	1.138	.367	6.650	4.648	-37.909	51.209
		Maxilloalveolar Length pr-alv	Equal variances assumed	4.723	.058	.336	9	.744	1.111	3.305	-6.366	8.588
			Equal variances not assumed			.620	6.392	.556	1.111	1.791	-3.206	5.429
		Maxilloalveolar Breadth ect-ect	Equal variances assumed	1.345	.262	.299	17	.768	1.676	5.603	-10.144	13.497
			Equal variances not assumed			.538	2.371	.637	1.676	3.117	-9.913	13.266
		Palatal Length ol-sta	Equal variances assumed	3.380	.084	.189	17	.852	.559	2.954	-5.673	6.791
			Equal variances not assumed			.505	12.301	.622	.559	1.106	-1.845	2.963
		Palatal Breadth enm-enm	Equal variances assumed	.468	.503	.855	17	.405	3.382	3.957	-4.966	11.730
			Equal variances not assumed			1.694	3.024	.188	3.382	1.996	-2.942	9.707
		Bicondylar Breadth cdl-cdl	Equal variances assumed	.	.	-.617	14	.547	-2.933	4.756	-13.135	7.268
			Equal variances not assumed			.	.	.	-2.933	.	.	.
		Bigonial Breadth go-go	Equal variances assumed	.343	.564	.449	21	.658	2.262	5.041	-8.220	12.744
			Equal variances not assumed			.594	1.401	.634	2.262	3.809	-23.072	27.596
		Height of Ascending Ramus Right go-cdl	Equal variances assumed	.255	.621	-1.026	15	.321	-3.933	3.833	-12.103	4.237
			Equal variances not assumed			-.762	1.133	.573	-3.933	5.159	-53.829	45.963
		Min Breadth of Ascending Ramus Right	Equal variances assumed	1.726	.206	.461	17	.651	.971	2.105	-3.470	5.411
			Equal variances not assumed			1.126	7.113	.297	.971	.862	-1.062	3.003
		Height at Mandibular Symphysis gn-idi	Equal variances assumed	.086	.773	.123	16	.904	.438	3.567	-7.124	7.999
			Equal variances not assumed			.135	1.342	.910	.438	3.230	-22.560	23.435
		Facial Height n-gn	Equal variances assumed	2.623	.124	1.174	17	.256	7.735	6.586	-6.160	21.631
			Equal variances not assumed			3.425	16.971	.003	7.735	2.258	2.970	12.500
		Facial Width zy-zy	Equal variances assumed	.806	.379	.696	22	.494	2.545	3.657	-5.039	10.130
			Equal variances not assumed			1.379	2.266	.288	2.545	1.846	-4.569	9.660
		Upper Facial Height n-pr	Equal variances assumed	.857	.364	1.225	24	.233	4.875	3.981	-3.341	13.091
			Equal variances not assumed			2.601	2.406	.101	4.875	1.875	-2.017	11.767
Male	English	Max Cranial Length	Equal variances assumed	2.208	.146	-.065	34	.949	-.353	5.453	-11.435	10.729
			Equal variances not assumed			-.215	6.704	.836	-.353	1.643	-4.274	3.568
		Max Cranial Breadth	Equal variances assumed	24.322	.000	-1.206	37	.235	-5.993	4.969	-16.061	4.075
			Equal variances not assumed			-.474	3.044	.667	-5.993	12.645	-45.908	33.922
		Cranial Height	Equal variances assumed	3.915	.057	.274	29	.786	1.143	4.178	-7.401	9.687
			Equal variances not assumed			.645	9.748	.534	1.143	1.771	-2.817	5.103
		FMT Width	Equal variances assumed	.356	.554	.035	38	.972	.083	2.383	-4.741	4.907
			Equal variances not assumed			.041	4.073	.969	.083	2.021	-5.487	5.654
		Maxilloalveolar Length pr-alv	Equal variances assumed	1.680	.207	-.115	24	.910	-.246	2.150	-4.684	4.192
			Equal variances not assumed			-.212	5.747	.839	-.246	1.162	-3.121	2.628
		Maxilloalveolar Breadth ect-ect	Equal variances assumed	.384	.539	1.241	38	.222	2.583	2.082	-1.631	6.797
			Equal variances not assumed			1.071	3.482	.353	2.583	2.411	-4.523	9.690

Measurement		F	Sig.	t	df	Sig. (2-tailed)	Mean Difference	Std. Error Difference	Lower	Upper
Palatal Length ol-sta	Equal variances assumed	1.026	.317	.474	42	.638	.900	1.897	-2.929	4.729
	Equal variances not assumed			.718	4.879	.506	.900	1.254	-2.347	4.147
Palatal Breadth enm-enm	Equal variances assumed	1.700	.200	.907	41	.370	1.667	1.838	-2.046	5.379
	Equal variances not assumed			.656	3.287	.555	1.667	2.541	-6.034	9.367
Bicondylar Breadth cdl-cdl	Equal variances assumed	3.153	.086	1.784	31	.084	6.433	3.606	-.921	13.788
	Equal variances not assumed			3.999	7.100	.005	6.433	1.609	2.640	10.226
Bigonial Breadth go-go	Equal variances assumed	.085	.772	.320	37	.751	1.493	4.672	-7.974	10.960
	Equal variances not assumed			.352	3.925	.743	1.493	4.243	-10.379	13.364
Height of Ascending Ramus Right go-cdl	Equal variances assumed	1.685	.202	2.031	39	.049	5.284	2.602	.020	10.547
	Equal variances not assumed			3.629	6.581	.009	5.284	1.456	1.796	8.771
Min Breadth of Ascending Ramus Right	Equal variances assumed	.092	.763	.497	40	.622	.763	1.534	-2.338	3.864
	Equal variances not assumed			.396	3.374	.716	.763	1.927	-5.001	6.528
Height at Mandibular Symphysis gn-idi	Equal variances assumed	.292	.592	.643	39	.524	1.176	1.829	-2.524	4.876
	Equal variances not assumed			.756	4.033	.491	1.176	1.555	-3.128	5.479
Facial Height n-gn	Equal variances assumed	.634	.433	2.571	25	.016	13.620	5.297	2.710	24.530
	Equal variances not assumed			3.592	1.375	.117	13.620	3.791	-12.329	39.569
Facial Width zy-zy	Equal variances assumed	.027	.870	1.238	24	.228	4.391	3.547	-2.930	11.713
	Equal variances not assumed			1.156	2.461	.347	4.391	3.799	-9.341	18.124
Upper Facial Height n-pr	Equal variances assumed	1.630	.211	1.539	33	.133	4.385	2.850	-1.413	10.184
	Equal variances not assumed			2.972	4.468	.036	4.385	1.475	.453	8.318
Macedonian Max Cranial Length	Equal variances assumed	.359	.554	1.830	26	.079	7.627	4.168	-.940	16.193
	Equal variances not assumed			1.518	2.314	.252	7.627	5.023	-11.400	26.654
Max Cranial Breadth	Equal variances assumed	2.699	.112	-.892	26	.381	-3.293	3.693	-10.884	4.297
	Equal variances not assumed			-.539	2.137	.641	-3.293	6.110	-28.028	21.441
Cranial Height	Equal variances assumed	.	.	.123	15	.904	.688	5.604	-11.258	12.633
	Equal variances not assumed			.	.	.	.688	.	.	.
Maxilloalveolar Breadth ect-ect	Equal variances assumed	.	.	-.883	15	.391	-5.125	5.805	-17.498	7.248
	Equal variances not assumed			.	.	.	-5.125	.	.	.
Palatal Length ol-sta	Equal variances assumed	.	.	-.488	15	.633	-2.563	5.256	-13.764	8.639
	Equal variances not assumed			.	.	.	-2.563	.	.	.
Palatal Breadth enm-enm	Equal variances assumed	.	.	.581	15	.570	4.188	7.203	-11.165	19.540
	Equal variances not assumed			.	.	.	4.188	.	.	.
Bigonial Breadth go-go	Equal variances assumed	.018	.895	.230	23	.820	.848	3.688	-6.781	8.478
	Equal variances not assumed			.238	2.630	.829	.848	3.571	-11.478	13.175
Height of Ascending Ramus Right go-cdl	Equal variances assumed	.	.	.159	15	.876	.813	5.122	-10.106	11.731
	Equal variances not assumed			.	.	.	.813	.	.	.
Min Breadth of Ascending Ramus Right	Equal variances assumed	1.488	.239	-.025	17	.981	-.059	2.398	-5.118	5.001
	Equal variances not assumed			-.046	2.610	.967	-.059	1.279	-4.496	4.378
Height at Mandibular Symphysis gn-idi	Equal variances assumed	1.767	.200	.017	18	.987	.056	3.253	-6.780	6.891
	Equal variances not assumed			.010	1.062	.994	.056	5.583	-61.823	61.935
Upper Facial Height n-pr	Equal variances assumed	.	.	-.667	19	.513	-2.750	4.124	-11.382	5.882
	Equal variances not assumed			.	.	.	-2.750	.	.	.

T-Test ectopic and impacted teeth

Independent Samples Test

Sex	MajorGeo			Levene's Test for Equality of Variances		t-test for Equality of Means					95% Confidence Interval of the Difference	
				F	Sig.	t	df	Sig. (2-tailed)	Mean Difference	Std. Error Difference	Lower	Upper
Female	English	Max Cranial Length	Equal variances assumed	2.654	.117	-.120	23	.906	-.607	5.069	-11.092	9.878
			Equal variances not assumed			-.195	9.697	.849	-.607	3.106	-7.556	6.342
		Max Cranial Breadth	Equal variances assumed	.664	.423	-.796	23	.434	-2.929	3.679	-10.540	4.683
			Equal variances not assumed			-1.030	5.777	.344	-2.929	2.842	-9.948	4.091
		Cranial Height	Equal variances assumed	37.299	.000	-2.083	17	.053	-13.854	6.650	-27.884	.176
			Equal variances not assumed			-.867	2.025	.476	-13.854	15.980	-81.808	54.100
		Facial Height n-gn	Equal variances assumed	5.088	.048	-.018	10	.986	-.100	5.623	-12.628	12.428
			Equal variances not assumed			-.041	9.000	.968	-.100	2.420	-5.574	5.374
		Facial Width zy-zy	Equal variances assumed	.	.	-.046	16	.964	-.353	7.743	-16.767	16.061
			Equal variances not assumed			.	.	.	-.353	.	.	.
		FMT Width	Equal variances assumed	.996	.328	.153	24	.880	.341	2.230	-4.262	4.944
			Equal variances not assumed			.213	6.360	.838	.341	1.600	-3.520	4.202
		Upper Facial Height n-pr	Equal variances assumed	3.695	.072	2.532	17	.021	6.765	2.671	1.129	12.400
			Equal variances not assumed			1.337	1.050	.401	6.765	5.061	-50.775	64.305
		Maxilloalveolar Length pr-alv	Equal variances assumed	.	.	-.790	16	.441	-2.765	3.500	-10.183	4.654
			Equal variances not assumed			.	.	.	-2.765	.	.	.
		Maxilloalveolar Breadth ect-ect	Equal variances assumed	1.089	.308	-.467	22	.645	-1.381	2.959	-7.517	4.756
			Equal variances not assumed			-.696	3.958	.525	-1.381	1.985	-6.916	4.155
		Palatal Length ol-sta	Equal variances assumed	2.312	.141	.039	24	.970	.091	2.358	-4.777	4.958
			Equal variances not assumed			.024	3.273	.982	.091	3.802	-11.455	11.637
		Palatal Breadth enm-enm	Equal variances assumed	.032	.860	.625	22	.538	1.571	2.515	-3.643	6.786
			Equal variances not assumed			.589	2.518	.604	1.571	2.667	-7.912	11.055
		Bicondylar Breadth cdl-cdl	Equal variances assumed	.916	.352	-.571	17	.576	-2.633	4.614	-12.367	7.101
			Equal variances not assumed			-.720	7.053	.495	-2.633	3.657	-11.269	6.002
		Bigonial Breadth go-go	Equal variances assumed	.069	.796	.465	20	.647	1.722	3.707	-6.011	9.456
			Equal variances not assumed			.524	5.140	.622	1.722	3.284	-6.652	10.096
		Height of Ascending Ramus Right go-cdl	Equal variances assumed	1.112	.305	.495	19	.626	1.059	2.137	-3.414	5.531
			Equal variances not assumed			.617	6.242	.559	1.059	1.716	-3.101	5.219
		Min Breadth of Ascending Ramus Right	Equal variances assumed	3.456	.078	-.294	20	.772	-.389	1.321	-3.145	2.367
			Equal variances not assumed			-.421	8.038	.685	-.389	.924	-2.518	1.740
		Height at Mandibular Symphysis gn-idi	Equal variances assumed	.714	.408	.545	20	.592	.806	1.479	-2.280	3.891
			Equal variances not assumed			.745	7.241	.480	.806	1.081	-1.733	3.345
	Macedonian	Max Cranial Length	Equal variances assumed	1.129	.298	1.665	26	.108	6.507	3.909	-1.528	14.541
			Equal variances not assumed			2.431	3.434	.082	6.507	2.676	-1.434	14.447
		Max Cranial Breadth	Equal variances assumed	.294	.592	2.230	26	.035	4.907	2.201	.383	9.430
			Equal variances not assumed			2.462	2.654	.102	4.907	1.993	-1.930	11.743
		Cranial Height	Equal variances assumed	.240	.632	.386	14	.705	1.641	4.254	-7.482	10.764
			Equal variances not assumed			.411	3.233	.707	1.641	3.990	-10.557	13.839
		Facial Height n-gn	Equal variances assumed	.002	.966	.934	17	.363	5.250	5.621	-6.609	17.109

154

		Measurement		F	Sig.	t	df	Sig. (2-tailed)	Mean Difference	Std. Error Difference	Lower	Upper
			Equal variances not assumed			.915	2.759	.433	5.250	5.741	-13.957	24.457
		Facial Width zy-zy	Equal variances assumed	6.977	.015	2.430	22	.024	6.667	2.743	.977	12.356
			Equal variances not assumed			1.246	2.092	.334	6.667	5.351	-15.418	28.751
		FMT Width	Equal variances assumed	.223	.642	1.544	20	.138	6.100	3.952	-2.143	14.343
			Equal variances not assumed			1.887	1.346	.257	6.100	3.232	-16.803	29.003
		Upper Facial Height n-pr	Equal variances assumed	.157	.695	1.250	24	.223	4.145	3.316	-2.699	10.989
			Equal variances not assumed			1.594	3.071	.207	4.145	2.601	-4.025	12.315
		Maxilloalveolar Breadth ect-ect	Equal variances assumed	1.382	.256	3.321	17	.004	14.529	4.375	5.299	23.760
			Equal variances not assumed			2.039	1.074	.277	14.529	7.126	-62.541	91.600
		Palatal Length ol-sta	Equal variances assumed	2.501	.132	.971	17	.345	2.794	2.878	-3.279	8.867
			Equal variances not assumed			2.578	11.902	.024	2.794	1.084	.430	5.158
		Palatal Breadth enm-enm	Equal variances assumed	35.428	.000	-1.988	17	.063	-7.235	3.640	-14.915	.444
			Equal variances not assumed			-.656	1.010	.629	-7.235	11.027	-144.169	129.699
		Bicondylar Breadth cdl-cdl	Equal variances assumed	.633	.439	.917	14	.375	3.143	3.427	-4.207	10.493
			Equal variances not assumed			1.128	1.536	.405	3.143	2.786	-13.088	19.373
		Bigonial Breadth go-go	Equal variances assumed	1.598	.220	.519	21	.610	2.183	4.211	-6.573	10.940
			Equal variances not assumed			.895	5.646	.407	2.183	2.438	-3.875	8.242
		Height of Ascending Ramus Right go-cdl	Equal variances assumed	.438	.518	2.350	15	.033	7.967	3.390	.741	15.193
			Equal variances not assumed			2.882	1.489	.142	7.967	2.764	-8.841	24.774
		Min Breadth of Ascending Ramus Right	Equal variances assumed	1.726	.206	.461	17	.651	.971	2.105	-3.470	5.411
			Equal variances not assumed			1.126	7.113	.297	.971	.862	-1.062	3.003
		Height at Mandibular Symphysis gn-idi	Equal variances assumed	.054	.820	1.109	16	.284	3.813	3.439	-3.478	11.103
			Equal variances not assumed			1.186	1.315	.407	3.813	3.214	-19.841	27.466
Male	English	Max Cranial Length	Equal variances assumed	3.199	.083	.834	34	.410	3.281	3.935	-4.715	11.278
			Equal variances not assumed			1.863	15.595	.081	3.281	1.761	-.460	7.022
		Max Cranial Breadth	Equal variances assumed	.447	.508	1.440	37	.158	7.100	4.929	-2.888	17.088
			Equal variances not assumed			1.272	3.525	.281	7.100	5.583	-9.262	23.462
		Cranial Height	Equal variances assumed	.876	.357	-.419	29	.678	-2.103	5.019	-12.368	8.161
			Equal variances not assumed			-.644	1.401	.609	-2.103	3.265	-23.805	19.598
		Facial Height n-gn	Equal variances assumed	1.011	.324	-.435	25	.667	-2.580	5.934	-14.802	9.642
			Equal variances not assumed			-.668	1.482	.593	-2.580	3.863	-26.230	21.070
		Facial Width zy-zy	Equal variances assumed	1.430	.243	1.126	24	.271	4.014	3.566	-3.345	11.374
			Equal variances not assumed			2.307	7.923	.050	4.014	1.740	-.005	8.034
		FMT Width	Equal variances assumed	.442	.510	1.602	38	.117	3.694	2.306	-.974	8.363
			Equal variances not assumed			2.040	4.320	.106	3.694	1.811	-1.191	8.580
		Upper Facial Height n-pr	Equal variances assumed	4.269	.047	.040	33	.968	.105	2.596	-5.177	5.386
			Equal variances not assumed			.089	15.248	.931	.105	1.184	-2.416	2.625
		Maxilloalveolar Length pr-alv	Equal variances assumed	.211	.650	.904	24	.375	2.292	2.536	-2.942	7.526
			Equal variances not assumed			1.080	1.266	.444	2.292	2.122	-14.370	18.953
		Maxilloalveolar Breadth ect-ect	Equal variances assumed	3.512	.069	-.354	38	.725	-.750	2.120	-5.041	3.541
			Equal variances not assumed			-.800	13.141	.438	-.750	.938	-2.774	1.274
		Palatal Length ol-sta	Equal variances assumed	.301	.586	1.065	42	.293	2.000	1.877	-1.789	5.789
			Equal variances not assumed			1.212	3.868	.294	2.000	1.650	-2.643	6.643
		Palatal Breadth enm-enm	Equal variances assumed	.629	.432	-.142	41	.888	-.263	1.856	-4.011	3.486

155

			Equal variances not assumed			-.183	4.249	.863	-.263	1.436	-4.158	3.632
	Bicondylar Breadth cdl-cdl	Equal variances assumed	3.917	.057	.315	31	.755	1.435	4.555	-7.854	10.725
		Equal variances not assumed			1.153	20.204	.262	1.435	1.245	-1.159	4.030
	Bigonial Breadth go-go	Equal variances assumed	3.004	.091	2.471	37	.018	12.194	4.935	2.195	22.194
		Equal variances not assumed			1.307	2.074	.317	12.194	9.328	-26.595	50.984
	Height of Ascending Ramus Right go-cdl	Equal variances assumed	1.796	.188	.312	39	.757	.851	2.733	-4.676	6.379
		Equal variances not assumed			.222	3.288	.838	.851	3.840	-10.785	12.488
	Min Breadth of Ascending Ramus Right	Equal variances assumed	3.332	.075	.679	40	.501	1.039	1.530	-2.054	4.133
		Equal variances not assumed			1.519	11.514	.156	1.039	.684	-.459	2.538
	Height at Mandibular Symphysis gn-idi	Equal variances assumed	1.014	.320	.339	39	.737	.622	1.836	-3.093	4.336
		Equal variances not assumed			.505	5.006	.635	.622	1.230	-2.539	3.782
Macedonian	Max Cranial Length	Equal variances assumed	.000	.990	-.848	26	.404	-2.991	3.527	-10.242	4.259
		Equal variances not assumed			-.783	5.458	.466	-2.991	3.820	-12.569	6.586
	Max Cranial Breadth	Equal variances assumed	.098	.757	-.569	26	.574	-1.875	3.293	-8.644	4.894
		Equal variances not assumed			-.520	3.826	.632	-1.875	3.606	-12.068	8.318
	Cranial Height	Equal variances assumed	.547	.471	-.360	15	.724	-1.115	3.097	-7.716	5.486
		Equal variances not assumed			-.324	4.361	.761	-1.115	3.438	-10.358	8.127
	Facial Height n-gn	Equal variances assumed	.778	.391	2.194	16	.043	7.893	3.598	.265	15.521
		Equal variances not assumed			1.788	3.892	.150	7.893	4.413	-4.496	20.282
	Facial Width zy-zy	Equal variances assumed	.939	.345	-.607	19	.551	-1.868	3.077	-8.308	4.573
		Equal variances not assumed			-.444	3.545	.682	-1.868	4.202	-14.148	10.413
	FMT Width	Equal variances assumed	.063	.805	-.974	15	.345	-6.524	6.698	-20.799	7.752
		Equal variances not assumed			-1.429	5.486	.207	-6.524	4.566	-17.954	4.907
	Upper Facial Height n-pr	Equal variances assumed	.241	.629	1.362	19	.189	2.941	2.160	-1.579	7.461
		Equal variances not assumed			1.171	3.935	.308	2.941	2.512	-4.080	9.962
	Maxilloalveolar Length pr-alv	Equal variances assumed	.278	.608	3.515	12	.004	5.848	1.664	2.223	9.474
		Equal variances not assumed			4.058	3.984	.016	5.848	1.441	1.840	9.857
	Maxilloalveolar Breadth ect-ect	Equal variances assumed	9.354	.008	-.610	15	.551	-2.214	3.630	-9.952	5.523
		Equal variances not assumed			-1.352	13.000	.200	-2.214	1.638	-5.753	1.325
	Palatal Length ol-sta	Equal variances assumed	.613	.446	.726	15	.479	2.333	3.213	-4.516	9.183
		Equal variances not assumed			1.194	7.681	.268	2.333	1.955	-2.208	6.874
	Palatal Breadth enm-enm	Equal variances assumed	3.978	.065	.346	15	.734	1.548	4.478	-7.996	11.092
		Equal variances not assumed			.756	13.652	.462	1.548	2.047	-2.853	5.948
	Bicondylar Breadth cdl-cdl	Equal variances assumed	.013	.912	.263	14	.796	1.145	4.358	-8.201	10.492
		Equal variances not assumed			.267	8.149	.796	1.145	4.282	-8.699	10.989
	Bigonial Breadth go-go	Equal variances assumed	.742	.398	-1.445	23	.162	-4.150	2.872	-10.092	1.792
		Equal variances not assumed			-1.175	5.072	.292	-4.150	3.532	-13.191	4.891
	Height of Ascending Ramus Right go-cdl	Equal variances assumed	.686	.420	.588	15	.565	1.654	2.812	-4.339	7.647
		Equal variances not assumed			.479	3.921	.658	1.654	3.455	-8.017	11.325
	Min Breadth of Ascending Ramus Right	Equal variances assumed	.961	.341	-.213	17	.834	-.383	1.803	-4.187	3.420
		Equal variances not assumed			-.187	4.122	.860	-.383	2.047	-6.001	5.234
	Height at Mandibular Symphysis gn-idi	Equal variances assumed	3.832	.066	1.084	18	.293	2.563	2.364	-2.404	7.529
		Equal variances not assumed			1.723	12.485	.110	2.563	1.487	-.664	5.789

T-Test Crowding

Independent Samples Test

Sex	MajorGeo			Levene's Test for Equality of Variances		t-test for Equality of Means					95% Confidence Interval of the Difference	
				F	Sig.	t	df	Sig. (2-tailed)	Mean Difference	Std. Error Difference	Lower	Upper
Female	English	Max Cranial Length	Equal variances assumed	.001	.974	.038	23	.970	.261	6.851	-13.912	14.434
			Equal variances not assumed			.036	1.158	.977	.261	7.262	-67.003	67.525
		Max Cranial Breadth	Equal variances assumed	1.919	.179	-1.602	23	.123	-6.394	3.991	-14.649	1.862
			Equal variances not assumed			-1.041	2.184	.399	-6.394	6.143	-30.806	18.018
		Cranial Height	Equal variances assumed	71.462	.000	-3.758	17	.002	-24.588	6.542	-38.392	-10.785
			Equal variances not assumed			-1.169	1.007	.450	-24.588	21.037	-287.524	238.348
		Facial Height n-gn	Equal variances assumed	3.835	.079	-.125	10	.903	-.700	5.618	-13.218	11.818
			Equal variances not assumed			-.284	9.628	.783	-.700	2.468	-6.227	4.827
		Facial Width zy-zy	Equal variances assumed	1.729	.207	.333	16	.743	1.875	5.624	-10.048	13.798
			Equal variances not assumed			.968	15.000	.348	1.875	1.936	-2.252	6.002
		FMT Width	Equal variances assumed	2.191	.152	1.171	24	.253	2.870	2.451	-2.189	7.928
			Equal variances not assumed			1.993	4.706	.106	2.870	1.440	-.903	6.642
		Upper Facial Height n-pr	Equal variances assumed	4.640	.046	1.640	17	.119	4.021	2.451	-1.151	9.193
			Equal variances not assumed			1.022	2.195	.406	4.021	3.935	-11.547	19.589
		Maxilloalveolar Length pr-alv	Equal variances assumed	.000	.992	-.938	16	.362	-2.375	2.531	-7.741	2.991
			Equal variances not assumed			-.900	1.238	.509	-2.375	2.638	-23.916	19.166
		Maxilloalveolar Breadth ect-ect	Equal variances assumed	1.089	.308	-.467	22	.645	-1.381	2.959	-7.517	4.756
			Equal variances not assumed			-.696	3.958	.525	-1.381	1.985	-6.916	4.155
		Palatal Length ol-sta	Equal variances assumed	2.656	.116	1.355	24	.188	3.478	2.567	-1.820	8.777
			Equal variances not assumed			.786	2.129	.510	3.478	4.428	-14.508	21.464
		Palatal Breadth enm-enm	Equal variances assumed	.002	.965	.780	22	.444	1.952	2.502	-3.237	7.142
			Equal variances not assumed			.762	2.571	.510	1.952	2.561	-7.023	10.928
		Bicondylar Breadth cdl-cdl	Equal variances assumed	.897	.357	-.516	17	.612	-2.667	5.167	-13.568	8.235
			Equal variances not assumed			-.697	4.082	.523	-2.667	3.826	-13.205	7.872
		Bigonial Breadth go-go	Equal variances assumed	.716	.407	.205	20	.839	.860	4.185	-7.869	9.589
			Equal variances not assumed			.304	4.217	.776	.860	2.829	-6.837	8.557
		Height of Ascending Ramus Right go-cdl	Equal variances assumed	1.942	.180	.416	19	.682	1.000	2.402	-4.028	6.028
			Equal variances not assumed			.670	5.307	.531	1.000	1.493	-2.772	4.772
		Min Breadth of Ascending Ramus Right	Equal variances assumed	.002	.967	-1.054	20	.305	-1.526	1.449	-4.548	1.495
			Equal variances not assumed			-.945	2.499	.427	-1.526	1.616	-7.303	4.251
		Height at Mandibular Symphysis gn-idi	Equal variances assumed	.398	.535	.283	20	.780	.474	1.671	-3.013	3.960
			Equal variances not assumed			.360	3.346	.741	.474	1.316	-3.481	4.429
	Macedonian	Max Cranial Length	Equal variances assumed	.052	.821	.260	26	.797	.762	2.933	-5.267	6.791
			Equal variances not assumed			.245	9.434	.811	.762	3.106	-6.215	7.739
		Max Cranial Breadth	Equal variances assumed	.030	.865	.334	26	.741	.571	1.712	-2.947	4.090
			Equal variances not assumed			.321	9.695	.755	.571	1.780	-3.412	4.555
		Cranial Height	Equal variances assumed	1.479	.244	-1.476	14	.162	-4.945	3.350	-12.129	2.239
			Equal variances not assumed			-1.699	11.144	.117	-4.945	2.911	-11.343	1.452
		Facial Height n-gn	Equal variances assumed	.438	.517	-.570	17	.576	-2.551	4.479	-12.001	6.898

157

				Equal variances not assumed			-.613	11.780	.552	-2.551	4.164	-11.644	6.541
		Facial Width zy-zy	Equal variances assumed	.000	.994	-1.738	22	.096	-3.664	2.108	-8.036	.708
			Equal variances not assumed			-1.816	12.390	.094	-3.664	2.018	-8.045	.717
		FMT Width	Equal variances assumed	1.330	.262	.214	20	.833	.667	3.112	-5.825	7.159
			Equal variances not assumed			.315	8.655	.760	.667	2.115	-4.147	5.481
		Upper Facial Height n-pr	Equal variances assumed	.102	.752	-.318	24	.753	-.782	2.460	-5.859	4.295
			Equal variances not assumed			-.305	9.952	.767	-.782	2.568	-6.507	4.943
		Maxilloalveolar Length pr-alv	Equal variances assumed	.469	.511	-.351	9	.734	-.929	2.649	-6.920	5.063
			Equal variances not assumed			-.367	7.296	.724	-.929	2.527	-6.855	4.998
		Maxilloalveolar Breadth ect-ect	Equal variances assumed	3.026	.100	-1.152	17	.265	-4.343	3.771	-12.298	3.613
			Equal variances not assumed			-1.604	15.364	.129	-4.343	2.708	-10.102	1.417
		Palatal Length ol-sta	Equal variances assumed	3.018	.100	-.667	17	.514	-1.357	2.034	-5.649	2.935
			Equal variances not assumed			-.518	5.026	.626	-1.357	2.618	-8.076	5.362
		Palatal Breadth enm-enm	Equal variances assumed	4.518	.048	.061	17	.952	.171	2.816	-5.770	6.112
			Equal variances not assumed			.103	13.558	.920	.171	1.668	-3.417	3.760
		Bicondylar Breadth cdl-cdl	Equal variances assumed	.474	.502	.733	14	.476	1.733	2.365	-3.340	6.807
			Equal variances not assumed			.693	8.934	.506	1.733	2.502	-3.933	7.400
		Bigonial Breadth go-go	Equal variances assumed	.134	.718	2.111	21	.047	5.946	2.817	.088	11.805
			Equal variances not assumed			2.133	11.789	.055	5.946	2.788	-.141	12.034
		Height of Ascending Ramus Right go-cdl	Equal variances assumed	.533	.477	-.096	15	.925	-.288	3.011	-6.706	6.129
			Equal variances not assumed			-.110	6.405	.916	-.288	2.623	-6.609	6.032
		Min Breadth of Ascending Ramus Right	Equal variances assumed	.076	.786	-.399	17	.695	-.586	1.469	-3.685	2.514
			Equal variances not assumed			-.442	8.719	.669	-.586	1.326	-3.599	2.428
		Height at Mandibular Symphysis gn-idi	Equal variances assumed	1.103	.309	-1.450	16	.166	-3.679	2.536	-9.055	1.698
			Equal variances not assumed			-1.877	7.949	.098	-3.679	1.960	-8.203	.846
Male	English	Max Cranial Length	Equal variances assumed	5.963	.020	1.510	34	.140	4.393	2.909	-1.518	10.304
			Equal variances not assumed			2.487	33.392	.018	4.393	1.766	.801	7.985
		Max Cranial Breadth	Equal variances assumed	.067	.798	1.387	37	.174	5.415	3.905	-2.496	13.327
			Equal variances not assumed			1.498	9.640	.166	5.415	3.614	-2.679	13.510
		Cranial Height	Equal variances assumed	.212	.649	.814	29	.422	2.520	3.095	-3.810	8.850
			Equal variances not assumed			.887	8.474	.399	2.520	2.840	-3.966	9.006
		Facial Height n-gn	Equal variances assumed	.219	.644	.423	25	.676	1.500	3.547	-5.805	8.805
			Equal variances not assumed			.449	11.802	.661	1.500	3.340	-5.790	8.790
		Facial Width zy-zy	Equal variances assumed	.770	.389	.797	24	.433	2.333	2.928	-3.709	8.375
			Equal variances not assumed			.606	4.821	.572	2.333	3.852	-7.679	12.346
		FMT Width	Equal variances assumed	.145	.706	1.300	38	.201	2.100	1.615	-1.170	5.370
			Equal variances not assumed			1.325	15.975	.204	2.100	1.585	-1.261	5.461
		Upper Facial Height n-pr	Equal variances assumed	.665	.421	.475	33	.638	.931	1.960	-3.058	4.919
			Equal variances not assumed			.539	14.252	.599	.931	1.728	-2.770	4.631
		Maxilloalveolar Length pr-alv	Equal variances assumed	.496	.488	-.115	24	.910	-.246	2.150	-4.684	4.192
			Equal variances not assumed			-.151	3.174	.889	-.246	1.633	-5.287	4.794
		Maxilloalveolar Breadth ect-ect	Equal variances assumed	.038	.847	.523	38	.604	.767	1.466	-2.201	3.734
			Equal variances not assumed			.531	15.881	.603	.767	1.443	-2.295	3.829
		Palatal Length ol-sta	Equal variances assumed	.063	.804	1.387	42	.173	1.771	1.276	-.805	4.346

			Equal variances not assumed			1.319	13.739	.209	1.771	1.342	-1.113	4.654
		Palatal Breadth enm-enm	Equal variances assumed	.208	.650	-.192	41	.848	-.245	1.276	-2.822	2.331
			Equal variances not assumed			-.209	17.092	.837	-.245	1.175	-2.723	2.233
		Bicondylar Breadth cdl-cdl	Equal variances assumed	.945	.339	-.470	31	.642	-1.190	2.531	-6.352	3.972
			Equal variances not assumed			-.515	13.949	.614	-1.190	2.309	-6.145	3.765
		Bigonial Breadth go-go	Equal variances assumed	1.174	.285	.916	37	.366	2.945	3.215	-3.568	9.458
			Equal variances not assumed			.766	12.118	.458	2.945	3.843	-5.419	11.309
		Height of Ascending Ramus Right go-cdl	Equal variances assumed	.076	.784	.541	39	.592	.988	1.826	-2.705	4.681
			Equal variances not assumed			.551	18.509	.588	.988	1.792	-2.769	4.744
		Min Breadth of Ascending Ramus Right	Equal variances assumed	1.194	.281	-.289	40	.774	-.296	1.027	-2.371	1.779
			Equal variances not assumed			-.250	14.118	.806	-.296	1.184	-2.833	2.241
		Height at Mandibular Symphysis gn-idi	Equal variances assumed	.023	.879	.935	39	.355	1.139	1.218	-1.324	3.603
			Equal variances not assumed			1.000	20.412	.329	1.139	1.140	-1.235	3.514
Macedonian	Max Cranial Length		Equal variances assumed	1.159	.292	.406	26	.688	1.156	2.849	-4.701	7.012
			Equal variances not assumed			.462	25.501	.648	1.156	2.501	-3.991	6.302
		Max Cranial Breadth	Equal variances assumed	.006	.938	-.005	26	.996	-.011	2.420	-4.985	4.963
			Equal variances not assumed			-.005	19.883	.996	-.011	2.370	-4.957	4.935
		Cranial Height	Equal variances assumed	.208	.655	.789	15	.443	2.071	2.627	-3.528	7.671
			Equal variances not assumed			.725	9.238	.486	2.071	2.857	-4.366	8.508
		Facial Height n-gn	Equal variances assumed	.003	.956	-.982	16	.341	-3.338	3.399	-10.543	3.867
			Equal variances not assumed			-.968	12.310	.352	-3.338	3.449	-10.831	4.155
		Facial Width zy-zy	Equal variances assumed	.511	.483	-1.355	19	.191	-3.250	2.399	-8.271	1.771
			Equal variances not assumed			-1.477	18.580	.156	-3.250	2.200	-7.861	1.361
		FMT Width	Equal variances assumed	1.507	.239	-.689	15	.501	-3.629	5.267	-14.855	7.597
			Equal variances not assumed			-.815	10.444	.434	-3.629	4.455	-13.498	6.241
		Upper Facial Height n-pr	Equal variances assumed	.319	.579	-2.036	19	.056	-3.282	1.612	-6.655	.092
			Equal variances not assumed			-2.019	17.697	.059	-3.282	1.626	-6.702	.138
		Maxilloalveolar Length pr-alv	Equal variances assumed	.022	.886	-.363	12	.723	-.733	2.019	-5.132	3.665
			Equal variances not assumed			-.353	7.709	.734	-.733	2.079	-5.559	4.092
		Maxilloalveolar Breadth ect-ect	Equal variances assumed	16.824	.001	-1.496	15	.155	-3.917	2.618	-9.497	1.664
			Equal variances not assumed			-1.551	12.315	.146	-3.917	2.526	-9.404	1.571
		Palatal Length ol-sta	Equal variances assumed	3.215	.093	-.312	15	.759	-.778	2.489	-6.083	4.527
			Equal variances not assumed			-.326	11.312	.750	-.778	2.387	-6.013	4.458
		Palatal Breadth enm-enm	Equal variances assumed	1.399	.255	-1.427	15	.174	-4.597	3.222	-11.464	2.270
			Equal variances not assumed			-1.381	10.758	.195	-4.597	3.328	-11.943	2.749
		Bicondylar Breadth cdl-cdl	Equal variances assumed	4.992	.042	-1.011	14	.329	-3.984	3.940	-12.436	4.467
			Equal variances not assumed			-1.077	13.311	.301	-3.984	3.700	-11.959	3.990
		Bigonial Breadth go-go	Equal variances assumed	.002	.968	.259	23	.798	.633	2.446	-4.426	5.693
			Equal variances not assumed			.266	21.052	.793	.633	2.384	-4.324	5.590
		Height of Ascending Ramus Right go-cdl	Equal variances assumed	.043	.839	-.991	15	.337	-2.424	2.445	-7.636	2.788
			Equal variances not assumed			-1.036	11.771	.321	-2.424	2.340	-7.534	2.686
		Min Breadth of Ascending Ramus Right	Equal variances assumed	1.175	.293	-1.622	17	.123	-2.250	1.387	-5.177	.677
			Equal variances not assumed			-1.537	12.017	.150	-2.250	1.464	-5.440	.940
		Height at Mandibular	Equal variances assumed	.007	.935	-2.341	18	.031	-4.083	1.744	-7.748	-.418

Symphysis gn-idi	Equal variances not assumed			-2.374	15.871	.031	-4.083	1.720	-7.732	-.435

d. Indices and ratios with anomalies, all skulls.

T-Test supplemental teeth

Independent Samples Test

		Levene's Test for Equality of Variances		t-test for Equality of Means					95% Confidence Interval of the Difference	
		F	Sig.	t	df	Sig. (2-tailed)	Mean Difference	Std. Error Difference	Lower	Upper
Cranial Index	Equal variances assumed	.001	.971	1.792	112	.076	6.0493	3.3749	-.6376	12.7362
	Equal variances not assumed			1.851	1.039	.308	6.0493	3.2673	-31.9970	44.0955
Total Facial Index	Equal variances assumed	.	.	1.091	65	.279	6.77921	6.21164	-5.62629	19.18471
	Equal variances not assumed			.	.	.	6.77921	.	.	.
Upper Facial Index	Equal variances assumed	.	.	1.765	80	.081	5.21769	2.95592	-.66477	11.10015
	Equal variances not assumed			.	.	.	5.21769	.	.	.
Maxilloalveolar Index	Equal variances assumed	.	.	-.179	63	.859	-2.03918	11.41842	-24.85708	20.77872
	Equal variances not assumed			.	.	.	-2.03918	.	.	.
Palatal Index	Equal variances assumed	1.665	.200	.293	99	.770	2.71369	9.26838	-15.67678	21.10416
	Equal variances not assumed			2.070	98.000	.041	2.71369	1.31088	.11229	5.31509
Palatal/max ratio	Equal variances assumed	.	.	.395	61	.694	.05008	.12674	-.20335	.30351
	Equal variances not assumed			.	.	.	.05008	.	.	.
TFHFMT	Equal variances assumed	.	.	.965	63	.338	11.41485	11.82875	-12.22301	35.05272
	Equal variances not assumed			.	.	.	11.41485	.	.	.
UFHFMT	Equal variances assumed	.438	.510	.468	85	.641	1.57958	3.37359	-5.12801	8.28717
	Equal variances not assumed			.312	1.020	.807	1.57958	5.06262	-59.78474	62.94390
MAXBCDL	Equal variances assumed	.	.	-.649	63	.519	-.03142	.04840	-.12813	.06530
	Equal variances not assumed			.	.	.	-.03142	.	.	.
cdlgo	Equal variances assumed	.	.	-.875	82	.384	-.05100	.05830	-.16697	.06498
	Equal variances not assumed			.	.	.	-.05100	.	.	.
ZYGFMT	Equal variances assumed	.	.	-.108	75	.914	-.00445	.04109	-.08631	.07740
	Equal variances not assumed			.	.	.	-.00445	.	.	.
UHTH	Equal variances assumed	.	.	.158	72	.875	.00589	.03723	-.06832	.08011
	Equal variances not assumed			.	.	.	.00589	.	.	.
FB	Equal variances assumed	.	.	1.309	58	.196	.05407	.04130	-.02860	.13674
	Equal variances not assumed			.	.	.	.05407	.	.	.
FB2	Equal variances assumed	.	.	-.857	66	.394	-.06262	.07304	-.20844	.08321
	Equal variances not assumed			.	.	.	-.06262	.	.	.
UFIMAI	Equal variances assumed	.	.	1.196	49	.237	.05647	.04721	-.03840	.15134
	Equal variances not assumed			.	.	.	.05647	.	.	.

T-Test Rotations

Independent Samples Test

		Levene's Test for Equality of Variances		t-test for Equality of Means					95% Confidence Interval of the Difference	
		F	Sig.	t	df	Sig. (2-tailed)	Mean Difference	Std. Error Difference	Lower	Upper
Cranial Index	Equal variances assumed	.756	.387	-1.127	112	.262	-1.1106	.9853	-3.0629	.8417
	Equal variances not assumed			-1.006	47.825	.319	-1.1106	1.1040	-3.3305	1.1093
Cranial Module	Equal variances assumed	.069	.794	1.465	76	.147	2.26509	1.54638	-.81479	5.34496
	Equal variances not assumed			1.454	40.674	.153	2.26509	1.55730	-.88071	5.41088
Cranial length-height Index	Equal variances assumed	.076	.784	.976	78	.332	1.00015	1.02461	-1.03970	3.04000
	Equal variances not assumed			.986	41.633	.330	1.00015	1.01415	-1.04702	3.04732
Cranial breadth-height Index	Equal variances assumed	1.336	.251	2.187	78	.032	3.02103	1.38148	.27071	5.77134
	Equal variances not assumed			1.987	35.764	.055	3.02103	1.52039	-.06318	6.10524

Total Facial Index	Equal variances assumed	2.766	.101	.593	65	.555	.90665	1.52989	-2.14875	3.96205
	Equal variances not assumed			.565	47.620	.575	.90665	1.60414	-2.31936	4.13266
Upper Facial Index	Equal variances assumed	.243	.624	.373	80	.710	.25597	.68595	-1.10911	1.62106
	Equal variances not assumed			.351	50.115	.727	.25597	.72981	-1.20981	1.72176
Maxilloalveolar Index	Equal variances assumed	.730	.396	-1.278	63	.206	-3.96453	3.10142	-10.16222	2.23316
	Equal variances not assumed			-1.394	37.181	.172	-3.96453	2.84467	-9.72744	1.79838
Palatal Index	Equal variances assumed	.827	.365	-.485	99	.629	-1.41376	2.91549	-7.19872	4.37120
	Equal variances not assumed			-.552	60.993	.583	-1.41376	2.56259	-6.53799	3.71047
Palatal/max ratio	Equal variances assumed	1.209	.276	.109	61	.914	.00388	.03573	-.06756	.07533
	Equal variances not assumed			.133	45.802	.894	.00388	.02908	-.05466	.06243
TFHFMT	Equal variances assumed	.004	.948	1.357	63	.180	4.10140	3.02325	-1.94008	10.14288
	Equal variances not assumed			1.501	58.969	.139	4.10140	2.73289	-1.36716	9.56995
UFHFMT	Equal variances assumed	1.899	.172	-.346	85	.730	-.37841	1.09348	-2.55254	1.79573
	Equal variances not assumed			-.380	63.452	.705	-.37841	.99545	-2.36738	1.61057
MAXBCDL	Equal variances assumed	.674	.415	-2.418	63	.019	-.02891	.01196	-.05280	-.00501
	Equal variances not assumed			-2.624	56.639	.011	-.02891	.01102	-.05097	-.00685
cdlgo	Equal variances assumed	1.159	.285	-1.729	82	.088	-.02288	.01324	-.04921	.00345
	Equal variances not assumed			-1.820	62.141	.074	-.02288	.01257	-.04801	.00224
ZYGFMT	Equal variances assumed	.157	.693	-.628	75	.532	-.00623	.00991	-.02597	.01352
	Equal variances not assumed			-.656	53.054	.515	-.00623	.00949	-.02527	.01282
UHTH	Equal variances assumed	.282	.597	-1.366	72	.176	-.01196	.00875	-.02940	.00549
	Equal variances not assumed			-1.326	51.794	.191	-.01196	.00902	-.03006	.00614
FB	Equal variances assumed	.014	.907	2.529	58	.014	.02628	.01039	.00548	.04708
	Equal variances not assumed			2.490	46.782	.016	.02628	.01056	.00504	.04752
FB2	Equal variances assumed	.126	.724	-2.123	66	.038	-.03881	.01828	-.07531	-.00230
	Equal variances not assumed			-2.320	52.211	.024	-.03881	.01673	-.07237	-.00524
UFIMAI	Equal variances assumed	.586	.448	1.361	49	.180	.01912	.01405	-.00911	.04735
	Equal variances not assumed			1.377	30.008	.179	.01912	.01388	-.00924	.04747

T-Test Reversals

Independent Samples Test

		Levene's Test for Equality of Variances		t-test for Equality of Means					95% Confidence Interval of the Difference	
		F	Sig.	t	df	Sig. (2-tailed)	Mean Difference	Std. Error Difference	Lower	Upper
Cranial Index	Equal variances assumed	.082	.775	-.795	112	.429	-2.7120	3.4133	-9.4751	4.0511
	Equal variances not assumed			-.996	1.058	.494	-2.7120	2.7217	-33.1364	27.7124
Cranial Module	Equal variances assumed	.591	.445	1.456	76	.150	6.49561	4.46181	-2.39085	15.38208
	Equal variances not assumed			2.497	1.172	.212	6.49561	2.60097	-17.05218	30.04340
Cranial length-height Index	Equal variances assumed	.173	.679	-1.478	78	.144	-4.35527	2.94741	-10.22311	1.51257
	Equal variances not assumed			-1.954	1.094	.284	-4.35527	2.22885	-27.52268	18.81214
Cranial breadth-height Index	Equal variances assumed	1.838	.179	-.592	78	.556	-2.46726	4.16802	-10.76515	5.83062
	Equal variances not assumed			-3.216	14.054	.006	-2.46726	.76728	-4.11233	-.82220
Total Facial Index	Equal variances assumed	1.904	.172	-.822	65	.414	-3.65186	4.44329	-12.52572	5.22200
	Equal variances not assumed			-3.156	3.235	.046	-3.65186	1.15708	-7.18758	-.11613
Upper Facial Index	Equal variances assumed	.478	.491	.201	80	.841	.43125	2.14319	-3.83385	4.69634
	Equal variances not assumed			.300	1.118	.811	.43125	1.43973	-13.86459	14.72708
Maxilloalveolar Index	Equal variances assumed	.045	.833	-.998	63	.322	-8.06052	8.07633	-24.19979	8.07875
	Equal variances not assumed			-.812	1.042	.561	-8.06052	9.92364	-122.83667	106.71563
Palatal Index	Equal variances assumed	.437	.510	-.218	99	.828	-2.02058	9.27016	-20.41460	16.37344
	Equal variances not assumed			-.455	1.199	.718	-2.02058	4.44567	-40.53035	36.48919
Palatal/max ratio	Equal variances assumed	.653	.422	.482	61	.631	.04355	.09029	-.13700	.22410

		F	Sig.	t	df	Sig. (2-tailed)	Mean Difference	Std. Error Difference	95% Confidence Interval of the Difference Lower	Upper
	Equal variances not assumed			1.657	2.591	.210	.04355	.02628	-.04806	.13516
TFHFMT	Equal variances assumed	.850	.360	-.511	63	.611	-4.33424	8.47481	-21.26980	12.60133
	Equal variances not assumed			-2.165	5.038	.082	-4.33424	2.00177	-9.46843	.79995
UFHFMT	Equal variances assumed	.878	.351	-.275	85	.784	-.93019	3.37643	-7.64343	5.78305
	Equal variances not assumed			-.471	1.151	.711	-.93019	1.97289	-19.42340	17.56302
MAXBCDL	Equal variances assumed	.757	.388	-.180	63	.857	-.00624	.03460	-.07538	.06290
	Equal variances not assumed			-.356	1.296	.771	-.00624	.01751	-.13832	.12584
cdlgo	Equal variances assumed	.179	.673	1.793	82	.077	.07329	.04087	-.00802	.15461
	Equal variances not assumed			1.943	1.058	.292	.07329	.03773	-.34783	.49442
ZYGFMT	Equal variances assumed	2.078	.154	.587	75	.559	.01714	.02918	-.04100	.07527
	Equal variances not assumed			3.400	41.121	.002	.01714	.00504	.00696	.02731
UHTH	Equal variances assumed	.901	.346	.819	72	.416	.02161	.02639	-.03100	.07422
	Equal variances not assumed			1.954	1.402	.241	.02161	.01106	-.05181	.09503
FB	Equal variances assumed	2.208	.143	-.766	58	.447	-.02279	.02974	-.08231	.03673
	Equal variances not assumed			-2.998	4.232	.037	-.02279	.00760	-.04344	-.00213
FB2	Equal variances assumed	1.967	.165	.679	66	.500	.03539	.05214	-.06872	.13950
	Equal variances not assumed			3.748	48.164	.000	.03539	.00944	.01640	.05437
UFIMAI	Equal variances assumed	.197	.659	.985	49	.330	.03336	.03388	-.03471	.10144
	Equal variances not assumed			.731	1.044	.594	.03336	.04567	-.49243	.55916

T-Test Misshapen teeth

Independent Samples Test

		Levene's Test for Equality of Variances		t-test for Equality of Means						
		F	Sig.	t	df	Sig. (2-tailed)	Mean Difference	Std. Error Difference	95% Confidence Interval of the Difference Lower	Upper
Cranial Index	Equal variances assumed	.901	.345	-.418	112	.677	-1.1722	2.8052	-6.7303	4.3859
	Equal variances not assumed			-.877	2.568	.455	-1.1722	1.3363	-5.8595	3.5151
Cranial Module	Equal variances assumed	.752	.389	-2.334	76	.022	-8.38222	3.59156	-15.53544	-1.22900
	Equal variances not assumed			-3.735	2.469	.046	-8.38222	2.24399	-16.47506	-.28938
Cranial length-height Index	Equal variances assumed	.769	.383	-.403	78	.688	-.98781	2.45325	-5.87184	3.89623
	Equal variances not assumed			-.734	2.623	.523	-.98781	1.34516	-5.63820	3.66258
Cranial breadth-height Index	Equal variances assumed	2.434	.123	-.027	78	.979	-.09219	3.43287	-6.92650	6.74212
	Equal variances not assumed			-.107	12.283	.917	-.09219	.86288	-1.96746	1.78308
Total Facial Index	Equal variances assumed	.182	.671	-1.192	65	.238	-5.26608	4.41830	-14.09003	3.55787
	Equal variances not assumed			-1.454	1.096	.368	-5.26608	3.62250	-42.80845	32.27629
Upper Facial Index	Equal variances assumed	.099	.754	.672	80	.503	1.43723	2.13771	-2.81694	5.69140
	Equal variances not assumed			.749	1.064	.585	1.43723	1.91849	-19.75144	22.62590
Palatal Index	Equal variances assumed	1.636	.204	-.100	99	.921	-.66072	6.62348	-13.80315	12.48171
	Equal variances not assumed			-.311	8.152	.763	-.66072	2.12120	-5.53643	4.21499
TFHFMT	Equal variances assumed	1.049	.310	-1.458	63	.150	-10.02117	6.87473	-23.75922	3.71688
	Equal variances not assumed			-5.163	11.503	.000	-10.02117	1.94106	-14.27075	-5.77159
UFHFMT	Equal variances assumed	2.361	.128	-.693	85	.490	-1.91799	2.76663	-7.41879	3.58281
	Equal variances not assumed			-1.742	3.300	.172	-1.91799	1.10123	-5.24924	1.41327
MAXBCDL	Equal variances assumed	.	.	.628	63	.532	.03039	.04841	-.06634	.12712
	Equal variances not assumed			.	.	.	.03039	.	.	.
cdlgo	Equal variances assumed	1.148	.287	-1.347	82	.182	-.04561	.03386	-.11297	.02174
	Equal variances not assumed			-1.878	2.314	.184	-.04561	.02429	-.13765	.04642
ZYGFMT	Equal variances assumed	.002	.964	1.117	75	.267	.03241	.02901	-.02538	.09021
	Equal variances not assumed			1.109	1.053	.460	.03241	.02922	-.29737	.36220
UHTH	Equal variances assumed	1.876	.175	1.901	72	.061	.03526	.01855	-.00172	.07225

		F	Sig.	t	df	Sig. (2-tailed)	Mean Difference	Std. Error Difference	Lower	Upper
	Equal variances not assumed			4.598	6.583	.003	.03526	.00767	.01689	.05363
FB	Equal variances assumed			-.160	58	.874	-.00669	.04190	-.09056	.07717
	Equal variances not assumed						-.00669			
FB2	Equal variances assumed	.162	.688	.021	66	.984	.00107	.05232	-.10340	.10554
	Equal variances not assumed			.016	1.037	.990	.00107	.06691	-.78143	.78357

T-Test Congenitally absent teeth

Independent Samples Test

		Levene's Test for Equality of Variances		t-test for Equality of Means					95% Confidence Interval of the Difference	
		F	Sig.	t	df	Sig. (2-tailed)	Mean Difference	Std. Error Difference	Lower	Upper
Cranial Index	Equal variances assumed	1.550	.216	.939	112	.350	2.2855	2.4327	-2.5347	7.1056
	Equal variances not assumed			.701	3.118	.532	2.2855	3.2614	-7.8754	12.4464
Cranial Module	Equal variances assumed	3.751	.056	-.328	76	.744	-1.21778	3.71542	-8.61767	6.18212
	Equal variances not assumed			-.172	2.040	.879	-1.21778	7.06132	-31.03574	28.60018
Cranial length-height Index	Equal variances assumed	.001	.971	-.176	78	.861	-.43255	2.45531	-5.32068	4.45559
	Equal variances not assumed			-.174	2.155	.877	-.43255	2.47953	-10.39671	9.53161
Cranial breadth-height Index	Equal variances assumed	.662	.418	-.199	78	.843	-.68351	3.43201	-7.51612	6.14910
	Equal variances not assumed			-.357	2.599	.748	-.68351	1.91328	-7.34064	5.97362
Total Facial Index	Equal variances assumed	.392	.533	-.164	65	.870	-.73320	4.46539	-9.65121	8.18480
	Equal variances not assumed			-.238	1.140	.847	-.73320	3.08006	-30.17629	28.70989
Upper Facial Index	Equal variances assumed	.042	.839	-.556	80	.580	-1.18931	2.13961	-5.44727	3.06865
	Equal variances not assumed			-.458	1.034	.725	-1.18931	2.59599	-31.73458	29.35596
Maxilloalveolar Index	Equal variances assumed	.344	.560	.639	63	.525	5.18178	8.11371	-11.03217	21.39574
	Equal variances not assumed			.443	1.030	.733	5.18178	11.70294	-133.75937	144.12294
Palatal Index	Equal variances assumed	.044	.835	1.038	99	.302	6.83800	6.58807	-6.23416	19.91016
	Equal variances not assumed			1.379	3.475	.250	6.83800	4.95879	-7.79095	21.46695
Palatal/max ratio	Equal variances assumed	.580	.449	.429	61	.670	.03872	.09033	-.14190	.21935
	Equal variances not assumed			1.333	2.104	.308	.03872	.02904	-.08049	.15794
TFHFMT	Equal variances assumed	.003	.954	-.130	63	.897	-1.10809	8.49124	-18.07647	15.86030
	Equal variances not assumed			-.142	1.077	.909	-1.10809	7.83010	-85.32350	83.10733
UFHFMT	Equal variances assumed	.081	.777	-1.251	85	.214	-2.99588	2.39522	-7.75823	1.76646
	Equal variances not assumed			-1.242	3.291	.296	-2.99588	2.41310	-10.30525	4.31348
MAXBCDL	Equal variances assumed	1.089	.301	1.808	63	.075	.06100	.03374	-.00643	.12843
	Equal variances not assumed			4.906	1.684	.055	.06100	.01243	-.00338	.12537
cdlgo	Equal variances assumed	3.835	.054	2.243	82	.028	.09072	.04045	.01026	.17118
	Equal variances not assumed			14.103	74.438	.000	.09072	.00643	.07790	.10354
ZYGFMT	Equal variances assumed	.003	.953	.630	75	.531	.01838	.02917	-.03974	.07650
	Equal variances not assumed			.634	1.055	.636	.01838	.02901	-.30797	.34474
UHTH	Equal variances assumed	1.092	.300	-.632	72	.529	-.01672	.02644	-.06943	.03598
	Equal variances not assumed			-1.737	1.586	.256	-.01672	.00963	-.07046	.03701
FB	Equal variances assumed	1.530	.221	-1.675	58	.099	-.04890	.02919	-.10732	.00953
	Equal variances not assumed			-4.578	1.788	.055	-.04890	.01068	-.10048	.00269
FB2	Equal variances assumed	.738	.393	1.143	66	.257	.05921	.05181	-.04424	.16266
	Equal variances not assumed			2.526	1.369	.182	.05921	.02344	-.10242	.22084
UFIMAI	Equal variances assumed			-2.504	49	.016	-.11290	.04510	-.20352	-.02228
	Equal variances not assumed						-.11290			

T-Test absent

Independent Samples Test

		Levene's Test for Equality of Variances		t-test for Equality of Means					
								95% Confidence Interval of the Difference	
		F	Sig.	t	df	Sig. (2-tailed)	Mean Difference	Std. Error Difference	Lower	Upper
Cranial Index	Equal variances assumed	17.722	.000	-1.374	112	.172	-2.1645	1.5753	-5.2858	.9569
	Equal variances not assumed			-.658	9.250	.527	-2.1645	3.2893	-9.5750	5.2460
Cranial Module	Equal variances assumed	2.476	.120	-.272	76	.786	-.88288	3.24002	-7.33594	5.57017
	Equal variances not assumed			-.164	3.105	.880	-.88288	5.39519	-17.72871	15.96295
Cranial length-height Index	Equal variances assumed	.811	.371	-.485	78	.629	-1.03664	2.13751	-5.29209	3.21880
	Equal variances not assumed			-.384	3.192	.725	-1.03664	2.69802	-9.33771	7.26443
Cranial breadth-height Index	Equal variances assumed	4.973	.029	1.370	78	.175	3.35170	2.44687	-1.51966	8.22305
	Equal variances not assumed			.817	5.239	.449	3.35170	4.10167	-7.04893	13.75233
Total Facial Index	Equal variances assumed	4.259	.043	1.204	65	.233	3.82122	3.17270	-2.51509	10.15753
	Equal variances not assumed			4.547	59.789	.000	3.82122	.84031	2.14022	5.50222
Upper Facial Index	Equal variances assumed	.077	.781	1.232	80	.222	1.87380	1.52080	-1.15269	4.90029
	Equal variances not assumed			1.386	3.411	.249	1.87380	1.35192	-2.14971	5.89732
Maxilloalveolar Index	Equal variances assumed	3.951	.051	1.014	63	.315	4.88408	4.81715	-4.74222	14.51037
	Equal variances not assumed			2.133	15.080	.050	4.88408	2.28995	.00541	9.76274
Palatal Index	Equal variances assumed	1.406	.239	1.012	99	.314	4.81602	4.75886	-4.62659	14.25863
	Equal variances not assumed			1.706	11.943	.114	4.81602	2.82306	-1.33818	10.97022
Palatal/max ratio	Equal variances assumed	1.927	.170	.025	61	.980	.00137	.05403	-.10667	.10941
	Equal variances not assumed			.063	29.428	.950	.00137	.02180	-.04319	.04592
TFHFMT	Equal variances assumed	.271	.604	1.232	63	.223	7.42889	6.03047	-4.62205	19.47983
	Equal variances not assumed			2.030	4.375	.106	7.42889	3.65884	-2.39535	17.25313
UFHFMT	Equal variances assumed	.295	.589	1.257	85	.212	2.70916	2.15518	-1.57592	6.99423
	Equal variances not assumed			1.416	4.661	.220	2.70916	1.91355	-2.31953	7.73784
MAXBCDL	Equal variances assumed	.023	.879	.084	63	.933	.00210	.02487	-.04759	.05179
	Equal variances not assumed			.087	3.430	.936	.00210	.02425	-.06987	.07407
cdlgo	Equal variances assumed	.073	.787	.512	82	.610	.01261	.02463	-.03638	.06160
	Equal variances not assumed			.482	5.689	.648	.01261	.02617	-.05229	.07751
ZYGFMT	Equal variances assumed	.280	.598	.081	75	.936	.00153	.01888	-.03608	.03914
	Equal variances not assumed			.072	4.439	.945	.00153	.02119	-.05507	.05813
UHTH	Equal variances assumed	.172	.679	-.721	72	.473	-.01366	.01894	-.05142	.02411
	Equal variances not assumed			-.909	3.601	.420	-.01366	.01502	-.05725	.02993
FB	Equal variances assumed	.484	.489	-.904	58	.370	-.02210	.02444	-.07103	.02683
	Equal variances not assumed			-.677	2.114	.565	-.02210	.03262	-.15548	.11128
FB2	Equal variances assumed	1.072	.304	-.560	66	.578	-.01740	.03110	-.07948	.04468
	Equal variances not assumed			-.792	7.495	.453	-.01740	.02196	-.06864	.03384
UFIMAI	Equal variances assumed	1.540	.221	.395	49	.695	.00973	.02466	-.03982	.05929
	Equal variances not assumed			.652	4.948	.544	.00973	.01493	-.02878	.04825

T-Test Ectopic, impacted teeth

Independent Samples Test

		Levene's Test for Equality of Variances		t-test for Equality of Means					
								95% Confidence Interval of the Difference	
		F	Sig.	t	df	Sig. (2-tailed)	Mean Difference	Std. Error Difference	Lower	Upper
Cranial Index	Equal variances assumed	1.288	.259	.144	112	.886	.1913	1.3293	-2.4425	2.8251
	Equal variances not assumed			.186	23.663	.854	.1913	1.0258	-1.9274	2.3099
Cranial Module	Equal variances assumed	1.102	.297	.023	76	.981	.04794	2.05433	-4.04361	4.13949
	Equal variances not assumed			.018	11.738	.986	.04794	2.61232	-5.65796	5.75385

		F	Sig.	t	df	Sig. (2-tailed)	Mean Difference	Std. Error Difference	Lower	Upper
Cranial length-height Index	Equal variances assumed	2.425	.123	-1.689	78	.095	-2.16707	1.28338	-4.72209	.38795
	Equal variances not assumed			-1.176	12.371	.262	-2.16707	1.84353	-6.17047	1.83632
Cranial breadth-height Index	Equal variances assumed	.009	.925	-1.247	78	.216	-2.33824	1.87525	-6.07157	1.39509
	Equal variances not assumed			-.993	11.762	.341	-2.33824	2.35478	-7.48043	2.80394
Total Facial Index	Equal variances assumed	1.246	.268	.618	65	.539	1.31327	2.12674	-2.93412	5.56066
	Equal variances not assumed			.521	11.033	.613	1.31327	2.52269	-4.23708	6.86362
Upper Facial Index	Equal variances assumed	.031	.860	.981	80	.330	.94596	.96452	-.97349	2.86541
	Equal variances not assumed			.977	13.254	.346	.94596	.96860	-1.14251	3.03443
Maxilloalveolar Index	Equal variances assumed	.348	.557	-2.066	63	.043	-9.71019	4.69967	-19.10173	-.31864
	Equal variances not assumed			-2.402	6.561	.050	-9.71019	4.04315	-19.40200	-.01837
Palatal Index	Equal variances assumed	.152	.698	-1.547	99	.125	-6.10460	3.94502	-13.93238	1.72317
	Equal variances not assumed			-1.337	13.107	.204	-6.10460	4.56494	-15.95835	3.74914
Palatal/max ratio	Equal variances assumed	1.873	.176	.730	61	.468	.03928	.05380	-.06830	.14685
	Equal variances not assumed			1.754	25.553	.091	.03928	.02239	-.00679	.08535
TFHFMT	Equal variances assumed	.015	.904	1.291	63	.201	5.40988	4.19113	-2.96543	13.78519
	Equal variances not assumed			1.630	13.491	.126	5.40988	3.31801	-1.73182	12.55158
UFHFMT	Equal variances assumed	.062	.805	1.533	85	.129	2.30293	1.50263	-.68471	5.29057
	Equal variances not assumed			1.474	12.750	.165	2.30293	1.56288	-1.08020	5.68606
MAXBCDL	Equal variances assumed	1.280	.262	.758	63	.451	.01306	.01723	-.02137	.04748
	Equal variances not assumed			.544	9.043	.600	.01306	.02400	-.04119	.06730
cdlgo	Equal variances assumed	3.777	.055	-.008	82	.993	-.00015	.01756	-.03509	.03479
	Equal variances not assumed			-.007	14.384	.995	-.00015	.02196	-.04713	.04683
ZYGFMT	Equal variances assumed	.122	.728	-1.064	75	.291	-.01529	.01437	-.04392	.01334
	Equal variances not assumed			-1.161	10.840	.270	-.01529	.01317	-.04433	.01374
UHTH	Equal variances assumed	.526	.471	.296	72	.768	.00357	.01208	-.02050	.02765
	Equal variances not assumed			.260	12.533	.799	.00357	.01376	-.02627	.03342
FB	Equal variances assumed	.237	.628	.197	58	.844	.00296	.01502	-.02710	.03302
	Equal variances not assumed			.225	12.534	.825	.00296	.01313	-.02551	.03143
FB2	Equal variances assumed	.024	.877	-.535	66	.594	-.01333	.02491	-.06306	.03640
	Equal variances not assumed			-.584	13.295	.569	-.01333	.02283	-.06254	.03588
UFIMAI	Equal variances assumed	.303	.585	2.170	49	.035	.04271	.01969	.00315	.08227
	Equal variances not assumed			2.095	6.283	.079	.04271	.02038	-.00663	.09205

T-Test Crowding

Independent Samples Test

		Levene's Test for Equality of Variances		t-test for Equality of Means					95% Confidence Interval of the Difference	
		F	Sig.	t	df	Sig. (2-tailed)	Mean Difference	Std. Error Difference	Lower	Upper
Cranial Index	Equal variances assumed	1.820	.180	-.003	112	.998	-.0033	1.0710	-2.1254	2.1187
	Equal variances not assumed			-.004	60.743	.997	-.0033	.8693	-1.7417	1.7350
Cranial Module	Equal variances assumed	.461	.499	-.223	76	.824	-.36437	1.63695	-3.62463	2.89590
	Equal variances not assumed			-.218	31.801	.829	-.36437	1.67398	-3.77499	3.04625
Cranial length-height Index	Equal variances assumed	.086	.770	-2.532	78	.013	-2.62228	1.03576	-4.68431	-.56024
	Equal variances not assumed			-2.160	25.995	.040	-2.62228	1.21396	-5.11763	-.12692
Cranial breadth-height Index	Equal variances assumed	.925	.339	-2.221	78	.029	-3.24367	1.46071	-6.15171	-.33563
	Equal variances not assumed			-2.198	32.060	.035	-3.24367	1.47558	-6.24912	-.23822
Total Facial Index	Equal variances assumed	.030	.862	.041	65	.967	.06965	1.68624	-3.29800	3.43729
	Equal variances not assumed			.039	29.424	.969	.06965	1.79109	-3.59125	3.73055
Upper Facial Index	Equal variances assumed	.351	.555	.326	80	.745	.24327	.74586	-1.24104	1.72757
	Equal variances not assumed			.317	35.523	.753	.24327	.76736	-1.31374	1.80028
Maxilloalveolar Index	Equal variances assumed	2.097	.153	-.203	63	.840	-.69261	3.41834	-7.52362	6.13840

		F	Sig.	t	df	Sig. (2-tailed)	Mean Difference	Std. Error Difference	Lower	Upper
	Equal variances not assumed			-.243	28.242	.809	-.69261	2.84617	-6.52047	5.13526
Palatal Index	Equal variances assumed	.200	.656	-1.570	99	.120	-4.64318	2.95668	-10.50987	1.22352
	Equal variances not assumed			-1.516	38.699	.138	-4.64318	3.06295	-10.84012	1.55377
Palatal/max ratio	Equal variances assumed	.464	.499	-.408	61	.685	-.01554	.03810	-.09172	.06065
	Equal variances not assumed			-.390	19.820	.700	-.01554	.03980	-.09860	.06753
TFHFMT	Equal variances assumed	2.511	.118	-.596	63	.553	-1.98421	3.32773	-8.63414	4.66573
	Equal variances not assumed			-.862	62.186	.392	-1.98421	2.30159	-6.58474	2.61632
UFHFMT	Equal variances assumed	.165	.685	-1.872	85	.065	-2.13648	1.14140	-4.40588	.13292
	Equal variances not assumed			-1.845	35.378	.073	-2.13648	1.15797	-4.48839	.21342
MAXBCDL	Equal variances assumed	2.071	.155	.406	63	.686	.00532	.01312	-.02090	.03155
	Equal variances not assumed			.487	52.289	.628	.00532	.01092	-.01659	.02724
cdlgo	Equal variances assumed	.152	.698	1.084	82	.281	.01514	.01396	-.01264	.04291
	Equal variances not assumed			1.143	47.660	.259	.01514	.01324	-.01149	.04177
ZYGFMT	Equal variances assumed	5.317	.024	2.105	75	.039	.02295	.01090	.00123	.04466
	Equal variances not assumed			3.154	62.007	.002	.02295	.00728	.00841	.03749
UHTH	Equal variances assumed	.004	.951	.961	72	.340	.00898	.00935	-.00965	.02761
	Equal variances not assumed			.963	39.830	.341	.00898	.00932	-.00986	.02783
FB	Equal variances assumed	11.114	.001	-.858	58	.394	-.00998	.01163	-.03327	.01330
	Equal variances not assumed			-1.116	57.304	.269	-.00998	.00895	-.02790	.00793
FB2	Equal variances assumed	6.200	.015	1.800	66	.076	.03521	.01956	-.00385	.07427
	Equal variances not assumed			2.582	65.259	.012	.03521	.01364	.00798	.06245
UFIMAI	Equal variances assumed	.004	.949	-.494	49	.623	-.00751	.01520	-.03805	.02303
	Equal variances not assumed			-.499	21.189	.623	-.00751	.01505	-.03879	.02377

e. By sex, Indices and ratios with anomalies
T-Test Supplemental teeth

Independent Samples Test

			Levene's Test for Equality of Variances		t-test for Equality of Means					95% Confidence Interval of the Difference	
Sex			F	Sig.	t	df	Sig. (2-tailed)	Mean Difference	Std. Error Difference	Lower	Upper
Male	Cranial Index	Equal variances assumed	.047	.830	1.557	60	.125	6.1578	3.9537	-1.7507	14.0663
		Equal variances not assumed			1.858	1.099	.297	6.1578	3.3139	-27.9593	40.2749
	Total Facial Index	Equal variances assumed	.	.	1.368	35	.180	7.21043	5.27181	-3.49191	17.91277
		Equal variances not assumed	.	.	.	.	.	7.21043	.	.	.
	Upper Facial Index	Equal variances assumed	.	.	1.813	41	.077	5.43266	2.99587	-.61762	11.48295
		Equal variances not assumed	.	.	.	.	.	5.43266	.	.	.
	Maxilloalveolar Index	Equal variances assumed	.	.	-.244	35	.808	-2.86065	11.70194	-26.61685	20.89555
		Equal variances not assumed	.	.	.	.	.	-2.86065	.	.	.
	Palatal Index	Equal variances assumed	1.501	.226	.227	56	.822	2.28351	10.07930	-17.90776	22.47479
		Equal variances not assumed			1.209	55.000	.232	2.28351	1.88862	-1.50136	6.06839
	Palatal/max ratio	Equal variances assumed	.	.	.422	34	.675	.06382	.15108	-.24321	.37084
		Equal variances not assumed	.	.	.	.	.	.06382	.	.	.
	TFHFMT	Equal variances assumed	.	.	.997	36	.325	13.56171	13.60245	-14.02535	41.14876
		Equal variances not assumed	.	.	.	.	.	13.56171	.	.	.
	UFHFMT	Equal variances assumed	.703	.406	.764	45	.449	2.46131	3.22336	-4.03088	8.95349
		Equal variances not assumed			.485	1.034	.711	2.46131	5.07927	-57.28509	62.20770
	MAXBCDL	Equal variances assumed	.	.	-.810	35	.423	-.03602	.04446	-.12628	.05423
		Equal variances not assumed	.	.	.	.	.	-.03602	.	.	.

					t	df	Sig. (2-tailed)	Mean Difference	Std. Error	Lower	Upper
cdlgo	Equal variances assumed				-.578	47	.566	-.03398	.05879	-.15225	.08429
	Equal variances not assumed							-.03398			
ZYGFMT	Equal variances assumed				-.417	39	.679	-.01495	.03583	-.08743	.05752
	Equal variances not assumed							-.01495			
UHTH	Equal variances assumed				.139	41	.891	.00489	.03531	-.06642	.07621
	Equal variances not assumed							.00489			
FB	Equal variances assumed				1.502	28	.144	.05032	.03350	-.01830	.11894
	Equal variances not assumed							.05032			
FB2	Equal variances assumed				-.867	36	.392	-.07304	.08422	-.24385	.09776
	Equal variances not assumed							-.07304			
UFIMAI	Equal variances assumed				1.251	26	.222	.06828	.05456	-.04386	.18042
	Equal variances not assumed							.06828			

a. No statistics are computed for one or more split files

T-Test Rotations

Independent Samples Test

			Levene's Test for Equality of Variances		t-test for Equality of Means						
										95% Confidence Interval of the Difference	
Sex			F	Sig.	t	df	Sig. (2-tailed)	Mean Difference	Std. Error Difference	Lower	Upper
Female	Cranial Index	Equal variances assumed	.090	.766	-1.752	50	.086	-1.8670	1.0658	-4.0077	.2737
		Equal variances not assumed			-1.759	32.114	.088	-1.8670	1.0616	-4.0291	.2951
	Cranial Module	Equal variances assumed	.175	.679	.675	32	.505	1.42556	2.11301	-2.87850	5.72962
		Equal variances not assumed			.685	20.606	.501	1.42556	2.07991	-2.90490	5.75602
	Cranial length-height Index	Equal variances assumed	.350	.558	.326	33	.747	.61731	1.89645	-3.24105	4.47566
		Equal variances not assumed			.356	24.351	.725	.61731	1.73615	-2.96321	4.19782
	Cranial breadth-height Index	Equal variances assumed	2.289	.140	1.162	32	.254	2.64150	2.27396	-1.99040	7.27341
		Equal variances not assumed			1.420	31.339	.166	2.64150	1.86082	-1.15201	6.43501
	Total Facial Index	Equal variances assumed	5.594	.025	.272	28	.787	.73616	2.70155	-4.79772	6.27003
		Equal variances not assumed			.298	23.518	.768	.73616	2.46703	-4.36107	5.83338
	Upper Facial Index	Equal variances assumed	.743	.394	-.876	37	.387	-.82824	.94516	-2.74332	1.08685
		Equal variances not assumed			-.850	29.002	.402	-.82824	.97387	-2.82002	1.16354
	Maxilloalveolar Index	Equal variances assumed	.469	.499	-3.029	26	.005	-11.99392	3.96025	-20.13433	-3.85352
		Equal variances not assumed			-3.332	20.200	.003	-11.99392	3.60009	-19.49882	-4.48902
	Palatal Index	Equal variances assumed	1.450	.235	-.868	41	.391	-3.28902	3.78979	-10.94265	4.36462
		Equal variances not assumed			-1.034	39.215	.307	-3.28902	3.18034	-9.72073	3.14270
	Palatal/max ratio	Equal variances assumed	1.755	.197	.614	25	.545	.02266	.03691	-.05337	.09868
		Equal variances not assumed			.829	24.959	.415	.02266	.02733	-.03364	.07895
	TFHFMT	Equal variances assumed	8.565	.007	-.017	25	.987	-.05554	3.25857	-6.76670	6.65561
		Equal variances not assumed			-.017	16.815	.987	-.05554	3.33942	-7.10700	6.99591
	UFHFMT	Equal variances assumed	2.644	.112	-1.213	38	.233	-1.94198	1.60098	-5.18299	1.29902
		Equal variances not assumed			-1.388	36.969	.173	-1.94198	1.39906	-4.77682	.89286
	MAXBCDL	Equal variances assumed	.022	.884	-2.086	26	.047	-.03962	.01899	-.07866	-.00059
		Equal variances not assumed			-2.121	25.857	.044	-.03962	.01868	-.07804	-.00121
	cdlgo	Equal variances assumed	.003	.955	-1.989	33	.055	-.03225	.01621	-.06524	.00074
		Equal variances not assumed			-2.008	31.273	.053	-.03225	.01607	-.06500	.00050
	ZYGFMT	Equal variances assumed	.505	.482	.188	34	.852	.00284	.01515	-.02794	.03363

		Equal variances not assumed			.198	32.340	.844	.00284	.01435	-.02638	.03206
	UHTH	Equal variances assumed	1.696	.203	-1.804	29	.082	-.02522	.01398	-.05382	.00337
		Equal variances not assumed			-1.856	28.757	.074	-.02522	.01359	-.05302	.00258
	FB	Equal variances assumed	.676	.418	2.395	28	.024	.03871	.01616	.00560	.07182
		Equal variances not assumed			2.395	26.779	.024	.03871	.01616	.00553	.07189
	FB2	Equal variances assumed	1.601	.216	-1.864	28	.073	-.03699	.01985	-.07765	.00367
		Equal variances not assumed			-1.819	21.745	.083	-.03699	.02034	-.07920	.00521
	UFIMAI	Equal variances assumed	1.088	.309	2.803	21	.011	.03472	.01239	.00896	.06048
		Equal variances not assumed			3.057	20.922	.006	.03472	.01136	.01110	.05835
Male	Cranial Index	Equal variances assumed	.673	.415	-.246	60	.807	-.3999	1.6276	-3.6555	2.8558
		Equal variances not assumed			-.201	19.619	.843	-.3999	1.9916	-4.5595	3.7598
	Cranial Module	Equal variances assumed	.000	.991	1.309	42	.198	2.27083	1.73486	-1.23026	5.77193
		Equal variances not assumed			1.208	17.172	.243	2.27083	1.88012	-1.69286	6.23452
	Cranial length-height Index	Equal variances assumed	2.489	.122	1.171	43	.248	1.25684	1.07361	-.90829	3.42197
		Equal variances not assumed			1.004	15.342	.331	1.25684	1.25183	-1.40619	3.91987
	Cranial breadth-height Index	Equal variances assumed	12.333	.001	1.862	44	.069	3.25801	1.74986	-.26860	6.78461
		Equal variances not assumed			1.341	13.647	.202	3.25801	2.43016	-1.96685	8.48286
	Total Facial Index	Equal variances assumed	.501	.484	.426	35	.672	.79709	1.86953	-2.99826	4.59243
		Equal variances not assumed			.464	27.159	.646	.79709	1.71769	-2.72636	4.32053
	Upper Facial Index	Equal variances assumed	.009	.924	1.320	41	.194	1.35272	1.02468	-.71667	3.42211
		Equal variances not assumed			1.238	17.792	.232	1.35272	1.09240	-.94424	3.64969
	Maxilloalveolar Index	Equal variances assumed	4.772	.036	.800	35	.429	3.50798	4.38680	-5.39769	12.41366
		Equal variances not assumed			1.083	26.502	.289	3.50798	3.23992	-3.14564	10.16161
	Palatal Index	Equal variances assumed	.148	.702	.130	56	.897	.57160	4.41159	-8.26588	9.40909
		Equal variances not assumed			.138	21.573	.891	.57160	4.13254	-8.00859	9.15180
	Palatal/max ratio	Equal variances assumed	.420	.521	-.260	34	.797	-.01491	.05743	-.13162	.10180
		Equal variances not assumed			-.316	20.683	.755	-.01491	.04723	-.11322	.08340
	TFHFMT	Equal variances assumed	.819	.371	1.245	36	.221	6.10992	4.90796	-3.84389	16.06373
		Equal variances not assumed			1.773	34.902	.085	6.10992	3.44517	-.88485	13.10470
	UFHFMT	Equal variances assumed	.061	.807	.570	45	.571	.83153	1.45865	-2.10635	3.76942
		Equal variances not assumed			.563	21.271	.579	.83153	1.47615	-2.23591	3.89898
	MAXBCDL	Equal variances assumed	3.411	.073	-1.054	35	.299	-.01701	.01613	-.04976	.01574
		Equal variances not assumed			-1.366	29.475	.182	-.01701	.01245	-.04245	.00843
	cdlgo	Equal variances assumed	1.480	.230	-1.638	47	.108	-.03010	.01838	-.06708	.00687
		Equal variances not assumed			-1.810	26.135	.082	-.03010	.01663	-.06429	.00408
	ZYGFMT	Equal variances assumed	.023	.881	-.792	39	.433	-.00982	.01240	-.03491	.01527
		Equal variances not assumed			-.760	16.572	.458	-.00982	.01293	-.03714	.01751
	UHTH	Equal variances assumed	.551	.462	-.014	41	.989	-.00018	.01220	-.02482	.02446
		Equal variances not assumed			-.015	19.114	.988	-.00018	.01160	-.02444	.02408
	FB	Equal variances assumed	.814	.375	1.386	28	.177	.01829	.01319	-.00873	.04532
		Equal variances not assumed			1.547	19.827	.138	.01829	.01182	-.00639	.04297
	FB2	Equal variances assumed	.002	.967	-1.172	36	.249	-.03558	.03036	-.09715	.02599
		Equal variances not assumed			-1.382	22.703	.180	-.03558	.02575	-.08888	.01772
	UFIMAI	Equal variances assumed	.028	.869	-.172	26	.864	-.00415	.02406	-.05361	.04531

| | | | Equal variances not assumed | | | -.172 | 10.261 | .867 | -.00415 | .02415 | -.05777 | .04947 |

T-Test Reversals

Independent Samples Test[a]

Sex				Levene's Test for Equality of Variances		t-test for Equality of Means					95% Confidence Interval of the Difference	
				F	Sig.	t	df	Sig. (2-tailed)	Mean Difference	Std. Error Difference	Lower	Upper
Female	Cranial Index	Equal variances assumed		.000	.985	-1.054	50	.297	-2.7908	2.6491	-8.1117	2.5300
		Equal variances not assumed				-1.021	1.076	.484	-2.7908	2.7335	-32.2173	26.6357
	Cranial Module	Equal variances assumed		.459	.503	.677	32	.503	2.84375	4.20099	-5.71339	11.40089
		Equal variances not assumed				1.052	1.366	.444	2.84375	2.70352	-15.84917	21.53667
	Cranial length-height Index	Equal variances assumed		.265	.610	-1.333	33	.192	-4.93232	3.70068	-12.46141	2.59677
		Equal variances not assumed				-2.094	1.363	.227	-4.93232	2.35529	-21.27888	11.41424
	Cranial breadth-height Index	Equal variances assumed		1.908	.177	-.677	32	.504	-3.10037	4.58288	-12.43539	6.23465
		Equal variances not assumed				-2.598	27.180	.015	-3.10037	1.19325	-5.54795	-.65279
	Total Facial Index	Equal variances assumed		2.174	.151	-.798	28	.431	-4.24193	5.31378	-15.12670	6.64285
		Equal variances not assumed				-2.586	10.502	.026	-4.24193	1.64037	-7.87334	-.61052
	Upper Facial Index	Equal variances assumed		.436	.513	.124	37	.902	.26652	2.15778	-4.10557	4.63861
		Equal variances not assumed				.180	1.262	.882	.26652	1.48407	-11.44531	11.97835
	Maxilloalveolar Index	Equal variances assumed		.079	.781	-.888	26	.383	-7.30983	8.22886	-24.22450	9.60485
		Equal variances not assumed				-.727	1.100	.591	-7.30983	10.06092	-110.62286	96.00321
	Palatal Index	Equal variances assumed		.477	.494	-.168	41	.867	-1.43326	8.50695	-18.61339	15.74687
		Equal variances not assumed				-.309	1.415	.796	-1.43326	4.63430	-31.79782	28.93129
	Palatal/max ratio	Equal variances assumed		.723	.403	.421	25	.678	.02717	.06461	-.10590	.16025
		Equal variances not assumed				.993	2.992	.394	.02717	.02736	-.06001	.11436
	TFHFMT	Equal variances assumed		2.061	.163	-1.247	25	.224	-7.52462	6.03210	-19.94796	4.89872
		Equal variances not assumed				-3.522	6.068	.012	-7.52462	2.13638	-12.73807	-2.31117
	UFHFMT	Equal variances assumed		.736	.396	-.552	38	.584	-1.96257	3.55668	-9.16269	5.23756
		Equal variances not assumed				-.949	1.386	.478	-1.96257	2.06701	-15.94387	12.01874
	MAXBCDL	Equal variances assumed		.860	.362	-.017	26	.987	-.00066	.03973	-.08233	.08102
		Equal variances not assumed				-.033	2.037	.976	-.00066	.01964	-.08373	.08242
	odlgo	Equal variances assumed		.019	.891	1.422	33	.165	.05048	.03551	-.02176	.12273
		Equal variances not assumed				1.323	1.106	.396	.05048	.03815	-.33693	.43790
	ZYGFMT	Equal variances assumed		1.917	.175	.941	34	.353	.02997	.03185	-.03475	.09468
		Equal variances not assumed				3.836	33.554	.001	.02997	.00781	.01408	.04585
	UHTH	Equal variances assumed		.772	.387	.813	29	.423	.02401	.02954	-.03640	.08442
		Equal variances not assumed				1.891	2.413	.177	.02401	.01270	-.02257	.07059
	FB	Equal variances assumed		2.102	.158	-.530	28	.600	-.01875	.03539	-.09124	.05373
		Equal variances not assumed				-1.754	12.443	.104	-.01875	.01069	-.04196	.00445
	FB2	Equal variances assumed		4.760	.038	1.232	28	.228	.04959	.04025	-.03287	.13205
		Equal variances not assumed				4.527	27.250	.000	.04959	.01095	.02713	.07206
	UFIMAI	Equal variances assumed		2.313	.143	.855	21	.402	.02114	.02472	-.03028	.07255
		Equal variances not assumed				.463	1.046	.721	.02114	.04569	-.50279	.54507

a. No statistics are computed for one or more split files

T-Test Misshapen teeth

Independent Samples Test[a]

Sex			Levene's Test for Equality of Variances		t-test for Equality of Means					95% Confidence Interval of the Difference	
			F	Sig.	t	df	Sig. (2-tailed)	Mean Difference	Std. Error Difference	Lower	Upper
Male	Cranial Index	Equal variances assumed	1.134	.291	-.357	60	.723	-1.1826	3.3171	-7.8177	5.4525
		Equal variances not assumed			-.812	3.618	.467	-1.1826	1.4572	-5.4026	3.0374
	Cranial Module	Equal variances assumed	.313	.579	-1.871	42	.068	-5.62060	3.00457	-11.68406	.44286
		Equal variances not assumed			-2.474	2.592	.103	-5.62060	2.27169	-13.53844	2.29725
	Cranial length-height Index	Equal variances assumed	.679	.414	-.353	43	.726	-.68193	1.93059	-4.57535	3.21148
		Equal variances not assumed			-.503	2.695	.653	-.68193	1.35445	-5.28221	3.91834
	Cranial breadth-height Index	Equal variances assumed	2.050	.159	.094	44	.926	.31024	3.31406	-6.36881	6.98929
		Equal variances not assumed			.304	19.410	.764	.31024	1.02017	-1.82195	2.44243
	Total Facial Index	Equal variances assumed	.052	.822	-1.332	35	.191	-5.04401	3.78550	-12.72899	2.64097
		Equal variances not assumed			-1.382	1.128	.379	-5.04401	3.64870	-40.67633	30.58832
	Upper Facial Index	Equal variances assumed	.099	.755	.736	41	.466	1.63026	2.21381	-2.84062	6.10114
		Equal variances not assumed			.837	1.133	.543	1.63026	1.94888	-17.23382	20.49434
	Palatal Index	Equal variances assumed	1.561	.217	-.161	56	.872	-1.17046	7.25957	-15.71313	13.37221
		Equal variances not assumed			-.458	15.686	.653	-1.17046	2.55738	-6.60070	4.25978
	TFHFMT	Equal variances assumed	.820	.371	-1.022	36	.314	-8.24391	8.06922	-24.60905	8.12123
		Equal variances not assumed			-3.127	23.930	.005	-8.24391	2.63675	-13.68675	-2.80107
	UFHFMT	Equal variances assumed	2.524	.119	-.415	45	.680	-1.10936	2.67368	-6.49443	4.27572
		Equal variances not assumed			-.932	4.466	.399	-1.10936	1.19069	-4.28353	2.06482
	MAXBCDL	Equal variances assumed	.	.	.594	35	.556	.02653	.04465	-.06412	.11717
		Equal variances not assumed			.	.	.	.02653	.	.	.
	cdlgo	Equal variances assumed	.749	.391	-.829	47	.411	-.02863	.03454	-.09812	.04086
		Equal variances not assumed			-1.147	2.580	.347	-.02863	.02496	-.11591	.05865
	ZYGFMT	Equal variances assumed	.018	.893	.883	39	.383	.02248	.02546	-.02903	.07398
		Equal variances not assumed			.765	1.077	.577	.02248	.02938	-.29354	.33849
	UHTH	Equal variances assumed	1.950	.170	2.041	41	.048	.03564	.01746	.00037	.07090
		Equal variances not assumed			4.266	8.947	.002	.03564	.00835	.01672	.05455
	FB	Equal variances assumed	.	.	-.331	28	.743	-.01149	.03475	-.08268	.05970
		Equal variances not assumed			.	.	.	-.01149	.	.	.
	FB2	Equal variances assumed	.064	.802	-.145	36	.885	-.00885	.06098	-.13253	.11483
		Equal variances not assumed			-.131	1.090	.916	-.00885	.06776	-.71839	.70070

a. No statistics are computed for one or more split files

T-Test Congenitally absent teeth

Independent Samples Test

Sex			Levene's Test for Equality of Variances		t-test for Equality of Means					95% Confidence Interval of the Difference	
			F	Sig.	t	df	Sig. (2-tailed)	Mean Difference	Std. Error Difference	Lower	Upper
Female	Cranial Index	Equal variances assumed	2.322	.134	.297	50	.768	.7949	2.6760	-4.5799	6.1697
		Equal variances not assumed			.150	1.019	.905	.7949	5.2903	-63.5738	65.1637
	Cranial Module	Equal variances assumed	.302	.586	.507	32	.616	2.13542	4.21409	-6.44840	10.71923
		Equal variances not assumed			.708	1.281	.585	2.13542	3.01495	-21.04087	25.31170

	Cranial length-height Index	Equal variances assumed	.103	.750	.272	33	.787	1.03343	3.79472	-6.68698	8.75384
		Equal variances not assumed			.346	1.216	.780	1.03343	2.98928	-24.19805	26.26491
	Cranial breadth-height Index	Equal variances assumed	.569	.456	-.007	32	.994	-.03261	4.61553	-9.43414	9.36892
		Equal variances not assumed			-.012	1.495	.992	-.03261	2.64911	-16.05301	15.98779
	Total Facial Index	Equal variances assumed	.	.	.257	28	.799	1.91734	7.45887	-13.36146	17.19615
		Equal variances not assumed			.	.	.	1.91734	.	.	.
	Upper Facial Index	Equal variances assumed	.	.	.426	37	.673	1.27915	3.00442	-4.80838	7.36668
		Equal variances not assumed			.	.	.	1.27915	.	.	.
	Maxilloalveolar Index	Equal variances assumed	.	.	-.501	26	.621	-5.77681	11.53634	-29.49009	17.93647
		Equal variances not assumed			.	.	.	-5.77681	.	.	.
	Palatal Index	Equal variances assumed	.001	.978	.508	41	.614	4.30761	8.48326	-12.82468	21.43990
		Equal variances not assumed			.505	1.099	.696	4.30761	8.53175	-83.60084	92.21606
	Palatal/max ratio	Equal variances assumed	.	.	-.042	25	.967	-.00375	.08992	-.18893	.18144
		Equal variances not assumed			.	.	.	-.00375	.	.	.
	TFHFMT	Equal variances assumed	.	.	.465	25	.646	3.99435	8.58433	-13.68541	21.67410
		Equal variances not assumed			.	.	.	3.99435	.	.	.
	UFHFMT	Equal variances assumed	.644	.427	-.144	38	.886	-.51359	3.56993	-7.74054	6.71336
		Equal variances not assumed			-.238	1.350	.843	-.51359	2.15539	-15.70509	14.67791
	MAXBCDL	Equal variances assumed	.	.	1.029	26	.313	.05563	.05405	-.05547	.16674
		Equal variances not assumed			.	.	.	.05563	.	.	.
	cdlgo	Equal variances assumed	.	.	1.309	33	.199	.06507	.04969	-.03603	.16618
		Equal variances not assumed			.	.	.	.06507	.	.	.
	ZYGFMT	Equal variances assumed	.	.	.020	34	.984	.00092	.04496	-.09046	.09229
		Equal variances not assumed			.	.	.	.00092	.	.	.
	UHTH	Equal variances assumed	.	.	-.156	29	.877	-.00647	.04152	-.09137	.07844
		Equal variances not assumed			.	.	.	-.00647	.	.	.
	FB	Equal variances assumed	.	.	-1.112	28	.276	-.05376	.04837	-.15284	.04531
		Equal variances not assumed			.	.	.	-.05376	.	.	.
	FB2	Equal variances assumed	.	.	.871	28	.391	.04938	.05667	-.06671	.16547
		Equal variances not assumed			.	.	.	.04938	.	.	.
Male	Cranial Index	Equal variances assumed	.368	.546	.940	60	.351	3.7646	4.0034	-4.2435	11.7726
		Equal variances not assumed			.672	1.033	.620	3.7646	5.5982	-62.1807	69.7098
	Cranial Module	Equal variances assumed	.	.	-2.490	42	.017	-12.29457	4.93712	-22.25809	-2.33105
		Equal variances not assumed			.	.	.	-12.29457	.	.	.
	Cranial length-height Index	Equal variances assumed	.	.	-1.172	43	.248	-3.77552	3.22068	-10.27065	2.71961
		Equal variances not assumed			.	.	.	-3.77552	.	.	.
	Cranial breadth-height Index	Equal variances assumed	.	.	-.467	44	.643	-2.61518	5.59781	-13.89682	8.66646
		Equal variances not assumed			.	.	.	-2.61518	.	.	.
	Total Facial Index	Equal variances assumed	.	.	-.641	35	.526	-3.44801	5.37938	-14.36873	7.47272
		Equal variances not assumed			.	.	.	-3.44801	.	.	.
	Upper Facial Index	Equal variances assumed	.	.	-1.198	41	.238	-3.66787	3.06055	-9.84877	2.51304
		Equal variances not assumed			.	.	.	-3.66787	.	.	.
	Maxilloalveolar Index	Equal variances assumed	.	.	1.432	35	.161	16.30514	11.38303	-6.80363	39.41391
		Equal variances not assumed			.	.	.	16.30514	.	.	.

			F	Sig.	t	df	Sig. (2-tailed)	Mean Difference	Std. Error Difference	Lower	Upper
	Palatal Index	Equal variances assumed	.073	.788	.951	56	.346	9.51397	10.00346	-10.52536	29.55330
		Equal variances not assumed			1.317	1.148	.392	9.51397	7.22620	-58.57050	77.59844
	Palatal/max ratio	Equal variances assumed			.507	34	.616	.07647	.15090	-.23021	.38314
		Equal variances not assumed						.07647			
	TFHFMT	Equal variances assumed			-.508	36	.615	-6.97883	13.73982	-34.84449	20.88682
		Equal variances not assumed						-6.97883			
	UFHFMT	Equal variances assumed	.192	.663	-1.790	45	.080	-5.60940	3.13456	-11.92273	.70393
		Equal variances not assumed			-2.027	1.119	.270	-5.60940	2.76718	-33.03383	21.81502
	MAXBCDL	Equal variances assumed			1.561	35	.127	.06775	.04339	-.02033	.15583
		Equal variances not assumed						.06775			
	cdlgo	Equal variances assumed			1.924	47	.060	.10929	.05680	-.00498	.22357
		Equal variances not assumed						.10929			
	ZYGFMT	Equal variances assumed			1.052	39	.299	.03724	.03541	-.03439	.10888
		Equal variances not assumed						.03724			
	UHTH	Equal variances assumed			-.755	41	.454	-.02650	.03508	-.09734	.04434
		Equal variances not assumed						-.02650			
	FB	Equal variances assumed			-1.302	28	.203	-.04403	.03381	-.11329	.02523
		Equal variances not assumed						-.04403			
	FB2	Equal variances assumed			.850	36	.401	.07160	.08426	-.09928	.24248
		Equal variances not assumed						.07160			
	UFIMAI	Equal variances assumed			-1.985	26	.058	-.10392	.05235	-.21152	.00368
		Equal variances not assumed						-.10392			

T-Test Absent M3

Independent Samples Test

			Levene's Test for Equality of Variances		t-test for Equality of Means					95% Confidence Interval of the Difference	
Sex			F	Sig.	t	df	Sig. (2-tailed)	Mean Difference	Std. Error Difference	Lower	Upper
Female	Cranial Index	Equal variances assumed	3.787	.057	1.592	50	.118	2.7129	1.7045	-.7107	6.1365
		Equal variances not assumed			1.001	4.272	.370	2.7129	2.7110	-4.6290	10.0548
	Cranial Module	Equal variances assumed	1.968	.170	.592	32	.558	2.48958	4.20801	-6.08185	11.06102
		Equal variances not assumed			2.163	17.591	.045	2.48958	1.15096	.06747	4.91169
	Cranial length-height Index	Equal variances assumed	.225	.638	.068	33	.946	.25853	3.79871	-7.47000	7.98707
		Equal variances not assumed			.053	1.071	.966	.25853	4.89895	-53.06737	53.58444
	Cranial breadth-height Index	Equal variances assumed	.008	.928	.365	32	.718	1.67967	4.60597	-7.70239	11.06173
		Equal variances not assumed			.338	1.109	.788	1.67967	4.96433	-48.50093	51.86028
	Total Facial Index	Equal variances assumed	2.163	.153	.683	28	.500	3.63927	5.32971	-7.27815	14.55670
		Equal variances not assumed			2.398	20.510	.026	3.63927	1.51775	.47835	6.80020
	Upper Facial Index	Equal variances assumed	.097	.757	1.321	37	.195	2.78588	2.10907	-1.48751	7.05927
		Equal variances not assumed			1.488	1.145	.354	2.78588	1.87217	-14.94472	20.51648
	Maxilloalveolar Index	Equal variances assumed	1.900	.180	1.118	26	.274	7.59226	6.79385	-6.37270	21.55722
		Equal variances not assumed			2.304	7.102	.054	7.59226	3.29483	-.17621	15.36073
	Palatal Index	Equal variances assumed	1.867	.179	.481	41	.633	3.37389	7.01485	-10.79290	17.54068
		Equal variances not assumed			1.414	12.874	.181	3.37389	2.38550	-1.78482	8.53260
	Palatal/max ratio	Equal variances assumed	1.814	.190	-.370	25	.714	-.01996	.05389	-.13094	.09102

			F	Sig.	t	df	Sig. (2-tailed)	Mean Difference	Std. Error Difference	Lower	Upper
		Equal variances not assumed			-.990	23.884	.332	-.01996	.02016	-.06158	.02166
	TFHFMT	Equal variances assumed	.414	.526	-.106	25	.917	-.65723	6.21560	-13.45851	12.14405
		Equal variances not assumed			-.138	1.316	.908	-.65723	4.76169	-35.66327	34.34881
	UFHFMT	Equal variances assumed	.160	.692	-.197	38	.845	-.70365	3.56908	-7.92887	6.52157
		Equal variances not assumed			-.152	1.061	.903	-.70365	4.63381	-52.17868	50.77138
	MAXBCDL	Equal variances assumed	.	.	1.415	26	.169	.07520	.05313	-.03402	.18441
		Equal variances not assumed			.	.	.	.07520	.	.	.
	cdlgo	Equal variances assumed	3.872	.058	.820	33	.418	.02462	.03003	-.03647	.08572
		Equal variances not assumed			2.189	13.240	.047	.02462	.01125	.00036	.04888
	ZYGFMT	Equal variances assumed	.034	.854	1.676	34	.103	.05196	.03100	-.01104	.11497
		Equal variances not assumed			1.854	1.152	.289	.05196	.02802	-.21020	.31413
	UHTH	Equal variances assumed	.262	.613	-.018	29	.986	-.00053	.02987	-.06162	.06057
		Equal variances not assumed			-.027	1.398	.982	-.00053	.01949	-.13054	.12949
	FB	Equal variances assumed	.	.	-1.298	28	.205	-.06231	.04800	-.16063	.03601
		Equal variances not assumed			.	.	.	-.06231	.	.	.
	FB2	Equal variances assumed	.758	.391	.769	28	.449	.02614	.03401	-.04353	.09580
		Equal variances not assumed			.889	2.679	.446	.02614	.02939	-.07408	.12636
	UFIMAI	Equal variances assumed	2.006	.171	-.004	21	.997	-.00010	.02515	-.05240	.05220
		Equal variances not assumed			-.011	7.861	.992	-.00010	.00923	-.02144	.02124
Male	Cranial Index	Equal variances assumed	20.224	.000	-2.835	60	.006	-6.9661	2.4574	-11.8818	-2.0505
		Equal variances not assumed			-1.244	4.085	.280	-6.9661	5.6000	-22.3878	8.4555
	Cranial Module	Equal variances assumed	5.542	.023	-1.372	42	.177	-5.07937	3.70214	-12.55058	2.39185
		Equal variances not assumed			-.573	1.014	.668	-5.07937	8.86427	-114.08076	103.92203
	Cranial length-height Index	Equal variances assumed	.856	.360	-1.043	43	.303	-2.41030	2.31117	-7.07123	2.25062
		Equal variances not assumed			-.643	1.033	.633	-2.41030	3.74738	-46.55409	41.73348
	Cranial breadth-height Index	Equal variances assumed	11.265	.002	1.542	44	.130	4.36187	2.82890	-1.33939	10.06314
		Equal variances not assumed			.713	3.080	.526	4.36187	6.11745	-14.82362	23.54737
	Total Facial Index	Equal variances assumed	2.653	.112	1.026	35	.312	3.92281	3.82326	-3.83881	11.68444
		Equal variances not assumed			4.295	34.982	.000	3.92281	.91326	2.06877	5.77686
	Upper Facial Index	Equal variances assumed	.006	.941	.427	41	.671	.95037	2.22345	-3.53999	5.44073
		Equal variances not assumed			.420	1.096	.742	.95037	2.26320	-22.48410	24.38483
	Maxilloalveolar Index	Equal variances assumed	2.412	.129	.366	35	.716	2.54315	6.94463	-11.55519	16.64150
		Equal variances not assumed			.749	4.741	.489	2.54315	3.39475	-6.32884	11.41514
	Palatal Index	Equal variances assumed	.348	.558	.861	56	.393	5.60891	6.51266	-7.43751	18.65533
		Equal variances not assumed			1.275	6.186	.248	5.60891	4.39823	-5.07527	16.29309
	Palatal/max ratio	Equal variances assumed	.625	.435	.193	34	.848	.01742	.09001	-.16552	.20035
		Equal variances not assumed			.446	6.745	.669	.01742	.03902	-.07556	.11039
	TFHFMT	Equal variances assumed	.752	.391	1.514	36	.139	14.51517	9.58416	-4.92241	33.95274
		Equal variances not assumed			6.301	34.402	.000	14.51517	2.30381	9.83527	19.19506
	UFHFMT	Equal variances assumed	1.543	.221	2.032	45	.048	5.21019	2.56373	.04658	10.37379
		Equal variances not assumed			3.743	3.310	.028	5.21019	1.39194	1.00591	9.41446
	MAXBCDL	Equal variances assumed	1.073	.307	-.987	35	.331	-.02595	.02630	-.07933	.02743
		Equal variances not assumed			-1.764	3.731	.158	-.02595	.01471	-.06798	.01608
	cdlgo	Equal variances assumed	.265	.609	-.182	47	.857	-.00632	.03478	-.07630	.06365

174

			F	Sig.	t	df	Sig. (2-tailed)	Mean Difference	Std. Error Difference	Lower	Upper
		Equal variances not assumed			-.140	2.149	.900	-.00632	.04505	-.18783	.17518
	ZYGFMT	Equal variances assumed	.027	.871	-1.725	39	.092	-.03537	.02050	-.07685	.00610
		Equal variances not assumed			-1.605	2.276	.235	-.03537	.02204	-.11996	.04922
	UHTH	Equal variances assumed	.000	.984	-1.049	41	.300	-.02617	.02495	-.07654	.02421
		Equal variances not assumed			-.988	1.088	.493	-.02617	.02648	-.30495	.25262
	FB	Equal variances assumed	1.096	.304	-.156	28	.877	-.00390	.02505	-.05520	.04741
		Equal variances not assumed			-.094	1.047	.940	-.00390	.04133	-.47632	.46852
	FB2	Equal variances assumed	.510	.480	-1.154	36	.256	-.05726	.04960	-.15786	.04334
		Equal variances not assumed			-2.213	4.081	.090	-.05726	.02587	-.12852	.01400
	UFIMAI	Equal variances assumed	.263	.613	.421	26	.677	.01697	.04034	-.06595	.09989
		Equal variances not assumed			.511	1.253	.685	.01697	.03320	-.24840	.28234

T-Test Ectopic and impacted teeth

Independent Samples Test

			Levene's Test for Equality of Variances		t-test for Equality of Means						
										95% Confidence Interval of the Difference	
Sex			F	Sig.	t	df	Sig. (2-tailed)	Mean Difference	Std. Error Difference	Lower	Upper
Female	Cranial Index	Equal variances assumed	3.641	.062	-.391	50	.697	-.5895	1.5068	-3.6159	2.4369
		Equal variances not assumed			-.720	21.625	.479	-.5895	.8187	-2.2890	1.1100
	Cranial Module	Equal variances assumed	4.863	.035	-.619	32	.540	-1.60714	2.59591	-6.89483	3.68054
		Equal variances not assumed			-.363	5.352	.730	-1.60714	4.42602	-12.76287	9.54858
	Cranial length-height Index	Equal variances assumed	3.948	.055	-1.678	33	.103	-3.76912	2.24584	-8.33832	.80008
		Equal variances not assumed			-1.040	5.448	.342	-3.76912	3.62541	-12.86279	5.32456
	Cranial breadth-height Index	Equal variances assumed	1.988	.168	-1.639	32	.111	-4.48409	2.73626	-10.05767	1.08950
		Equal variances not assumed			-1.048	5.512	.338	-4.48409	4.27696	-15.17804	6.20987
	Total Facial Index	Equal variances assumed	.257	.616	-.227	28	.822	-.89400	3.93975	-8.96421	7.17621
		Equal variances not assumed			-.268	4.584	.800	-.89400	3.33249	-9.69947	7.91147
	Upper Facial Index	Equal variances assumed	.242	.626	.615	37	.542	.95984	1.56114	-2.20333	4.12301
		Equal variances not assumed			.761	4.262	.487	.95984	1.26175	-2.45999	4.37967
	Maxilloalveolar Index	Equal variances assumed	.	.	.055	26	.957	.63624	11.59116	-23.18973	24.46222
		Equal variances not assumed			.	.	.	.63624	.	.	.
	Palatal Index	Equal variances assumed	7.524	.009	-1.713	41	.094	-9.25260	5.40057	-20.15927	1.65407
		Equal variances not assumed			-.904	4.181	.415	-9.25260	10.23743	-37.19677	18.69157
	Palatal/max ratio	Equal variances assumed	.	.	.305	25	.763	.02737	.08975	-.15748	.21221
		Equal variances not assumed			.	.	.	.02737	.	.	.
	TFHFMT	Equal variances assumed	.991	.329	.638	25	.529	2.90025	4.54638	-6.46319	12.26368
		Equal variances not assumed			.876	5.987	.415	2.90025	3.31080	-5.20539	11.00588
	UFHFMT	Equal variances assumed	.048	.827	1.993	38	.053	4.92049	2.46835	-.07642	9.91740
		Equal variances not assumed			1.958	3.668	.128	4.92049	2.51329	-2.31348	12.15446
	MAXBCDL	Equal variances assumed	6.452	.017	2.170	26	.039	.05839	.02691	.00308	.11370
		Equal variances not assumed			1.193	3.173	.314	.05839	.04896	-.09272	.20951
	cdlgo	Equal variances assumed	.274	.604	.581	33	.565	.01303	.02242	-.03258	.05863
		Equal variances not assumed			.494	6.339	.638	.01303	.02638	-.05069	.07674
	ZYGFMT	Equal variances assumed	.988	.327	-.455	34	.652	-.01213	.02665	-.06630	.04203
		Equal variances not assumed			-.903	4.582	.411	-.01213	.01343	-.04763	.02336

	Variable		F	Sig.	t	df	Sig. (2-tailed)	Mean Difference	Std. Error Difference	95% CI Lower	95% CI Upper
	UHTH	Equal variances assumed	.122	.729	1.685	29	.103	.03208	.01904	-.00686	.07103
		Equal variances not assumed			1.441	5.032	.209	.03208	.02226	-.02503	.08919
	FB	Equal variances assumed	.042	.839	.316	28	.755	.00932	.02952	-.05115	.06978
		Equal variances not assumed			.352	2.617	.751	.00932	.02647	-.08233	.10096
	FB2	Equal variances assumed	.083	.776	.265	28	.793	.00732	.02763	-.04928	.06392
		Equal variances not assumed			.263	5.673	.802	.00732	.02789	-.06188	.07652
	UFIMAI	Equal variances assumed	.	.	.350	21	.730	.01213	.03465	-.05992	.08419
		Equal variances not assumed			.	.	.	.01213	.	.	.
Male	Cranial Index	Equal variances assumed	.141	.709	.410	60	.684	.8693	2.1225	-3.3764	5.1149
		Equal variances not assumed			.481	10.472	.641	.8693	1.8088	-3.1364	4.8750
	Cranial Module	Equal variances assumed	.443	.510	.054	42	.957	.13333	2.48359	-4.87876	5.14543
		Equal variances not assumed			.071	6.362	.945	.13333	1.87367	-4.38883	4.65550
	Cranial length-height Index	Equal variances assumed	.066	.799	-.531	43	.598	-.75097	1.41409	-3.60276	2.10082
		Equal variances not assumed			-.618	7.527	.555	-.75097	1.21527	-3.58432	2.08238
	Cranial breadth-height Index	Equal variances assumed	1.439	.237	-.103	44	.918	-.27111	2.62887	-5.56925	5.02703
		Equal variances not assumed			-.197	11.583	.847	-.27111	1.37802	-3.28558	2.74336
	Total Facial Index	Equal variances assumed	7.743	.009	1.250	35	.220	2.91063	2.32907	-1.81762	7.63888
		Equal variances not assumed			.785	5.466	.465	2.91063	3.70991	-6.38670	12.20797
	Upper Facial Index	Equal variances assumed	.272	.605	.806	41	.425	1.01671	1.26120	-1.53034	3.56377
		Equal variances not assumed			.721	7.780	.492	1.01671	1.41011	-2.25104	4.28447
	Maxilloalveolar Index	Equal variances assumed	.740	.396	-2.555	35	.015	-13.03083	5.10015	-23.38469	-2.67697
		Equal variances not assumed			-2.859	5.835	.030	-13.03083	4.55774	-24.26017	-1.80149
	Palatal Index	Equal variances assumed	.547	.463	-.687	56	.495	-3.86415	5.62447	-15.13132	7.40302
		Equal variances not assumed			-1.075	12.641	.302	-3.86415	3.59310	-11.64906	3.92076
	Palatal/max ratio	Equal variances assumed	1.530	.225	.760	34	.452	.05427	.07137	-.09079	.19932
		Equal variances not assumed			1.639	27.484	.113	.05427	.03311	-.01362	.12215
	TFHFMT	Equal variances assumed	.061	.806	1.106	36	.276	7.09966	6.42155	-5.92385	20.12317
		Equal variances not assumed			1.271	5.914	.252	7.09966	5.58695	-6.61970	20.81902
	UFHFMT	Equal variances assumed	.410	.525	.576	45	.568	1.05517	1.83254	-2.63575	4.74609
		Equal variances not assumed			.626	8.881	.547	1.05517	1.68531	-2.76504	4.87539
	MAXBCDL	Equal variances assumed	.918	.345	-1.080	35	.287	-.02262	.02094	-.06512	.01989
		Equal variances not assumed			-1.545	7.936	.161	-.02262	.01463	-.05641	.01118
	cdlgo	Equal variances assumed	2.678	.108	-.634	47	.529	-.01506	.02374	-.06281	.03270
		Equal variances not assumed			-.490	7.011	.639	-.01506	.03070	-.08762	.05751
	ZYGFMT	Equal variances assumed	.056	.813	-1.465	39	.151	-.02236	.01526	-.05322	.00851
		Equal variances not assumed			-1.192	6.006	.278	-.02236	.01875	-.06822	.02351
	UHTH	Equal variances assumed	.004	.949	-1.287	41	.205	-.01939	.01506	-.04981	.01103
		Equal variances not assumed			-1.357	7.014	.217	-.01939	.01428	-.05315	.01437
	FB	Equal variances assumed	.011	.918	-.215	28	.832	-.00335	.01561	-.03534	.02863
		Equal variances not assumed			-.210	7.521	.839	-.00335	.01594	-.04053	.03383
	FB2	Equal variances assumed	.003	.956	-.758	36	.453	-.03031	.03998	-.11139	.05077
		Equal variances not assumed			-.791	5.450	.462	-.03031	.03833	-.12644	.06581
	UFIMAI	Equal variances assumed	.177	.677	2.540	26	.017	.06188	.02436	.01180	.11196
		Equal variances not assumed			2.430	5.631	.054	.06188	.02547	-.00144	.12520

T-Test Crowding

Independent Samples Test

Sex			Levene's Test for Equality of Variances		t-test for Equality of Means					95% Confidence Interval of the Difference	
			F	Sig.	t	df	Sig. (2-tailed)	Mean Difference	Std. Error Difference	Lower	Upper
Female	Cranial Index	Equal variances assumed	.631	.431	-.669	50	.507	-.9067	1.3554	-3.6292	1.8157
		Equal variances not assumed			-.821	15.074	.424	-.9067	1.1039	-3.2588	1.4453
	Cranial Module	Equal variances assumed	1.840	.184	-.920	32	.364	-2.23633	2.43011	-7.18631	2.71364
		Equal variances not assumed			-.623	6.784	.553	-2.23633	3.58819	-10.77618	6.30351
	Cranial length-height Index	Equal variances assumed	1.296	.263	-3.600	33	.001	-6.72485	1.86800	-10.52532	-2.92437
		Equal variances not assumed			-2.617	7.046	.034	-6.72485	2.56960	-12.79290	-.65680
	Cranial breadth-height Index	Equal variances assumed	1.609	.214	-3.606	32	.001	-8.16635	2.26489	-12.77978	-3.55292
		Equal variances not assumed			-2.659	7.121	.032	-8.16635	3.07138	-15.40415	-.92856
	Total Facial Index	Equal variances assumed	1.774	.194	.680	28	.502	2.13637	3.14354	-4.30288	8.57561
		Equal variances not assumed			.530	7.492	.611	2.13637	4.02711	-7.26102	11.53375
	Upper Facial Index	Equal variances assumed	.050	.824	.587	37	.561	.66044	1.12465	-1.61832	2.93919
		Equal variances not assumed			.539	11.747	.600	.66044	1.22526	-2.01556	3.33643
	Maxilloalveolar Index	Equal variances assumed	.413	.526	-.785	26	.439	-4.06908	5.18151	-14.71984	6.58167
		Equal variances not assumed			-.959	11.182	.358	-4.06908	4.24131	-13.38561	5.24744
	Palatal Index	Equal variances assumed	.202	.656	-.200	41	.843	-.91858	4.60300	-10.21453	8.37737
		Equal variances not assumed			-.238	13.294	.815	-.91858	3.85628	-9.23090	7.39373
	Palatal/max ratio	Equal variances assumed	1.320	.261	1.102	25	.281	.04398	.03989	-.03817	.12613
		Equal variances not assumed			1.715	21.820	.100	.04398	.02564	-.00921	.09717
	TFHFMT	Equal variances assumed	1.189	.286	-1.498	25	.147	-6.01354	4.01524	-14.28308	2.25600
		Equal variances not assumed			-2.006	9.410	.074	-6.01354	2.99782	-12.75026	.72318
	UFHFMT	Equal variances assumed	.225	.638	-.653	38	.518	-1.32958	2.03684	-5.45295	2.79379
		Equal variances not assumed			-.539	7.493	.605	-1.32958	2.46491	-7.08128	4.42212
	MAXBCDL	Equal variances assumed	.778	.386	-.044	26	.965	-.00104	.02363	-.04961	.04754
		Equal variances not assumed			-.056	17.451	.956	-.00104	.01856	-.04012	.03804
	cdlgo	Equal variances assumed	4.823	.035	1.501	33	.143	.02821	.01880	-.01004	.06645
		Equal variances not assumed			1.910	23.927	.068	.02821	.01477	-.00228	.05870
	ZYGFMT	Equal variances assumed	2.146	.152	1.639	34	.110	.03129	.01909	-.00750	.07008
		Equal variances not assumed			2.671	17.142	.016	.03129	.01171	.00659	.05599
	UHTH	Equal variances assumed	.081	.779	1.815	29	.080	.02884	.01589	-.00366	.06134
		Equal variances not assumed			1.677	10.782	.122	.02884	.01719	-.00909	.06678
	FB	Equal variances assumed	10.593	.003	-.158	28	.876	-.00316	.02005	-.04423	.03792
		Equal variances not assumed			-.249	25.786	.805	-.00316	.01266	-.02919	.02288
	FB2	Equal variances assumed	4.774	.037	1.722	28	.096	.04221	.02451	-.00799	.09242
		Equal variances not assumed			2.522	16.200	.022	.04221	.01674	.00677	.07766
	UFIMAI	Equal variances assumed	1.044	.319	-.094	21	.926	-.00152	.01614	-.03508	.03203
		Equal variances not assumed			-.083	7.164	.936	-.00152	.01846	-.04498	.04193
Male	Cranial Index	Equal variances assumed	1.742	.192	.344	60	.732	.5496	1.5957	-2.6422	3.7414
		Equal variances not assumed			.425	46.984	.673	.5496	1.2933	-2.0521	3.1514
	Cranial Module	Equal variances assumed	.687	.412	1.164	42	.251	1.98015	1.70043	-1.45147	5.41177
		Equal variances not assumed			1.243	26.250	.225	1.98015	1.59356	-1.29394	5.25424

		F	Sig.	t	df	Sig. (2-tailed)	Mean Difference	Std. Error Difference	95% CI Lower	95% CI Upper
Cranial length-height Index	Equal variances assumed	.007	.935	-.042	43	.966	-.04520	1.06402	-2.19100	2.10060
	Equal variances not assumed			-.043	22.580	.966	-.04520	1.05794	-2.23596	2.14557
Cranial breadth-height Index	Equal variances assumed	1.416	.240	-.113	44	.910	-.20619	1.81722	-3.86855	3.45616
	Equal variances not assumed			-.146	39.941	.884	-.20619	1.40879	-3.05359	2.64120
Total Facial Index	Equal variances assumed	1.115	.298	-.621	35	.539	-1.15696	1.86415	-4.94138	2.62746
	Equal variances not assumed			-.695	29.184	.493	-1.15696	1.66455	-4.56042	2.24650
Upper Facial Index	Equal variances assumed	.540	.467	-.020	41	.984	-.02070	1.02180	-2.08427	2.04287
	Equal variances not assumed			-.020	22.964	.984	-.02070	1.02007	-2.13106	2.08965
Maxilloalveolar Index	Equal variances assumed	2.110	.155	.399	35	.692	1.83715	4.60309	-7.50763	11.18192
	Equal variances not assumed			.498	16.529	.625	1.83715	3.69202	-5.96928	9.64357
Palatal Index	Equal variances assumed	.528	.470	-1.782	56	.080	-7.00592	3.93233	-14.88333	.87149
	Equal variances not assumed			-1.662	26.002	.109	-7.00592	4.21632	-15.67265	1.66081
Palatal/max ratio	Equal variances assumed	1.147	.292	-1.020	34	.315	-.06017	.05898	-.18003	.05969
	Equal variances not assumed			-.952	10.360	.363	-.06017	.06318	-.20029	.07995
TFHFMT	Equal variances assumed	1.927	.174	.240	36	.812	1.13821	4.74470	-8.48449	10.76090
	Equal variances not assumed			.326	34.195	.746	1.13821	3.48924	-5.95129	8.22771
UFHFMT	Equal variances assumed	1.134	.293	-1.570	45	.123	-2.14716	1.36782	-4.90209	.60777
	Equal variances not assumed			-1.651	31.230	.109	-2.14716	1.30059	-4.79895	.50462
MAXBCDL	Equal variances assumed	1.357	.252	.523	35	.604	.00810	.01548	-.02333	.03954
	Equal variances not assumed			.604	31.263	.550	.00810	.01342	-.01926	.03546
cdlgo	Equal variances assumed	.219	.642	.597	47	.554	.01076	.01803	-.02552	.04704
	Equal variances not assumed			.627	30.296	.535	.01076	.01715	-.02425	.04578
ZYGFMT	Equal variances assumed	3.304	.077	1.059	39	.296	.01305	.01233	-.01188	.03799
	Equal variances not assumed			1.428	35.514	.162	.01305	.00914	-.00549	.03160
UHTH	Equal variances assumed	.273	.604	-.330	41	.743	-.00374	.01135	-.02666	.01917
	Equal variances not assumed			-.349	29.887	.729	-.00374	.01072	-.02564	.01816
FB	Equal variances assumed	.863	.361	-1.359	28	.185	-.01745	.01284	-.04376	.00886
	Equal variances not assumed			-1.460	21.916	.159	-.01745	.01196	-.04225	.00735
FB2	Equal variances assumed	3.622	.065	.934	36	.357	.02703	.02896	-.03169	.08576
	Equal variances not assumed			1.261	34.603	.216	.02703	.02143	-.01649	.07056
UFIMAI	Equal variances assumed	.336	.567	-.551	26	.587	-.01318	.02394	-.06238	.03602
	Equal variances not assumed			-.594	11.867	.564	-.01318	.02218	-.06156	.03521

f. By sex and population, indices and ratios with anomalies

T-Test Supplemental teeth

Independent Samples Test

				Levene's Test for Equality of Variances		t-test for Equality of Means					
Sex	MajorGeo			F	Sig.	t	df	Sig. (2-tailed)	Mean Difference	Std. Error Difference	95% CI Lower	95% CI Upper
Male	English	Cranial Index	Equal variances assumed	.056	.814	1.495	33	.144	6.5095	4.3545	-2.3498	15.3688
			Equal variances not assumed			1.913	1.220	.270	6.5095	3.4019	-22.0206	35.0396
		Total Facial Index	Equal variances assumed	.	.	1.752	18	.097	8.70677	4.96953	-1.73382	19.14735
			Equal variances not assumed			.	.	.	8.70677	.	.	.
		Upper Facial Index	Equal variances assumed	.	.	1.803	22	.085	5.44930	3.02266	-.81932	11.71792
			Equal variances not assumed			.	.	.	5.44930	.	.	.

			F	Sig.	t	df	Sig. (2-tailed)	Mean Difference	Std. Error Difference	Lower	Upper
Maxilloalveolar Index	Equal variances assumed		.	.	-.293	22	.772	-3.31222	11.30249	-26.75216	20.12772
	Equal variances not assumed				.	.	.	-3.31222		.	.
Palatal Index	Equal variances assumed		3.344	.075	-.141	40	.888	-.90144	6.37956	-13.79501	11.99213
	Equal variances not assumed				-.639	39.000	.526	-.90144	1.40987	-3.75317	1.95029
Palatal/max ratio	Equal variances assumed		.	.	.432	22	.670	.02822	.06525	-.10710	.16353
	Equal variances not assumed				.	.	.	.02822		.	.
TFHFMT	Equal variances assumed		.	.	1.843	23	.078	13.39386	7.26912	-1.64346	28.43118
	Equal variances not assumed				.	.	.	13.39386		.	.
UFHFMT	Equal variances assumed		.821	.372	.575	31	.569	1.84662	3.21032	-4.70088	8.39411
	Equal variances not assumed				.362	1.047	.777	1.84662	5.09542	-56.40467	60.09790
MAXBCDL	Equal variances assumed		.	.	-.861	27	.397	-.03494	.04058	-.11821	.04833
	Equal variances not assumed				.	.	.	-.03494		.	.
cdlgo	Equal variances assumed		.	.	-.676	31	.504	-.03572	.05287	-.14355	.07211
	Equal variances not assumed				.	.	.	-.03572		.	.
ZYGFMT	Equal variances assumed		.	.	-.450	24	.657	-.01622	.03608	-.09068	.05824
	Equal variances not assumed				.	.	.	-.01622		.	.
UHTH	Equal variances assumed		.	.	-.247	25	.807	-.00888	.03591	-.08285	.06509
	Equal variances not assumed				.	.	.	-.00888		.	.
FB	Equal variances assumed		.	.	1.552	16	.140	.04922	.03173	-.01803	.11648
	Equal variances not assumed				.	.	.	.04922		.	.
FB2	Equal variances assumed		.	.	-1.188	26	.246	-.06078	.05115	-.16593	.04437
	Equal variances not assumed				.	.	.	-.06078		.	.
UFIMAI	Equal variances assumed		.	.	1.781	15	.095	.07066	.03967	-.01389	.15521
	Equal variances not assumed				.	.	.	.07066		.	.

a. No statistics are computed for one or more split files

T-Test Rotations

Independent Samples Test

Sex	MajorGeo			Levene's Test for Equality of Variances		t-test for Equality of Means					95% Confidence Interval of the Difference	
				F	Sig.	t	df	Sig. (2-tailed)	Mean Difference	Std. Error Difference	Lower	Upper
Female	English	Cranial Index	Equal variances assumed	2.463	.131	-1.393	22	.178	-2.5715	1.8466	-6.4012	1.2582
			Equal variances not assumed			-1.192	8.480	.266	-2.5715	2.1573	-7.4976	2.3546
		Cranial Module	Equal variances assumed	.891	.359	.416	16	.683	1.38889	3.33481	-5.68059	8.45837
			Equal variances not assumed			.416	10.061	.686	1.38889	3.34005	-6.04713	8.82491
		Cranial length-height Index	Equal variances assumed	.073	.790	.375	17	.712	1.15757	3.08838	-5.35834	7.67347
			Equal variances not assumed			.417	12.883	.683	1.15757	2.77426	-4.84139	7.15652
		Cranial breadth-height Index	Equal variances assumed	1.428	.249	1.198	16	.249	4.26335	3.56006	-3.28364	11.81034
			Equal variances not assumed			1.527	15.889	.146	4.26335	2.79171	-1.65818	10.18488
		Total Facial Index	Equal variances assumed	1.179	.306	.000	9	1.000	-.00088	3.61702	-8.18315	8.18139
			Equal variances not assumed			.000	8.709	1.000	-.00088	3.19210	-7.25887	7.25711
		Upper Facial Index	Equal variances assumed	.136	.718	-.445	14	.663	-.50930	1.14568	-2.96653	1.94793
			Equal variances not assumed			-.445	13.331	.664	-.50930	1.14568	-2.97815	1.95955
		Maxilloalveolar Index	Equal variances assumed	2.280	.151	-2.109	16	.051	-10.26347	4.86720	-20.58147	.05453
			Equal variances not assumed			-2.440	15.275	.027	-10.26347	4.20562	-19.21349	-1.31344

	Palatal Index	Equal variances assumed	1.780	.196	-1.268	22	.218	-5.31572	4.19253	-14.01049	3.37905
		Equal variances not assumed			-1.512	17.189	.149	-5.31572	3.51621	-12.72805	2.09661
	Palatal/max ratio	Equal variances assumed	1.885	.190	-.009	15	.993	-.00046	.04872	-.10430	.10339
		Equal variances not assumed			-.012	13.189	.990	-.00046	.03769	-.08176	.08085
	TFHFMT	Equal variances assumed	4.612	.057	.077	10	.940	.38036	4.96107	-10.67358	11.43431
		Equal variances not assumed			.089	7.568	.931	.38036	4.27338	-9.57277	10.33350
	UFHFMT	Equal variances assumed	.118	.736	-1.281	17	.217	-2.48714	1.94087	-6.58201	1.60773
		Equal variances not assumed			-1.305	16.139	.210	-2.48714	1.90622	-6.52533	1.55105
	MAXBCDL	Equal variances assumed	1.277	.276	-1.533	15	.146	-.02836	.01850	-.06780	.01107
		Equal variances not assumed			-1.500	12.293	.159	-.02836	.01891	-.06946	.01274
	cdlgo	Equal variances assumed	.007	.934	-1.015	17	.324	-.02320	.02286	-.07144	.02504
		Equal variances not assumed			-1.030	15.982	.319	-.02320	.02253	-.07097	.02457
	ZYGFMT	Equal variances assumed	.908	.355	.934	16	.364	.02102	.02250	-.02669	.06873
		Equal variances not assumed			.996	14.342	.336	.02102	.02110	-.02414	.06618
	UHTH	Equal variances assumed	.933	.357	-1.457	10	.176	-.03231	.02217	-.08171	.01709
		Equal variances not assumed			-1.325	5.838	.235	-.03231	.02439	-.09240	.02778
	FB	Equal variances assumed	.582	.460	1.294	12	.220	.03407	.02632	-.02328	.09141
		Equal variances not assumed			1.350	11.986	.202	.03407	.02524	-.02094	.08907
	FB2	Equal variances assumed	.051	.824	-1.564	16	.137	-.03623	.02317	-.08534	.01289
		Equal variances not assumed			-1.585	15.766	.133	-.03623	.02285	-.08473	.01228
	UFIMAI	Equal variances assumed	.826	.381	2.739	12	.018	.02951	.01077	.00604	.05298
		Equal variances not assumed			2.739	10.912	.019	.02951	.01077	.00578	.05324
Macedonian	Cranial Index	Equal variances assumed	1.242	.275	-.925	26	.363	-1.0546	1.1399	-3.3977	1.2886
		Equal variances not assumed			-1.053	25.492	.302	-1.0546	1.0011	-3.1142	1.0051
	Cranial Module	Equal variances assumed	.905	.358	.870	14	.399	1.69697	1.94997	-2.48530	5.87924
		Equal variances not assumed			1.001	11.144	.338	1.69697	1.69489	-2.02759	5.42153
	Cranial length-height Index	Equal variances assumed	.294	.596	-.024	14	.981	-.04704	1.93839	-4.20447	4.11039
		Equal variances not assumed			-.026	9.677	.979	-.04704	1.77939	-4.02980	3.93573
	Cranial breadth-height Index	Equal variances assumed	1.322	.270	.250	14	.807	.71114	2.84979	-5.40105	6.82334
		Equal variances not assumed			.298	12.238	.770	.71114	2.38239	-4.46845	5.89074
	Total Facial Index	Equal variances assumed	5.528	.031	.262	17	.797	1.00947	3.86023	-7.13489	9.15383
		Equal variances not assumed			.272	11.967	.790	1.00947	3.70625	-7.06824	9.08718
	Upper Facial Index	Equal variances assumed	.425	.521	-.790	21	.438	-1.12748	1.42682	-4.09471	1.83975
		Equal variances not assumed			-.743	14.173	.469	-1.12748	1.51668	-4.37671	2.12175
	Maxilloalveolar Index	Equal variances assumed	.537	.485	-2.583	8	.032	-19.14309	7.41246	-36.23625	-2.04994
		Equal variances not assumed			-2.027	1.257	.250	-19.14309	9.44543	-94.24624	55.96006
	Palatal Index	Equal variances assumed	.357	.558	.012	17	.991	.07594	6.52419	-13.68889	13.84078
		Equal variances not assumed			.013	16.998	.989	.07594	5.66334	-11.87277	12.02466
	Palatal/max ratio	Equal variances assumed	1.374	.275	1.312	8	.226	.07895	.06019	-.05986	.21775
		Equal variances not assumed			2.560	7.994	.034	.07895	.03084	.00782	.15008
	TFHFMT	Equal variances assumed	2.766	.120	-.275	13	.788	-1.28514	4.67101	-11.37625	8.80597
		Equal variances not assumed			-.241	6.695	.816	-1.28514	5.32444	-13.99250	11.42222
	UFHFMT	Equal variances assumed	6.142	.023	-.816	19	.425	-2.08932	2.56019	-7.44787	3.26923
		Equal variances not assumed			-1.145	18.982	.267	-2.08932	1.82525	-5.90986	1.73122

		MAXBCDL	Equal variances assumed	.820	.389	-1.440	9	.184	-.05602	.03891	-.14405	.03201
			Equal variances not assumed			-1.507	8.388	.169	-.05602	.03717	-.14106	.02902
		cdlgo	Equal variances assumed	.022	.885	-1.781	14	.097	-.04305	.02417	-.09490	.00879
			Equal variances not assumed			-1.780	13.020	.098	-.04305	.02418	-.09529	.00919
		ZYGFMT	Equal variances assumed	.262	.616	-.706	16	.490	-.01448	.02050	-.05793	.02897
			Equal variances not assumed			-.649	8.207	.534	-.01448	.02230	-.06568	.03672
		UHTH	Equal variances assumed	5.550	.031	-1.118	17	.279	-.02118	.01893	-.06113	.01877
			Equal variances not assumed			-1.165	12.000	.267	-.02118	.01818	-.06079	.01844
		FB	Equal variances assumed	.623	.443	2.763	14	.015	.02975	.01077	.00666	.05285
			Equal variances not assumed			2.844	13.964	.013	.02975	.01046	.00731	.05220
		FB2	Equal variances assumed	1.273	.286	-.789	10	.449	-.02516	.03189	-.09622	.04591
			Equal variances not assumed			-.669	4.217	.538	-.02516	.03760	-.12748	.07716
		UFIMAI	Equal variances assumed	.016	.902	1.489	7	.180	.04994	.03354	-.02938	.12926
			Equal variances not assumed			1.524	1.683	.289	.04994	.03277	-.11976	.21964
Male	English	Cranial Index	Equal variances assumed	2.394	.131	-1.017	33	.317	-2.3146	2.2765	-6.9462	2.3169
			Equal variances not assumed			-.775	10.872	.455	-2.3146	2.9876	-8.8997	4.2704
		Cranial Module	Equal variances assumed	.119	.733	.911	26	.371	2.11306	2.31973	-2.65520	6.88132
			Equal variances not assumed			.832	12.818	.420	2.11306	2.53890	-3.37981	7.60593
		Cranial length-height Index	Equal variances assumed	3.791	.062	1.247	26	.223	1.65007	1.32311	-1.06962	4.36975
			Equal variances not assumed			1.052	10.958	.316	1.65007	1.56898	-1.80486	5.10500
		Cranial breadth-height Index	Equal variances assumed	7.404	.011	1.906	28	.067	4.43369	2.32664	-.33221	9.19958
			Equal variances not assumed			1.482	10.578	.167	4.43369	2.99074	-2.18108	11.04845
		Total Facial Index	Equal variances assumed	.011	.916	.878	18	.391	2.11306	2.40575	-2.94123	7.16735
			Equal variances not assumed			.854	11.452	.411	2.11306	2.47531	-3.30896	7.53508
		Upper Facial Index	Equal variances assumed	.864	.363	1.719	22	.100	2.21595	1.28882	-.45689	4.88879
			Equal variances not assumed			1.579	11.423	.142	2.21595	1.40316	-.85848	5.29038
		Maxilloalveolar Index	Equal variances assumed	3.481	.075	.337	22	.739	1.75659	5.21260	-9.05368	12.56686
			Equal variances not assumed			.488	20.067	.631	1.75659	3.60159	-5.75458	9.26777
		Palatal Index	Equal variances assumed	1.679	.203	.144	40	.886	.46008	3.18975	-5.98664	6.90680
			Equal variances not assumed			.186	25.532	.854	.46008	2.47668	-4.63535	5.55550
		Palatal/max ratio	Equal variances assumed	2.954	.100	-.450	22	.657	-.01354	.03010	-.07597	.04888
			Equal variances not assumed			-.587	15.536	.565	-.01354	.02306	-.06255	.03546
		TFHFMT	Equal variances assumed	.089	.769	1.428	23	.167	4.64991	3.25736	-2.08845	11.38827
			Equal variances not assumed			1.452	11.377	.173	4.64991	3.20208	-2.36944	11.66926
		UFHFMT	Equal variances assumed	.097	.758	.915	31	.367	1.51299	1.65348	-1.85930	4.88529
			Equal variances not assumed			.929	17.816	.365	1.51299	1.62833	-1.91054	4.93653
		MAXBCDL	Equal variances assumed	1.959	.173	-1.336	27	.193	-.02099	.01571	-.05323	.01125
			Equal variances not assumed			-1.622	24.824	.117	-.02099	.01294	-.04765	.00567
		cdlgo	Equal variances assumed	1.359	.253	-.851	31	.401	-.01724	.02026	-.05857	.02409
			Equal variances not assumed			-.970	19.229	.344	-.01724	.01777	-.05441	.01993
		ZYGFMT	Equal variances assumed	.844	.367	-.379	24	.708	-.00571	.01505	-.03678	.02535
			Equal variances not assumed			-.334	10.366	.745	-.00571	.01712	-.04367	.03225
		UHTH	Equal variances assumed	.000	.994	-.138	25	.892	-.00213	.01549	-.03403	.02977
			Equal variances not assumed			-.148	12.054	.885	-.00213	.01443	-.03357	.02930

			F	Sig.	t	df	Sig. (2-tailed)	Mean Difference	Std. Error Difference	Lower	Upper
	FB	Equal variances assumed	.575	.459	.103	16	.919	.00170	.01653	-.03334	.03674
		Equal variances not assumed			.115	13.569	.910	.00170	.01477	-.03008	.03348
	FB2	Equal variances assumed	1.426	.243	-.974	26	.339	-.02065	.02119	-.06421	.02292
		Equal variances not assumed			-.859	10.316	.410	-.02065	.02403	-.07397	.03267
	UFIMAI	Equal variances assumed	.518	.483	.911	15	.377	.01999	.02195	-.02679	.06677
		Equal variances not assumed			1.047	10.545	.319	.01999	.01910	-.02226	.06224
Macedonian	Cranial Index	Equal variances assumed	1.476	.236	1.157	25	.258	2.6106	2.2573	-2.0384	7.2595
		Equal variances not assumed			1.631	16.695	.122	2.6106	1.6008	-.7716	5.9927
	Cranial Module	Equal variances assumed	1.282	.277	1.035	14	.318	2.78632	2.69305	-2.98970	8.56235
		Equal variances not assumed			1.662	7.848	.136	2.78632	1.67606	-1.09172	6.66437
	Cranial length-height Index	Equal variances assumed	5.539	.033	-.317	15	.756	-.58895	1.85745	-4.54800	3.37010
		Equal variances not assumed			-.649	14.956	.526	-.58895	.90735	-2.52342	1.34552
	Cranial breadth-height Index	Equal variances assumed	.338	.570	-.771	14	.453	-1.45928	1.89219	-5.51762	2.59907
		Equal variances not assumed			-1.010	4.515	.364	-1.45928	1.44534	-5.29809	2.37953
	Total Facial Index	Equal variances assumed	1.025	.327	-.173	15	.865	-.49525	2.86044	-6.59214	5.60164
		Equal variances not assumed			-.223	13.827	.827	-.49525	2.22230	-5.26720	4.27670
	Upper Facial Index	Equal variances assumed	.020	.889	-.065	17	.949	-.11513	1.76239	-3.83344	3.60318
		Equal variances not assumed			-.065	4.756	.950	-.11513	1.75801	-4.70481	4.47455
	Maxilloalveolar Index	Equal variances assumed	.502	.493	.803	11	.439	6.84977	8.53373	-11.93284	25.63238
		Equal variances not assumed			.957	4.541	.387	6.84977	7.15751	-12.12350	25.82303
	Palatal Index	Equal variances assumed	.136	.717	-.127	14	.901	-1.74339	13.75619	-31.24749	27.76071
		Equal variances not assumed			-.111	2.666	.919	-1.74339	15.65894	-55.30749	51.82072
	Palatal/max ratio	Equal variances assumed	.308	.591	-.110	10	.915	-.01764	.16042	-.37507	.33980
		Equal variances not assumed			-.134	5.174	.899	-.01764	.13185	-.35316	.31789
	TFHFMT	Equal variances assumed	.890	.366	.645	11	.532	9.16855	14.20624	-22.09916	40.43627
		Equal variances not assumed			1.168	10.313	.269	9.16855	7.85213	-8.25543	26.59253
	UFHFMT	Equal variances assumed	.048	.829	-.651	12	.528	-1.92874	2.96485	-8.38860	4.53111
		Equal variances not assumed			-.679	3.382	.541	-1.92874	2.84142	-10.42014	6.56265
	MAXBCDL	Equal variances assumed	.	.	.223	6	.831	.01507	.06765	-.15047	.18061
		Equal variances not assumed			.	.	.	.01507	.	.	.
	cdlgo	Equal variances assumed	.381	.547	-1.494	14	.157	-.05857	.03920	-.14263	.02550
		Equal variances not assumed			-1.625	6.033	.155	-.05857	.03603	-.14661	.02948
	ZYGFMT	Equal variances assumed	1.488	.244	-.879	13	.395	-.02092	.02379	-.07232	.03047
		Equal variances not assumed			-1.640	12.895	.125	-.02092	.01276	-.04850	.00666
	UHTH	Equal variances assumed	.665	.428	.176	14	.863	.00209	.01188	-.02339	.02757
		Equal variances not assumed			.158	4.433	.881	.00209	.01321	-.03323	.03741
	FB	Equal variances assumed	2.742	.129	2.197	10	.053	.04676	.02128	-.00067	.09418
		Equal variances not assumed			2.849	6.137	.028	.04676	.01641	.00682	.08670
	FB2	Equal variances assumed	.133	.725	-.639	8	.541	-.07136	.11175	-.32906	.18635
		Equal variances not assumed			-.863	2.584	.461	-.07136	.08266	-.36011	.21739
	UFIMAI	Equal variances assumed	.369	.559	-.984	9	.351	-.05565	.05656	-.18360	.07230
		Equal variances not assumed			-.763	1.227	.565	-.05565	.07292	-.66073	.54943

T-Test Reversals

Independent Samples Test[a]

Sex	MajorGeo			Levene's Test for Equality of Variances		t-test for Equality of Means					95% Confidence Interval of the Difference	
				F	Sig.	t	df	Sig. (2-tailed)	Mean Difference	Std. Error Difference	Lower	Upper
Female	Macedonian	Cranial Index	Equal variances assumed	.161	.692	-.853	26	.402	-1.8132	2.1259	-6.1831	2.5567
			Equal variances not assumed			-.661	1.089	.621	-1.8132	2.7415	-30.5969	26.9704
		Cranial Module	Equal variances assumed	.081	.780	.136	14	.894	.38095	2.80404	-5.63312	6.39502
			Equal variances not assumed			.142	1.339	.906	.38095	2.69068	-18.83100	19.59291
		Cranial length-height Index	Equal variances assumed	.225	.643	-1.548	14	.144	-3.88538	2.51048	-9.26983	1.49907
			Equal variances not assumed			-1.650	1.360	.295	-3.88538	2.35490	-20.27948	12.50872
		Cranial breadth-height Index	Equal variances assumed	2.582	.130	-.710	14	.489	-2.79337	3.93270	-11.22819	5.64144
			Equal variances not assumed			-1.871	13.995	.082	-2.79337	1.49304	-5.99573	.40898
		Total Facial Index	Equal variances assumed	2.330	.145	-.657	17	.520	-4.08092	6.21480	-17.19300	9.03117
			Equal variances not assumed			-1.815	14.927	.090	-4.08092	2.24832	-8.87516	.71333
		Upper Facial Index	Equal variances assumed	.487	.493	.219	21	.829	.55613	2.54440	-4.73523	5.84750
			Equal variances not assumed			.349	1.674	.766	.55613	1.59429	-7.75488	8.86715
		Maxilloalveolar Index	Equal variances assumed	.058	.816	-.790	8	.453	-7.63412	9.66782	-29.92816	14.65992
			Equal variances not assumed			-.714	1.399	.575	-7.63412	10.69610	-78.91699	63.64875
		Palatal Index	Equal variances assumed	.476	.500	.228	17	.823	2.32993	10.23925	-19.27299	23.93285
			Equal variances not assumed			.428	2.629	.701	2.32993	5.44442	-16.46343	21.12329
		Palatal/max ratio	Equal variances assumed	1.053	.335	.520	8	.617	.03391	.06526	-.11658	.18439
			Equal variances not assumed			.911	6.115	.397	.03391	.03723	-.05677	.12458
		TFHFMT	Equal variances assumed	2.383	.147	-1.036	13	.319	-6.72051	6.48881	-20.73873	7.29771
			Equal variances not assumed			-2.403	9.922	.037	-6.72051	2.79671	-12.95859	-.48243
		UFHFMT	Equal variances assumed	1.206	.286	-.243	19	.811	-.97120	4.00232	-9.34814	7.40575
			Equal variances not assumed			-.425	2.046	.711	-.97120	2.28413	-10.59011	8.64772
		MAXBCDL	Equal variances assumed	.939	.358	-.394	9	.703	-.02175	.05525	-.14673	.10322
			Equal variances not assumed			-.731	6.539	.490	-.02175	.02977	-.09317	.04966
		cdlgo	Equal variances assumed	.000	.995	1.383	14	.188	.05209	.03767	-.02870	.13287
			Equal variances not assumed			1.319	1.269	.376	.05209	.03949	-.25672	.36089
		ZYGFMT	Equal variances assumed	2.408	.140	.836	16	.415	.02555	.03056	-.03924	.09033
			Equal variances not assumed			2.396	15.649	.029	.02555	.01066	.00291	.04818
		UHTH	Equal variances assumed	1.104	.308	.832	17	.417	.02604	.03129	-.03997	.09205
			Equal variances not assumed			1.789	3.943	.149	.02604	.01456	-.01461	.06669
		FB	Equal variances assumed	2.076	.172	.507	14	.620	.01008	.01990	-.03259	.05275
			Equal variances not assumed			1.121	6.600	.301	.01008	.00899	-.01144	.03160
		FB2	Equal variances assumed	2.190	.170	.514	10	.618	.02110	.04104	-.07034	.11255
			Equal variances not assumed			1.180	9.411	.267	.02110	.01788	-.01908	.06129
		UFIMAI	Equal variances assumed	.540	.486	.803	7	.448	.02957	.03683	-.05752	.11666
			Equal variances not assumed			.617	1.262	.630	.02957	.04791	-.34884	.40798

a. No statistics are computed for one or more split files

T-Test Misshapen teeth

Independent Samples Test[a]

Sex	MajorGeo			Levene's Test for Equality of Variances		t-test for Equality of Means					95% Confidence Interval of the Difference	
				F	Sig.	t	df	Sig. (2-tailed)	Mean Difference	Std. Error Difference	Lower	Upper
Male	English	Cranial Index	Equal variances assumed	1.143	.293	-.278	33	.783	-1.0357	3.7264	-8.6173	6.5458
			Equal variances not assumed			-.615	6.211	.560	-1.0357	1.6832	-5.1206	3.0491
		Cranial Module	Equal variances assumed	.497	.487	-1.754	26	.091	-5.90222	3.36462	-12.81829	1.01385
			Equal variances not assumed			-2.451	3.256	.085	-5.90222	2.40823	-13.23688	1.43244
		Cranial length-height Index	Equal variances assumed	.678	.418	-.680	26	.503	-1.38561	2.03870	-5.57622	2.80500
			Equal variances not assumed			-.969	3.332	.398	-1.38561	1.43041	-5.69161	2.92039
		Cranial breadth-height Index	Equal variances assumed	2.460	.128	-.204	28	.840	-.79104	3.88293	-8.74486	7.16278
			Equal variances not assumed			-.572	25.486	.572	-.79104	1.38294	-3.63651	2.05442
		Total Facial Index	Equal variances assumed	.333	.571	-1.029	18	.317	-3.90609	3.79595	-11.88108	4.06890
			Equal variances not assumed			-1.045	1.243	.458	-3.90609	3.73905	-34.24197	26.42979
		Upper Facial Index	Equal variances assumed	.058	.811	.693	22	.496	1.60403	2.31614	-3.19935	6.40741
			Equal variances not assumed			.800	1.269	.546	1.60403	2.00543	-14.07524	17.28329
		Palatal Index	Equal variances assumed	2.493	.122	-1.004	40	.321	-4.59019	4.57213	-13.83080	4.65043
			Equal variances not assumed			-2.086	9.107	.066	-4.59019	2.20010	-9.55828	.37791
		TFHFMT	Equal variances assumed	2.405	.135	-2.097	23	.047	-9.02249	4.30250	-17.92289	-.12209
			Equal variances not assumed			-4.551	10.816	.001	-9.02249	1.98256	-13.39516	-4.64981
		UFHFMT	Equal variances assumed	2.517	.123	-.687	31	.497	-1.82646	2.65857	-7.24864	3.59573
			Equal variances not assumed			-1.433	5.721	.204	-1.82646	1.27419	-4.98158	1.32867
		MAXBCDL	Equal variances assumed	.	.	.689	27	.497	.02809	.04078	-.05559	.11176
			Equal variances not assumed						.02809			
		cdlgo	Equal variances assumed	.576	.454	-.993	31	.328	-.03105	.03126	-.09482	.03271
			Equal variances not assumed			-1.228	2.715	.315	-.03105	.02529	-.11653	.05442
		ZYGFMT	Equal variances assumed	.009	.926	.857	24	.400	.02207	.02576	-.03109	.07523
			Equal variances not assumed			.743	1.124	.582	.02207	.02970	-.26977	.31391
		UHTH	Equal variances assumed	1.452	.239	1.199	25	.242	.02230	.01859	-.01599	.06058
			Equal variances not assumed			2.267	13.986	.040	.02230	.00984	.00120	.04339
		FB	Equal variances assumed	.	.	-.415	16	.684	-.01404	.03385	-.08579	.05771
			Equal variances not assumed						-.01404			
		FB2	Equal variances assumed	1.877	.182	.118	26	.907	.00445	.03784	-.07333	.08222
			Equal variances not assumed			.066	1.043	.957	.00445	.06701	-.76898	.77787

a. No statistics are computed for one or more split files

T-Test Congenitally absent teeth

Independent Samples Test[a]

Sex	MajorGeo			Levene's Test for Equality of Variances		t-test for Equality of Means					95% Confidence Interval of the Difference	
				F	Sig.	t	df	Sig. (2-tailed)	Mean Difference	Std. Error Difference	Lower	Upper
Female	English	Cranial Index	Equal variances assumed	1.400	.249	-.139	22	.891	-.4386	3.1665	-7.0056	6.1283
			Equal variances not assumed			-.082	1.055	.947	-.4386	5.3370	-60.4192	59.5420
		Cranial Module	Equal variances assumed	.285	.601	.940	16	.361	4.60417	4.89576	-5.77439	14.98272
			Equal variances not assumed			1.401	1.796	.309	4.60417	3.28658	-11.19187	20.40020

		Cranial length-height Index	Equal variances assumed	.134	.718	-.019	17	.985	-.08818	4.69700	-9.99799	9.82163
			Equal variances not assumed			-.027	1.673	.981	-.08818	3.24198	-17.00010	16.82373
		Cranial breadth-height Index	Equal variances assumed	.554	.467	-.091	16	.928	-.50832	5.57283	-12.32219	11.30555
			Equal variances not assumed			-.166	2.598	.880	-.50832	3.06085	-11.15886	10.14222
		Total Facial Index	Equal variances assumed	.	.	.241	9	.815	1.45398	6.03300	-12.19361	15.10157
			Equal variances not assumed			.	.	.	1.45398	.	.	.
		Upper Facial Index	Equal variances assumed	.	.	.396	14	.698	.93856	2.36990	-4.14438	6.02150
			Equal variances not assumed			.	.	.	.93856	.	.	.
		Maxilloalveolar Index	Equal variances assumed	.	.	-.543	16	.595	-6.29840	11.60348	-30.89669	18.29989
			Equal variances not assumed			.	.	.	-6.29840	.	.	.
		Palatal Index	Equal variances assumed	.035	.854	.210	22	.835	1.50000	7.13513	-13.29735	16.29735
			Equal variances not assumed			.175	1.123	.887	1.50000	8.57837	-83.01044	86.01044
		Palatal/max ratio	Equal variances assumed	.	.	-.051	15	.960	-.00506	.09894	-.21596	.20583
			Equal variances not assumed			.	.	.	-.00506	.	.	.
		TFHFMT	Equal variances assumed	.	.	.299	10	.771	2.63772	8.81259	-16.99796	22.27339
			Equal variances not assumed			.	.	.	2.63772	.	.	.
		UFHFMT	Equal variances assumed	.464	.505	-.544	17	.594	-1.76299	3.24172	-8.60242	5.07645
			Equal variances not assumed			-.777	1.647	.533	-1.76299	2.26779	-13.82474	10.29877
		MAXBCDL	Equal variances assumed	.	.	1.797	15	.092	.06882	.03829	-.01279	.15043
			Equal variances not assumed			.	.	.	.06882	.	.	.
		odlgo	Equal variances assumed	.	.	1.389	17	.183	.06853	.04934	-.03556	.17262
			Equal variances not assumed			.	.	.	.06853	.	.	.
		ZYGFMT	Equal variances assumed	.	.	.137	16	.893	.00687	.05010	-.09935	.11308
			Equal variances not assumed			.	.	.	.00687	.	.	.
		UHTH	Equal variances assumed	.	.	-.190	10	.853	-.00827	.04347	-.10512	.08858
			Equal variances not assumed			.	.	.	-.00827	.	.	.
		FB	Equal variances assumed	.	.	-1.857	12	.088	-.08837	.04758	-.19203	.01530
			Equal variances not assumed			.	.	.	-.08837	.	.	.
		FB2	Equal variances assumed	.	.	1.389	16	.184	.07080	.05097	-.03726	.17886
			Equal variances not assumed			.	.	.	.07080	.	.	.
Male	English	Cranial Index	Equal variances assumed	.	.	1.598	33	.120	9.6498	6.0398	-2.6382	21.9378
			Equal variances not assumed			.	.	.	9.6498	.	.	.
		Palatal Index	Equal variances assumed	.	.	-.099	40	.922	-.87945	8.91250	-18.89228	17.13337
			Equal variances not assumed			.	.	.	-.87945	.	.	.
		UFHFMT	Equal variances assumed	.	.	-.765	31	.450	-3.40560	4.45053	-12.48252	5.67131
			Equal variances not assumed			.	.	.	-3.40560	.	.	.
	Macedonian	Cranial Index	Equal variances assumed	.	.	-.438	25	.665	-2.2231	5.0809	-12.6875	8.2413
			Equal variances not assumed			.	.	.	-2.2231	.	.	.
		Cranial Module	Equal variances assumed	.	.	-4.330	14	.001	-12.75556	2.94562	-19.07328	-6.43783
			Equal variances not assumed			.	.	.	-12.75556	.	.	.
		Cranial length-height Index	Equal variances assumed	.	.	-.981	15	.342	-2.87115	2.92705	-9.11002	3.36772
			Equal variances not assumed			.	.	.	-2.87115	.	.	.
		Cranial breadth-height Index	Equal variances assumed	.	.	-.233	14	.819	-.72499	3.10917	-7.39349	5.94351
			Equal variances not assumed			.	.	.	-.72499	.	.	.

Variable				t	df	Sig.	Mean Difference	Std. Error Difference	Lower	Upper
Total Facial Index	Equal variances assumed	.	.	-.954	15	.355	-5.13434	5.38394	-16.60994	6.34127
	Equal variances not assumed	.	.	.	.	.	-5.13434	.	.	.
Upper Facial Index	Equal variances assumed	.	.	-1.187	17	.252	-3.66949	3.09256	-10.19422	2.85523
	Equal variances not assumed	.	.	.	.	.	-3.66949	.	.	.
Maxilloalveolar Index	Equal variances assumed	.	.	1.406	11	.187	17.96824	12.78179	-10.16428	46.10076
	Equal variances not assumed	.	.	.	.	.	17.96824	.	.	.
Palatal Index	Equal variances assumed	.	.	1.224	14	.241	25.82204	21.09367	-19.41938	71.06346
	Equal variances not assumed	.	.	.	.	.	25.82204	.	.	.
Palatal/max ratio	Equal variances assumed	.	.	.639	10	.537	.15747	.24650	-.39176	.70670
	Equal variances not assumed	.	.	.	.	.	.15747	.	.	.
TFHFMT	Equal variances assumed	.	.	-.291	11	.776	-6.63912	22.79563	-56.81197	43.53372
	Equal variances not assumed	.	.	.	.	.	-6.63912	.	.	.
UFHFMT	Equal variances assumed	.	.	-1.634	12	.128	-7.10235	4.34710	-16.57386	2.36916
	Equal variances not assumed	.	.	.	.	.	-7.10235	.	.	.
MAXBCDL	Equal variances assumed	.	.	1.134	6	.300	.06991	.06164	-.08093	.22074
	Equal variances not assumed	.	.	.	.	.	.06991	.	.	.
cdlgo	Equal variances assumed	.	.	1.706	14	.110	.11718	.06870	-.03017	.26453
	Equal variances not assumed	.	.	.	.	.	.11718	.	.	.
ZYGFMT	Equal variances assumed	.	.	1.085	13	.298	.04080	.03760	-.04043	.12203
	Equal variances not assumed	.	.	.	.	.	.04080	.	.	.
UHTH	Equal variances assumed	.	.	-.170	14	.867	-.00362	.02125	-.04920	.04197
	Equal variances not assumed	.	.	.	.	.	-.00362	.	.	.
FB	Equal variances assumed	.	.	-1.121	10	.288	-.04290	.03827	-.12817	.04237
	Equal variances not assumed	.	.	.	.	.	-.04290	.	.	.
FB2	Equal variances assumed	.	.	.253	8	.806	.03853	.15215	-.31232	.38938
	Equal variances not assumed	.	.	.	.	.	.03853	.	.	.
UFIMAI	Equal variances assumed	.	.	-1.575	9	.150	-.11137	.07071	-.27132	.04859
	Equal variances not assumed	.	.	.	.	.	-.11137	.	.	.

a. No statistics are computed for one or more split files

T-Test Absent M3

Independent Samples Test

Sex	MajorGeo			Levene's Test for Equality of Variances		t-test for Equality of Means					95% Confidence Interval of the Difference	
				F	Sig.	t	df	Sig. (2-tailed)	Mean Difference	Std. Error Difference	Lower	Upper
Female	English	Cranial Index	Equal variances assumed	1.444	.242	1.951	22	.064	4.7695	2.4444	-.2999	9.8388
			Equal variances not assumed			1.281	2.195	.319	4.7695	3.7228	-9.9572	19.4961
		Cranial Module	Equal variances assumed	.	.	.609	16	.551	4.15686	6.82137	-10.30380	18.61753
			Equal variances not assumed			.	.	.	4.15686	.	.	.
		Cranial length-height Index	Equal variances assumed	.	.	.664	17	.516	4.22900	6.37348	-9.21786	17.67586
			Equal variances not assumed			.	.	.	4.22900	.	.	.
		Cranial breadth-height Index	Equal variances assumed	.	.	.849	16	.409	6.35023	7.48125	-9.50932	22.20979
			Equal variances not assumed			.	.	.	6.35023	.	.	.
		Maxilloalveolar Index	Equal variances assumed	.	.	.914	16	.374	10.43037	11.41581	-13.77006	34.63080
			Equal variances not assumed			.	.	.	10.43037	.	.	.
		Palatal Index	Equal variances assumed	.	.	.145	22	.886	1.43478	9.87397	-19.04257	21.91213
			Equal variances not assumed			.	.	.	1.43478	.	.	.
		Palatal/max ratio	Equal variances assumed	.	.	-.361	15	.723	-.03558	.09853	-.24559	.17442
			Equal variances not assumed			.	.	.	-.03558	.	.	.
		cdlgo	Equal variances assumed	3.494	.079	.816	17	.426	.03032	.03716	-.04808	.10872
			Equal variances not assumed			1.873	5.196	.118	.03032	.01618	-.01082	.07146
		FB2	Equal variances assumed	4.298	.055	.473	16	.643	.01848	.03906	-.06432	.10127
			Equal variances not assumed			.984	3.871	.382	.01848	.01877	-.03433	.07129
	Macedonian	Cranial Index	Equal variances assumed	2.003	.169	-.441	26	.663	-.9473	2.1475	-5.3614	3.4669
			Equal variances not assumed			-1.328	7.972	.221	-.9473	.7133	-2.5931	.6985
		Cranial Module	Equal variances assumed	.	.	.139	14	.891	.53333	3.83092	-7.68318	8.74985
			Equal variances not assumed			.	.	.	.53333	.	.	.
		Cranial length-height Index	Equal variances assumed	.	.	-.987	14	.340	-3.54284	3.58901	-11.24050	4.15483
			Equal variances not assumed			.	.	.	-3.54284	.	.	.
		Cranial breadth-height Index	Equal variances assumed	.	.	-.549	14	.592	-2.96860	5.41120	-14.57447	8.63727
			Equal variances not assumed			.	.	.	-2.96860	.	.	.
		Maxilloalveolar Index	Equal variances assumed	2.593	.146	.738	8	.482	7.16769	9.71235	-15.22903	29.56442
			Equal variances not assumed			1.331	6.762	.226	7.16769	5.38697	-5.66206	19.99744
		Palatal Index	Equal variances assumed	.828	.376	.674	17	.509	6.82368	10.12040	-14.52850	28.17586
			Equal variances not assumed			1.656	7.372	.140	6.82368	4.12053	-2.82115	16.46851
		Palatal/max ratio	Equal variances assumed	2.447	.156	-.160	8	.877	-.01060	.06624	-.16336	.14216
			Equal variances not assumed			-.333	7.126	.749	-.01060	.03181	-.08555	.06436
		cdlgo	Equal variances assumed	.	.	.286	14	.779	.01565	.05471	-.10169	.13298
			Equal variances not assumed			.	.	.	.01565	.	.	.
		FB2	Equal variances assumed	.	.	.962	10	.359	.05159	.05364	-.06793	.17111
			Equal variances not assumed			.	.	.	.05159	.	.	.
		Total Facial Index	Equal variances assumed	1.910	.185	.666	17	.514	4.14026	6.21249	-8.96695	17.24747
			Equal variances not assumed			1.919	16.937	.072	4.14026	2.15746	-.41288	8.69340
		Upper Facial Index	Equal variances assumed	.120	.732	1.295	21	.209	3.17393	2.45132	-1.92387	8.27174

			Equal variances not assumed			1.626	1.350	.300	3.17393	1.95155	-10.57823	16.92609
		TFHFMT	Equal variances assumed	.503	.491	.091	13	.929	.61645	6.74905	-13.96399	15.19688
			Equal variances not assumed			.121	1.728	.916	.61645	5.10731	-25.02858	26.26148
		UFHFMT	Equal variances assumed	.038	.847	.087	19	.931	.35067	4.00771	-8.03756	8.73889
			Equal variances not assumed			.074	1.148	.952	.35067	4.72657	-44.17290	44.87423
		MAXBCDL	Equal variances assumed	.	.	.846	9	.420	.06085	.07195	-.10192	.22362
			Equal variances not assumed			.	.	.	.06085	.	.	.
		ZYGFMT	Equal variances assumed	.025	.877	1.703	16	.108	.04892	.02872	-.01197	.10981
			Equal variances not assumed			1.705	1.265	.297	.04892	.02869	-.17664	.27448
		UHTH	Equal variances assumed	.408	.532	.012	17	.990	.00039	.03192	-.06696	.06773
			Equal variances not assumed			.019	1.802	.987	.00039	.02080	-.09923	.10001
		FB	Equal variances assumed	.	.	-1.409	14	.181	-.03617	.02567	-.09123	.01889
			Equal variances not assumed			.	.	.	-.03617	.	.	.
		UFIMAI	Equal variances assumed	4.507	.071	.121	7	.907	.00464	.03845	-.08628	.09556
			Equal variances not assumed			.229	6.687	.826	.00464	.02024	-.04367	.05295
Male	English	Cranial Index	Equal variances assumed	32.896	.000	-2.323	33	.026	-9.6910	4.1713	-18.1776	-1.2044
			Equal variances not assumed			-.658	1.006	.629	-9.6910	14.7187	-194.2186	174.8366
		Cranial Module	Equal variances assumed	.	.	-2.718	26	.012	-14.22222	5.23339	-24.97962	-3.46483
			Equal variances not assumed			.	.	.	-14.22222	.	.	.
		Cranial length-height Index	Equal variances assumed	.	.	.246	26	.807	.84312	3.42390	-6.19480	7.88105
			Equal variances not assumed			.	.	.	.84312	.	.	.
		Cranial breadth-height Index	Equal variances assumed	11.435	.002	1.476	28	.151	5.52421	3.74294	-2.14285	13.19127
			Equal variances not assumed			.675	2.058	.567	5.52421	8.17822	-28.73475	39.78317
		Maxilloalveolar Index	Equal variances assumed	2.108	.161	.326	22	.748	2.22409	6.82604	-11.93224	16.38043
			Equal variances not assumed			.601	6.381	.569	2.22409	3.70371	-6.70895	11.15714
		Palatal Index	Equal variances assumed	.161	.690	.457	40	.650	2.11094	4.61733	-7.22103	11.44291
			Equal variances not assumed			.400	3.475	.712	2.11094	5.27272	-13.44416	17.66604
		Palatal/max ratio	Equal variances assumed	.623	.438	-.553	22	.586	-.02176	.03932	-.10330	.05978
			Equal variances not assumed			-.684	3.097	.541	-.02176	.03179	-.12115	.07764
		cdlgo	Equal variances assumed	.743	.395	-.253	31	.802	-.00802	.03172	-.07272	.05668
			Equal variances not assumed			-.177	2.176	.874	-.00802	.04519	-.18816	.17212
		FB2	Equal variances assumed	.668	.421	-1.489	26	.148	-.04505	.03025	-.10724	.01713
			Equal variances not assumed			-1.891	2.955	.156	-.04505	.02382	-.12152	.03141
		Total Facial Index	Equal variances assumed	4.731	.043	1.498	18	.151	5.51850	3.68307	-2.21934	13.25633
			Equal variances not assumed			4.572	17.432	.000	5.51850	1.20701	2.97673	8.06026
		Upper Facial Index	Equal variances assumed	.001	.981	.384	22	.704	.89682	2.33343	-3.94241	5.73606
			Equal variances not assumed			.388	1.194	.756	.89682	2.31225	-19.29733	21.09097
		TFHFMT	Equal variances assumed	2.796	.108	3.078	23	.005	14.57010	4.73374	4.77761	24.36260
			Equal variances not assumed			9.805	17.932	.000	14.57010	1.48601	11.44725	17.69295
		UFHFMT	Equal variances assumed	1.418	.243	1.841	31	.075	4.68133	2.54335	-.50588	9.86854
			Equal variances not assumed			3.214	3.938	.033	4.68133	1.45652	.61193	8.75073
		MAXBCDL	Equal variances assumed	.691	.413	-1.040	27	.308	-.02513	.02417	-.07472	.02445
			Equal variances not assumed			-1.689	3.893	.169	-.02513	.01489	-.06691	.01664
		ZYGFMT	Equal variances assumed	.046	.832	-1.876	24	.073	-.03820	.02037	-.08023	.00384

Sex	MajorGeo	Variable	Variance	F	Sig.	t	df	Sig. (2-tailed)	Mean Difference	Std. Error Difference	Lower	Upper
			Equal variances not assumed			-1.705	2.430	.208	-.03820	.02240	-.11995	.04355
		UHTH	Equal variances assumed	.009	.924	-1.682	25	.105	-.04134	.02458	-.09196	.00928
			Equal variances not assumed			-1.544	1.136	.344	-.04134	.02678	-.29889	.21621
		FB	Equal variances assumed	1.608	.223	-.263	16	.796	-.00652	.02475	-.05898	.04595
			Equal variances not assumed			-.157	1.071	.900	-.00652	.04157	-.45834	.44531
		UFIMAI	Equal variances assumed	.026	.875	.591	15	.564	.01861	.03152	-.04857	.08580
			Equal variances not assumed			.561	1.248	.659	.01861	.03317	-.24842	.28565
	Macedonian	Cranial Index	Equal variances assumed	2.894	.101	-1.836	25	.078	-5.2816	2.8772	-11.2072	.6440
			Equal variances not assumed			-1.008	2.107	.415	-5.2816	5.2379	-26.7524	16.1892
		Cranial Module	Equal variances assumed	.	.	.990	14	.339	4.31111	4.35556	-5.03063	13.65285
			Equal variances not assumed			.	.	.	4.31111	.	.	.
		Cranial length-height Index	Equal variances assumed	.	.	-1.990	15	.065	-5.34511	2.68562	-11.06937	.37914
			Equal variances not assumed			.	.	.	-5.34511	.	.	.
		Cranial breadth-height Index	Equal variances assumed	.	.	-.038	14	.970	-.11973	3.11504	-6.80081	6.56136
			Equal variances not assumed			.	.	.	-.11973	.	.	.
		Palatal Index	Equal variances assumed	.	.	.673	14	.512	14.69366	21.84372	-32.15646	61.54379
			Equal variances not assumed			.	.	.	14.69366	.	.	.

T-Test Ectopic and impacted teeth

Independent Samples Test

Sex	MajorGeo	Variable	Variance	Levene's Test for Equality of Variances		t-test for Equality of Means					95% Confidence Interval of the Difference	
				F	Sig.	t	df	Sig. (2-tailed)	Mean Difference	Std. Error Difference	Lower	Upper
Female	English	Cranial Index	Equal variances assumed	1.197	.286	-.624	22	.539	-1.4522	2.3289	-6.2820	3.3776
			Equal variances not assumed			-1.069	12.109	.306	-1.4522	1.3580	-4.4080	1.5036
		Cranial Module	Equal variances assumed	10.907	.004	-1.616	16	.126	-6.35556	3.93216	-14.69135	1.98024
			Equal variances not assumed			-.858	2.107	.477	-6.35556	7.41017	-36.73485	24.02374
		Cranial length-height Index	Equal variances assumed	18.191	.001	-1.785	17	.092	-6.47410	3.62794	-14.12838	1.18018
			Equal variances not assumed			-.853	2.067	.481	-6.47410	7.58555	-38.11996	25.17176
		Cranial breadth-height Index	Equal variances assumed	14.230	.002	-1.857	16	.082	-7.91597	4.26376	-16.95473	1.12279
			Equal variances not assumed			-.896	2.067	.462	-7.91597	8.83351	-44.77309	28.94115
		Total Facial Index	Equal variances assumed	.	.	-.001	9	1.000	-.00367	6.05243	-13.69523	13.68789
			Equal variances not assumed			.	.	.	-.00367	.	.	.
		Upper Facial Index	Equal variances assumed	.	.	.768	14	.455	1.79211	2.33452	-3.21493	6.79915
			Equal variances not assumed			.	.	.	1.79211	.	.	.
		Maxilloalveolar Index	Equal variances assumed	.	.	.021	16	.983	.24937	11.70967	-24.57401	25.07276
			Equal variances not assumed			.	.	.	.24937	.	.	.
		Palatal Index	Equal variances assumed	5.177	.033	-.243	22	.810	-1.45144	5.96086	-13.81351	10.91064
			Equal variances not assumed			-.563	15.914	.581	-1.45144	2.57795	-6.91886	4.01598
		Palatal/max ratio	Equal variances assumed	.	.	.271	15	.790	.02677	.09871	-.18363	.23717
			Equal variances not assumed			.	.	.	.02677	.	.	.
		TFHFMT	Equal variances assumed	1.050	.330	.175	10	.864	1.14843	6.55475	-13.45646	15.75332
			Equal variances not assumed			.309	4.460	.771	1.14843	3.71890	-8.77022	11.06708
		UFHFMT	Equal variances assumed	.232	.636	2.574	17	.020	7.13989	2.77360	1.28810	12.99169
			Equal variances not assumed			2.001	1.133	.272	7.13989	3.56877	-27.37367	41.65345

	MAXBCDL	Equal variances assumed	.227	.641	.836	15	.416	.02130	.02547	-.03298	.07557
		Equal variances not assumed			.689	2.511	.549	.02130	.03093	-.08892	.13151
	cdlgo	Equal variances assumed	1.349	.262	.996	17	.333	.02760	.02772	-.03088	.08607
		Equal variances not assumed			.713	3.527	.520	.02760	.03870	-.08577	.14096
	ZYGFMT	Equal variances assumed	.	.	-.316	16	.756	-.01577	.04998	-.12172	.09017
		Equal variances not assumed			.	.	.	-.01577	.	.	.
	UHTH	Equal variances assumed	7.692	.020	2.964	10	.014	.06984	.02356	.01735	.12234
		Equal variances not assumed			1.476	1.050	.371	.06984	.04731	-.46736	.60704
	FB	Equal variances assumed	.	.	.559	12	.586	.02980	.05330	-.08633	.14592
		Equal variances not assumed			.	.	.	.02980	.	.	.
	FB2	Equal variances assumed	.337	.569	.863	16	.401	.02508	.02906	-.03652	.08669
		Equal variances not assumed			.726	4.002	.508	.02508	.03455	-.07081	.12098
	UFIMAI	Equal variances assumed	.	.	.375	12	.714	.00994	.02651	-.04782	.06769
		Equal variances not assumed			.	.	.	.00994	.	.	.
Macedonian	Cranial Index	Equal variances assumed	2.199	.150	-.082	26	.935	-.1480	1.7946	-3.8368	3.5407
		Equal variances not assumed			-.178	8.285	.863	-.1480	.8335	-2.0586	1.7625
	Cranial Module	Equal variances assumed	.000	.988	1.310	14	.211	2.94017	2.24387	-1.87245	7.75279
		Equal variances not assumed			1.263	2.891	.299	2.94017	2.32860	-4.63056	10.51090
	Cranial length-height Index	Equal variances assumed	.001	.971	-.320	14	.754	-.73428	2.29359	-5.65353	4.18498
		Equal variances not assumed			-.308	2.885	.779	-.73428	2.38543	-8.49964	7.03109
	Cranial breadth-height Index	Equal variances assumed	.578	.460	-.268	14	.793	-.90618	3.38311	-8.16222	6.34987
		Equal variances not assumed			-.355	4.641	.738	-.90618	2.55077	-7.61886	5.80651
	Total Facial Index	Equal variances assumed	.077	.784	-.202	17	.842	-1.07039	5.29009	-12.23149	10.09072
		Equal variances not assumed			-.228	3.150	.834	-1.07039	4.70086	-15.63514	13.49436
	Upper Facial Index	Equal variances assumed	.221	.643	.391	21	.700	.82946	2.12352	-3.58664	5.24555
		Equal variances not assumed			.481	3.154	.662	.82946	1.72269	-4.50443	6.16335
	Palatal Index	Equal variances assumed	40.673	.000	-2.426	17	.027	-21.44083	8.83854	-40.08851	-2.79314
		Equal variances not assumed			-.825	1.011	.560	-21.44083	25.98234	-342.94606	300.06441
	TFHFMT	Equal variances assumed	.012	.914	.642	13	.532	4.26743	6.64666	-10.09180	18.62666
		Equal variances not assumed			.630	1.313	.620	4.26743	6.76960	-45.66958	54.20444
	UFHFMT	Equal variances assumed	1.074	.313	.659	19	.518	2.61372	3.96341	-5.68180	10.90923
		Equal variances not assumed			1.140	2.001	.372	2.61372	2.29202	-7.24454	12.47197
	MAXBCDL	Equal variances assumed	.	.	4.046	9	.003	.18015	.04453	.07942	.28088
		Equal variances not assumed			.	.	.	.18015	.	.	.
	cdlgo	Equal variances assumed	.534	.477	-.280	14	.784	-.01121	.04005	-.09710	.07468
		Equal variances not assumed			-.433	2.097	.705	-.01121	.02587	-.11770	.09529
	ZYGFMT	Equal variances assumed	.544	.472	-.436	16	.669	-.01353	.03103	-.07932	.05226
		Equal variances not assumed			-.676	1.905	.572	-.01353	.02001	-.10387	.07680
	UHTH	Equal variances assumed	.856	.368	.266	17	.794	.00712	.02681	-.04944	.06368
		Equal variances not assumed			.428	6.098	.683	.00712	.01663	-.03340	.04765
	FB	Equal variances assumed	2.640	.127	.577	14	.573	.01146	.01984	-.03110	.05402
		Equal variances not assumed			1.473	13.413	.164	.01146	.00778	-.00529	.02821
	FB2	Equal variances assumed	.	.	.006	10	.996	.00032	.05607	-.12460	.12525
		Equal variances not assumed			.	.	.	.00032	.	.	.

Sex	Ethnicity	Variable	Test	F	Sig.	t	df	Sig. (2-tailed)	Mean Difference	Std. Error Difference	Lower	Upper
Male	English	Cranial Index	Equal variances assumed	.000	.992	.842	33	.406	2.7357	3.2479	-3.8723	9.3437
			Equal variances not assumed			.930	4.066	.404	2.7357	2.9419	-5.3808	10.8521
		Cranial Module	Equal variances assumed	.544	.467	.282	26	.780	1.20513	4.26667	-7.56514	9.97540
			Equal variances not assumed			.438	1.469	.717	1.20513	2.75374	-15.85493	18.26519
		Cranial length-height Index	Equal variances assumed	.106	.748	-.733	26	.470	-1.79304	2.44490	-6.81860	3.23252
			Equal variances not assumed			-.822	1.208	.542	-1.79304	2.18138	-20.41318	16.82709
		Cranial breadth-height Index	Equal variances assumed	.943	.340	-.618	28	.541	-2.86967	4.64179	-12.37794	6.63861
			Equal variances not assumed			-1.512	2.840	.233	-2.86967	1.89813	-9.10793	3.36860
		Total Facial Index	Equal variances assumed	.681	.420	-1.189	18	.250	-4.47362	3.76098	-12.37516	3.42791
			Equal variances not assumed			-1.373	1.336	.356	-4.47362	3.25857	-27.83725	18.89001
		Upper Facial Index	Equal variances assumed	3.791	.064	-.250	22	.805	-.48808	1.95384	-4.54010	3.56393
			Equal variances not assumed			-.649	21.914	.523	-.48808	.75203	-2.04805	1.07188
		Maxilloalveolar Index	Equal variances assumed	.181	.675	-.550	22	.588	-4.47093	8.13195	-21.33556	12.39370
			Equal variances not assumed			-.639	1.273	.618	-4.47093	6.99581	-58.84483	49.90297
		Palatal Index	Equal variances assumed	.041	.841	-.860	40	.395	-3.94600	4.58714	-13.21695	5.32495
			Equal variances not assumed			-.850	3.642	.448	-3.94600	4.64201	-17.34958	9.45758
		Palatal/max ratio	Equal variances assumed	.039	.844	-.215	22	.832	-.01018	.04732	-.10833	.08796
			Equal variances not assumed			-.210	1.179	.864	-.01018	.04848	-.44371	.42334
		TFHFMT	Equal variances assumed	.803	.379	-.710	23	.485	-3.95152	5.56411	-15.46176	7.55872
			Equal variances not assumed			-1.069	1.507	.427	-3.95152	3.69547	-26.04066	18.13762
		UFHFMT	Equal variances assumed	4.405	.044	-.695	31	.492	-1.62800	2.34132	-6.40315	3.14715
			Equal variances not assumed			-1.468	14.705	.163	-1.62800	1.10910	-3.99612	.74012
		MAXBCDL	Equal variances assumed	.922	.345	-.228	27	.821	-.00675	.02959	-.06747	.05397
			Equal variances not assumed			-.518	2.467	.647	-.00675	.01303	-.05378	.04028
		cdlgo	Equal variances assumed	.760	.390	.594	31	.557	.02261	.03805	-.05499	.10020
			Equal variances not assumed			.380	1.049	.767	.02261	.05952	-.65555	.70076
		ZYGFMT	Equal variances assumed	4.603	.042	-.392	24	.699	-.00851	.02174	-.05338	.03636
			Equal variances not assumed			-1.039	23.684	.309	-.00851	.00819	-.02543	.00841
		UHTH	Equal variances assumed	.047	.830	.296	25	.770	.00767	.02588	-.04564	.06098
			Equal variances not assumed			.341	1.233	.782	.00767	.02246	-.17722	.19256
		FB	Equal variances assumed	1.179	.294	-.630	16	.538	-.01543	.02450	-.06736	.03651
			Equal variances not assumed			-1.141	2.570	.349	-.01543	.01352	-.06282	.03197
		FB2	Equal variances assumed	5.349	.029	.301	26	.766	.01135	.03778	-.06631	.08902
			Equal variances not assumed			1.003	17.408	.330	.01135	.01132	-.01249	.03520
		UFIMAI	Equal variances assumed	.171	.685	.728	15	.478	.02281	.03134	-.04398	.08961
			Equal variances not assumed			.764	1.321	.558	.02281	.02987	-.19541	.24104
	Macedonian	Cranial Index	Equal variances assumed	.255	.618	-.418	25	.680	-1.1289	2.7020	-6.6937	4.4360
			Equal variances not assumed			-.522	5.180	.624	-1.1289	2.1647	-6.6355	4.3778
		Cranial Module	Equal variances assumed	.051	.824	-.227	14	.824	-.63248	2.78900	-6.61428	5.34933
			Equal variances not assumed			-.223	2.956	.838	-.63248	2.83140	-9.71998	8.45502
		Cranial length-height Index	Equal variances assumed	.117	.737	.428	15	.675	.71301	1.66475	-2.83533	4.26135
			Equal variances not assumed			.420	4.875	.692	.71301	1.69643	-3.68174	5.10776
		Cranial breadth-height Index	Equal variances assumed	.003	.958	1.841	14	.087	3.19203	1.73341	-.52576	6.90982
			Equal variances not assumed			2.078	3.489	.116	3.19203	1.53585	-1.33009	7.71414

191

			F	Sig.	t	df	Sig. (2-tailed)	Mean Difference	Std. Error Difference	Lower	Upper
Total Facial Index	Equal variances assumed	12.694	.003	2.416	15	.029	6.30507	2.60951	.74304	11.86710
	Equal variances not assumed			1.520	3.272	.218	6.30507	4.14818	-6.29597	18.90610
Upper Facial Index	Equal variances assumed	6.242	.023	1.407	17	.177	2.34720	1.66815	-1.17228	5.86668
	Equal variances not assumed			.970	3.451	.395	2.34720	2.41995	-4.81448	9.50888
Maxilloalveolar Index	Equal variances assumed	6.629	.026	-3.215	11	.008	-20.26689	6.30470	-34.14345	-6.39033
	Equal variances not assumed			-4.379	6.368	.004	-20.26689	4.62866	-31.43595	-9.09783
Palatal Index	Equal variances assumed	2.953	.108	.071	14	.945	.97086	13.76164	-28.54491	30.48664
	Equal variances not assumed			.137	13.795	.893	.97086	7.10083	-14.28017	16.22189
Palatal/max ratio	Equal variances assumed	6.018	.034	1.157	10	.274	.17436	.15075	-.16152	.51025
	Equal variances not assumed			2.064	8.079	.073	.17436	.08446	-.02007	.36880
TFHFMT	Equal variances assumed	.330	.577	1.262	11	.233	17.07555	13.52599	-12.69495	46.84605
	Equal variances not assumed			1.892	8.473	.093	17.07555	9.02371	-3.53262	37.68372
UFHFMT	Equal variances assumed	.781	.394	2.373	12	.035	5.90495	2.48890	.48210	11.32780
	Equal variances not assumed			1.723	2.388	.206	5.90495	3.42809	-6.76977	18.57967
MAXBCDL	Equal variances assumed	1.918	.215	-1.250	6	.258	-.05166	.04134	-.15280	.04949
	Equal variances not assumed			-1.472	5.989	.191	-.05166	.03509	-.13755	.03423
cdlgo	Equal variances assumed	.514	.485	-.924	14	.371	-.03536	.03828	-.11746	.04674
	Equal variances not assumed			-.855	6.598	.423	-.03536	.04136	-.13439	.06367
ZYGFMT	Equal variances assumed	11.036	.006	-1.685	13	.116	-.03738	.02219	-.08530	.01055
	Equal variances not assumed			-.969	2.144	.429	-.03738	.03858	-.19311	.11836
UHTH	Equal variances assumed	4.892	.044	-1.546	14	.144	-.01699	.01099	-.04057	.00658
	Equal variances not assumed			-2.476	13.988	.027	-.01699	.00686	-.03172	-.00227
FB	Equal variances assumed	.024	.880	.316	10	.759	.00748	.02369	-.04530	.06026
	Equal variances not assumed			.295	5.171	.779	.00748	.02533	-.05700	.07196
FB2	Equal variances assumed	.033	.860	-1.205	8	.263	-.11085	.09200	-.32301	.10131
	Equal variances not assumed			-1.356	5.107	.232	-.11085	.08177	-.31972	.09803
UFIMAI	Equal variances assumed	.235	.639	2.425	9	.038	.09723	.04009	.00654	.18791
	Equal variances not assumed			2.539	3.976	.064	.09723	.03829	-.00934	.20379

T-Test Crowding

Independent Samples Test

Sex	MajorGeo			Levene's Test for Equality of Variances		t-test for Equality of Means					95% Confidence Interval of the Difference	
				F	Sig.	t	df	Sig. (2-tailed)	Mean Difference	Std. Error Difference	Lower	Upper
Female	English	Cranial Index	Equal variances assumed	.910	.351	-.326	22	.747	-1.0316	3.1603	-7.5856	5.5224
			Equal variances not assumed			-.733	3.069	.516	-1.0316	1.4083	-5.4571	3.3939
		Cranial Module	Equal variances assumed	21.368	.000	-1.972	16	.066	-8.89583	4.51081	-18.45832	.66666
			Equal variances not assumed			-.748	1.018	.589	-8.89583	11.88581	-153.80196	136.01029
		Cranial length-height Index	Equal variances assumed	14.488	.001	-3.863	17	.001	-13.24153	3.42758	-20.47309	-6.00998
			Equal variances not assumed			-1.555	1.022	.360	-13.24153	8.51407	-116.05902	89.57596
		Cranial breadth-height Index	Equal variances assumed	11.836	.003	-4.137	16	.001	-16.02982	3.87464	-24.24370	-7.81594
			Equal variances not assumed			-1.732	1.026	.329	-16.02982	9.25429	-126.91152	94.85188
		Total Facial Index	Equal variances assumed	.	.	-.394	9	.702	-2.36650	6.00081	-15.94128	11.20827
			Equal variances not assumed			.	.	.	-2.36650	.	.	.
		Upper Facial Index	Equal variances assumed	5.109	.040	-.206	14	.840	-.35840	1.74165	-4.09387	3.37707

			F	Sig.	t	df	Sig. (2-tailed)	Mean Difference	Std. Error Difference	95% CI Lower	95% CI Upper
		Equal variances not assumed			-.476	8.378	.646	-.35840	.75271	-2.08062	1.36382
	Maxilloalveolar Index	Equal variances assumed	.313	.584	-.153	16	.880	-1.30490	8.52870	-19.38493	16.77513
		Equal variances not assumed			-.205	1.580	.861	-1.30490	6.36317	-36.98110	34.37131
	Palatal Index	Equal variances assumed	.034	.854	-.332	22	.743	-1.97818	5.95397	-14.32596	10.36960
		Equal variances not assumed			-.329	2.592	.767	-1.97818	6.00963	-22.92518	18.96882
	Palatal/max ratio	Equal variances assumed	.050	.826	.333	15	.744	.02396	.07200	-.12951	.17742
		Equal variances not assumed			.438	1.598	.713	.02396	.05468	-.27815	.32606
	TFHFMT	Equal variances assumed	2.683	.132	-.177	10	.863	-1.15926	6.55456	-15.76373	13.44521
		Equal variances not assumed			-.404	9.537	.695	-1.15926	2.86853	-7.59309	5.27457
	UFHFMT	Equal variances assumed	2.008	.175	1.032	17	.316	2.75624	2.66952	-2.87596	8.38843
		Equal variances not assumed			.705	2.262	.546	2.75624	3.90701	-12.31717	17.82964
	MAXBCDL	Equal variances assumed	.121	.733	.862	15	.402	.02193	.02543	-.03227	.07613
		Equal variances not assumed			.769	2.654	.504	.02193	.02850	-.07583	.11969
	cdlgo	Equal variances assumed	.751	.398	.707	17	.489	.02222	.03142	-.04407	.08852
		Equal variances not assumed			.862	3.475	.444	.02222	.02579	-.05387	.09832
	ZYGFMT	Equal variances assumed	.473	.501	.359	16	.724	.01308	.03639	-.06408	.09023
		Equal variances not assumed			.645	2.514	.573	.01308	.02027	-.05909	.08524
	UHTH	Equal variances assumed	10.596	.009	2.416	10	.036	.06200	.02566	.00483	.11918
		Equal variances not assumed			1.152	1.042	.449	.06200	.05381	-.56007	.68408
	FB	Equal variances assumed	3.052	.106	-.667	12	.517	-.02603	.03902	-.11104	.05898
		Equal variances not assumed			-1.637	11.937	.128	-.02603	.01591	-.06071	.00864
	FB2	Equal variances assumed	1.145	.300	1.592	16	.131	.04905	.03082	-.01628	.11437
		Equal variances not assumed			1.821	3.309	.157	.04905	.02693	-.03230	.13039
	UFIMAI	Equal variances assumed	.389	.544	-.233	12	.819	-.00457	.01958	-.04723	.03809
		Equal variances not assumed			-.176	1.168	.886	-.00457	.02592	-.24072	.23158
Macedonian	Cranial Index	Equal variances assumed	.254	.618	-.028	26	.978	-.0365	1.2820	-2.6716	2.5987
		Equal variances not assumed			-.027	9.664	.979	-.0365	1.3358	-3.0270	2.9540
	Cranial Module	Equal variances assumed	.058	.813	-.614	14	.549	-1.21212	1.97564	-5.44944	3.02520
		Equal variances not assumed			-.666	9.572	.521	-1.21212	1.82118	-5.29468	2.87044
	Cranial length-height Index	Equal variances assumed	.844	.374	-1.603	14	.131	-2.85571	1.78186	-6.67741	.96600
		Equal variances not assumed			-1.763	9.921	.109	-2.85571	1.62012	-6.46947	.75806
	Cranial breadth-height Index	Equal variances assumed	1.684	.215	-1.724	14	.107	-4.47162	2.59407	-10.03534	1.09210
		Equal variances not assumed			-2.060	12.207	.061	-4.47162	2.17110	-9.19316	.24992
	Total Facial Index	Equal variances assumed	1.906	.185	.896	17	.383	3.63719	4.06015	-4.92898	12.20336
		Equal variances not assumed			.752	6.858	.477	3.63719	4.83953	-7.85484	15.12921
	Upper Facial Index	Equal variances assumed	.081	.779	.837	21	.412	1.28369	1.53453	-1.90755	4.47492
		Equal variances not assumed			.777	9.854	.455	1.28369	1.65142	-2.40330	4.97068
	Maxilloalveolar Index	Equal variances assumed	.082	.781	-.786	8	.454	-6.20726	7.89630	-24.41616	12.00165
		Equal variances not assumed			-.851	7.939	.420	-6.20726	7.29705	-23.05699	10.64248
	Palatal Index	Equal variances assumed	.106	.749	.315	17	.757	2.24495	7.12615	-12.78991	17.27980
		Equal variances not assumed			.380	10.729	.711	2.24495	5.90082	-10.78287	15.27276
	Palatal/max ratio	Equal variances assumed	3.207	.111	1.458	8	.183	.07020	.04815	-.04084	.18125
		Equal variances not assumed			1.769	6.003	.127	.07020	.03968	-.02688	.16729
	TFHFMT	Equal variances assumed	2.403	.145	-1.782	13	.098	-9.16504	5.14361	-20.27713	1.94705

			Equal variances not assumed			-3.058	10.762	.011	-9.16504	2.99728	-15.77988	-2.55021
		UFHFMT	Equal variances assumed	.906	.353	-1.525	19	.144	-4.31333	2.82844	-10.23333	1.60666
			Equal variances not assumed			-2.007	6.979	.085	-4.31333	2.14954	-9.39927	.77260
		MAXBCDL	Equal variances assumed	1.467	.257	-.870	9	.407	-.03732	.04291	-.13439	.05974
			Equal variances not assumed			-1.083	8.471	.309	-.03732	.03445	-.11601	.04136
		cdlgo	Equal variances assumed	3.037	.103	1.289	14	.218	.03344	.02594	-.02218	.08907
			Equal variances not assumed			1.495	13.936	.157	.03344	.02238	-.01457	.08146
		ZYGFMT	Equal variances assumed	2.955	.105	1.827	16	.086	.03922	.02147	-.00629	.08472
			Equal variances not assumed			3.182	15.998	.006	.03922	.01233	.01309	.06535
		UHTH	Equal variances assumed	.734	.404	.828	17	.419	.01710	.02066	-.02649	.06070
			Equal variances not assumed			.953	14.028	.357	.01710	.01795	-.02138	.05559
		FB	Equal variances assumed	1.970	.182	3.147	14	.007	.03303	.01050	.01052	.05555
			Equal variances not assumed			3.646	13.940	.003	.03303	.00906	.01359	.05247
		FB2	Equal variances assumed	3.962	.075	.651	10	.530	.02280	.03505	-.05530	.10091
			Equal variances not assumed			1.160	8.119	.279	.02280	.01966	-.02242	.06803
		UFIMAI	Equal variances assumed	.042	.843	.156	7	.881	.00501	.03215	-.07101	.08102
			Equal variances not assumed			.155	6.419	.882	.00501	.03233	-.07287	.08288
Male	English	Cranial Index	Equal variances assumed	.039	.845	.410	33	.684	1.0688	2.6044	-4.2299	6.3674
			Equal variances not assumed			.486	11.907	.635	1.0688	2.1972	-3.7226	5.8601
		Cranial Module	Equal variances assumed	1.679	.206	1.253	26	.221	3.26263	2.60462	-2.09125	8.61651
			Equal variances not assumed			1.794	16.669	.091	3.26263	1.81818	-.57920	7.10446
		Cranial length-height Index	Equal variances assumed	.257	.617	.120	26	.905	.18665	1.54989	-2.99919	3.37249
			Equal variances not assumed			.112	7.265	.914	.18665	1.67056	-3.73460	4.10791
		Cranial breadth-height Index	Equal variances assumed	1.314	.261	.239	28	.813	.69559	2.91139	-5.26812	6.65930
			Equal variances not assumed			.370	19.147	.715	.69559	1.87847	-3.23405	4.62523
		Total Facial Index	Equal variances assumed	.523	.479	-1.018	18	.322	-2.67974	2.63142	-8.20814	2.84866
			Equal variances not assumed			-1.069	7.500	.318	-2.67974	2.50793	-8.53090	3.17142
		Upper Facial Index	Equal variances assumed	1.035	.320	.742	22	.466	1.16846	1.57376	-2.09532	4.43223
			Equal variances not assumed			.567	4.878	.596	1.16846	2.06071	-4.16871	6.50562
		Maxilloalveolar Index	Equal variances assumed	3.794	.064	.752	22	.460	5.07745	6.75631	-8.93429	19.08919
			Equal variances not assumed			1.877	21.268	.074	5.07745	2.70495	-.54348	10.69838
		Palatal Index	Equal variances assumed	2.084	.157	-.979	40	.333	-3.20527	3.27281	-9.81986	3.40932
			Equal variances not assumed			-1.273	20.636	.217	-3.20527	2.51784	-8.44704	2.03650
		Palatal/max ratio	Equal variances assumed	.394	.537	-.063	22	.950	-.00250	.03959	-.08460	.07959
			Equal variances not assumed			-.075	2.963	.945	-.00250	.03349	-.10984	.10483
		TFHFMT	Equal variances assumed	3.221	.086	-.178	23	.860	-.60466	3.39626	-7.63035	6.42104
			Equal variances not assumed			-.223	18.761	.826	-.60466	2.71025	-6.28216	5.07284
		UFHFMT	Equal variances assumed	1.669	.206	-.048	31	.962	-.08712	1.79688	-3.75187	3.57764
			Equal variances not assumed			-.055	15.109	.957	-.08712	1.57707	-3.44644	3.27220
		MAXBCDL	Equal variances assumed	1.277	.268	.601	27	.553	.01048	.01742	-.02528	.04623
			Equal variances not assumed			.793	18.410	.438	.01048	.01321	-.01724	.03819
		cdlgo	Equal variances assumed	.000	.985	.005	31	.996	.00010	.02130	-.04334	.04355
			Equal variances not assumed			.005	11.253	.996	.00010	.02202	-.04823	.04844
		ZYGFMT	Equal variances assumed	3.997	.057	.111	24	.913	.00196	.01767	-.03452	.03844

			Equal variances not assumed			.174	15.083	.864	.00196	.01126	-.02203	.02595
		UHTH	Equal variances assumed	.295	.592	.448	25	.658	.00692	.01543	-.02487	.03870
			Equal variances not assumed			.516	14.066	.614	.00692	.01341	-.02184	.03568
		FB	Equal variances assumed	1.696	.211	-.817	16	.426	-.01501	.01837	-.05395	.02393
			Equal variances not assumed			-1.121	9.268	.291	-.01501	.01340	-.04519	.01516
		FB2	Equal variances assumed	10.119	.004	.964	26	.344	.02131	.02212	-.02415	.06678
			Equal variances not assumed			1.375	23.237	.182	.02131	.01550	-.01074	.05337
		UFIMAI	Equal variances assumed	4.207	.058	-.945	15	.360	-.02473	.02618	-.08054	.03107
			Equal variances not assumed			-1.838	13.728	.088	-.02473	.01346	-.05364	.00418
Macedonian	Cranial Index	Equal variances assumed	2.664	.115	-.021	25	.983	-.0424	1.9946	-4.1504	4.0656
			Equal variances not assumed			-.025	24.851	.980	-.0424	1.7137	-3.5729	3.4881
	Cranial Module	Equal variances assumed	.643	.436	.343	14	.737	.75132	2.18921	-3.94406	5.44671
			Equal variances not assumed			.320	8.831	.757	.75132	2.35133	-4.58328	6.08593
	Cranial length-height Index	Equal variances assumed	.481	.498	.342	15	.737	.49146	1.43800	-2.57356	3.55647
			Equal variances not assumed			.346	13.588	.735	.49146	1.42136	-2.56576	3.54868
	Cranial breadth-height Index	Equal variances assumed	.357	.560	.315	14	.758	.47671	1.51471	-2.77203	3.72544
			Equal variances not assumed			.318	13.496	.755	.47671	1.49916	-2.74997	3.70339
	Total Facial Index	Equal variances assumed	3.151	.096	-.312	15	.759	-.82447	2.64234	-6.45648	4.80754
			Equal variances not assumed			-.355	13.069	.728	-.82447	2.32408	-5.84264	4.19371
	Upper Facial Index	Equal variances assumed	3.073	.098	-.659	17	.519	-.94647	1.43721	-3.97872	2.08577
			Equal variances not assumed			-.722	15.971	.481	-.94647	1.31180	-3.72778	1.83483
	Maxilloalveolar Index	Equal variances assumed	1.908	.195	.027	11	.979	.20362	7.60353	-16.53164	16.93887
			Equal variances not assumed			.029	10.801	.977	.20362	6.94577	-15.11831	15.52555
	Palatal Index	Equal variances assumed	.007	.933	-.583	14	.569	-6.19164	10.61639	-28.96153	16.57826
			Equal variances not assumed			-.583	13.895	.569	-6.19164	10.61639	-28.97766	16.59439
	Palatal/max ratio	Equal variances assumed	.006	.942	-.300	10	.770	-.04210	.14035	-.35482	.27062
			Equal variances not assumed			-.318	9.986	.757	-.04210	.13236	-.33709	.25288
	TFHFMT	Equal variances assumed	1.429	.257	.347	11	.735	4.32235	12.46579	-23.11467	31.75937
			Equal variances not assumed			.434	8.198	.675	4.32235	9.95862	-18.54609	27.19080
	UFHFMT	Equal variances assumed	1.064	.323	-2.204	12	.048	-4.60417	2.08860	-9.15485	-.05350
			Equal variances not assumed			-2.204	10.632	.051	-4.60417	2.08860	-9.22065	.01230
	MAXBCDL	Equal variances assumed	3.593	.107	-.052	6	.960	-.00240	.04639	-.11592	.11113
			Equal variances not assumed			-.043	2.557	.969	-.00240	.05617	-.19999	.19519
	cdlgo	Equal variances assumed	2.049	.174	.849	14	.410	.03050	.03593	-.04656	.10755
			Equal variances not assumed			.894	13.737	.387	.03050	.03410	-.04277	.10376
	ZYGFMT	Equal variances assumed	.509	.488	1.552	13	.145	.02850	.01837	-.01118	.06817
			Equal variances not assumed			1.773	12.203	.101	.02850	.01608	-.00647	.06346
	UHTH	Equal variances assumed	1.076	.317	-.173	14	.865	-.00179	.01037	-.02404	.02045
			Equal variances not assumed			-.180	13.993	.860	-.00179	.00998	-.02321	.01962
	FB	Equal variances assumed	.127	.729	-.909	10	.385	-.01962	.02157	-.06768	.02845
			Equal variances not assumed			-.909	9.861	.385	-.01962	.02157	-.06777	.02854
	FB2	Equal variances assumed	5.810	.042	.098	8	.924	.00899	.09160	-.20223	.22022
			Equal variances not assumed			.098	4.262	.926	.00899	.09160	-.23928	.25726
	UFIMAI	Equal variances assumed	.154	.704	-.084	9	.935	-.00401	.04771	-.11193	.10391

| | Equal variances not assumed | | | -.089 | 7.471 | .932 | -.00401 | .04513 | -.10937 | .10135 |